Psoriasis and Psoriatic Arthritis: How to Treat in the Era of Biologics and Small Molecule Inhibitors?

Psoriasis and Psoriatic Arthritis: How to Treat in the Era of Biologics and Small Molecule Inhibitors?

Editor

Mayumi Komine

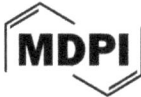

Basel • Beijing • Wuhan • Barcelona • Belgrade • Novi Sad • Cluj • Manchester

Editor
Mayumi Komine
Department of Dermatology
Jichi Medical University
Tochigi
Japan

Editorial Office
MDPI AG
Grosspeteranlage 5
4052 Basel, Switzerland

This is a reprint of articles from the Special Issue published online in the open access journal *Journal of Clinical Medicine* (ISSN 2077-0383) (available at: https://www.mdpi.com/journal/jcm/special_issues/Psoriasis_Psoriatic_Arthritis).

For citation purposes, cite each article independently as indicated on the article page online and as indicated below:

Lastname, A.A.; Lastname, B.B. Article Title. *Journal Name* **Year**, *Volume Number*, Page Range.

ISBN 978-3-7258-1879-2 (Hbk)
ISBN 978-3-7258-1880-8 (PDF)
doi.org/10.3390/books978-3-7258-1880-8

Cover image courtesy of Mayumi Komine

© 2024 by the authors. Articles in this book are Open Access and distributed under the Creative Commons Attribution (CC BY) license. The book as a whole is distributed by MDPI under the terms and conditions of the Creative Commons Attribution-NonCommercial-NoDerivs (CC BY-NC-ND) license.

Contents

About the Editor vii

Masaru Honma and Hiroyoshi Nozaki
Molecular Pathogenesis of Psoriasis and Biomarkers Reflecting Disease Activity
Reprinted from: *J. Clin. Med.* **2021**, *10*, 3199, doi:10.3390/jcm10153199 1

Trung T. Vu, Hanako Koguchi-Yoshioka and Rei Watanabe
Skin-Resident Memory T Cells: Pathogenesis and Implication for the Treatment of Psoriasis
Reprinted from: *J. Clin. Med.* **2021**, *10*, 3822, doi:10.3390/jcm10173822 20

Naoko Kanda, Toshihiko Hoashi and Hidehisa Saeki
The Defect in Regulatory T Cells in Psoriasis and Therapeutic Approaches
Reprinted from: *J. Clin. Med.* **2021**, *10*, 3880, doi:10.3390/jcm10173880 32

**Tomoyo Matsuda-Taniguchi, Masaki Takemura, Takeshi Nakahara,
Akiko Hashimoto-Hachiya, Ayako Takai-Yumine, Masutaka Furue and Gaku Tsuji**
The Antidiabetic Agent Metformin Inhibits IL-23 Production in Murine Bone-Marrow-Derived Dendritic Cells
Reprinted from: *J. Clin. Med.* **2021**, *10*, 5610, doi:10.3390/jcm10235610 45

Akimasa Adachi and Tetsuya Honda
Regulatory Roles of Estrogens in Psoriasis
Reprinted from: *J. Clin. Med.* **2022**, *11*, 4890, doi:10.3390/jcm11164890 56

**Eugenia Piragine, Davide Petri, Alma Martelli, Agata Janowska, Valentina Dini,
Marco Romanelli, et al.**
Adherence and Persistence to Biological Drugs for Psoriasis: Systematic Review with Meta-Analysis
Reprinted from: *J. Clin. Med.* **2022**, *11*, 1506, doi:10.3390/jcm11061506 67

Sylwia Słuczanowska-Głąbowska, Anna Ziegler-Krawczyk, Kamila Szumilas and Andrzej Pawlik
Role of Janus Kinase Inhibitors in Therapy of Psoriasis
Reprinted from: *J. Clin. Med.* **2021**, *10*, 4307, doi:10.3390/jcm10194307 86

Tomoyuki Hioki, Mayumi Komine and Mamitaro Ohtsuki
Diagnosis and Intervention in Early Psoriatic Arthritis
Reprinted from: *J. Clin. Med.* **2022**, *11*, 2051, doi:10.3390/jcm11072051 101

Koji Kamiya, Mayumi Komine and Mamitaro Ohtsuki
Biologics for Psoriasis during the COVID-19 Pandemic
Reprinted from: *J. Clin. Med.* **2021**, *10*, 1390, doi:10.3390/jcm10071390 112

**Lidia Rudnicka, Małgorzata Olszewska, Mohamad Goldust, Anna Waśkiel-Burnat,
Olga Warszawik-Hendzel, Przemysław Dorożyński, et al.**
Efficacy and Safety of Different Formulations of Calcipotriol/Betamethasone Dipropionate in Psoriasis: Gel, Foam, and Ointment
Reprinted from: *J. Clin. Med.* **2021**, *10*, 5589, doi:10.3390/jcm10235589 122

Tal Gazitt, Muhanad Abu Elhija, Amir Haddad, Idit Lavi, Muna Elias and Devy Zisman
Implementation of the Treat-to-Target Concept in Evaluation of Psoriatic Arthritis Patients
Reprinted from: *J. Clin. Med.* **2021**, *10*, 5659, doi:10.3390/jcm10235659 133

Yukari Okubo, Ann Chuo Tang, Sachie Inoue, Hitoe Torisu-Itakura and Mamitaro Ohtsuki
Comparison of Treatment Goals between Users of Biological and Non-Biological Therapies for Treatment of Psoriasis in Japan
Reprinted from: *J. Clin. Med.* **2021**, *10*, 5732, doi:10.3390/jcm10245732 . . . . **144**

About the Editor

Mayumi Komine

Dr. Mayumi Komine is generally interested in any events that occur in the natural world, from daily weather to events in the wider universe; her interest covers all living things, such as bacteria, fungi, plants, birds, and mammals, including humans, as well as environmental issues. She works as a Japanese dermatologist who specializes in psoriasis and psoriatic arthritis and sees many patients in this role. Her particular interests in dermatology include the special distribution of inflammatory and regulatory molecules in psoriatic plaques and their surrounding skin, and the mechanisms of action of small-molecule inhibitors—including JAK inhibitors and PDE4 inhibitors—in psoriasis and in alopecia and vitiligo. She has received the Husic Prize from the Ronald O. Perelman Department of Dermatology, New York University School of Medicine; the Galderma Award from Galdema Pharmaceutical Company; the JSID Shiseido Award from JSID; and an Excellent Paper Award from Jichi Medical University (as a corresponding author). She belongs to many academic associations, such as the Japanese Dermatological Association, the Japanese Society for Investigative Dermatology, the Japanese Society for Psoriatic Research, the Society for Investigative Dermatology, among many other societies. She is a member of the Board of Directors for the Asian Society for Psoriasis, as well as for the Women Physicians Committee within Tochigi Medical Association. On top of this, she is a member of the Board of Representatives for the Japanese Dermatological Association and the Japanese Society for Cutaneous Immunology and Allergy. She also serves as Councilor for the Japanese Society for Investigative Dermatology, the Japanese Society for Psoriatic Research, and the Japanese Society of vitiligo.

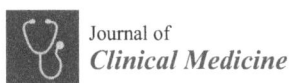

Review

Molecular Pathogenesis of Psoriasis and Biomarkers Reflecting Disease Activity

Masaru Honma [1,2,*] and Hiroyoshi Nozaki [1]

[1] Department of Dermatology, Asahikawa Medical University Hospital, 2-1-1-1 Midorigaoka-Higashi, Asahikawa 0788510, Japan; hnozaki@asahikawa-med.ac.jp
[2] International Medical Support Center, Asahikawa Medical University Hospital, 2-1-1-1 Midorigaoka-Higashi, Asahikawa 0788510, Japan
* Correspondence: wanwan@asahikawa-med.ac.jp; Tel.: +81-166-68-2523

Abstract: Psoriasis is a chronic inflammatory skin disease induced by multifactorial causes and is characterized by bothersome, scaly reddish plaques, especially on frequently chafed body parts, such as extensor sites of the extremities. The latest advances in molecular-targeted therapies using biologics or small-molecule inhibitors help to sufficiently treat even the most severe psoriatic symptoms and the extra cutaneous comorbidities of psoriatic arthritis. The excellent clinical effects of these therapies provide a deeper understanding of the impaired quality of life caused by this disease and the detailed molecular mechanism in which the interleukin (IL)-23/IL-17 axis plays an essential role. To establish standardized therapeutic strategies, biomarkers that define deep remission are indispensable. Several molecules, such as cytokines, chemokines, antimicrobial peptides, and proteinase inhibitors, have been recognized as potent biomarker candidates. In particular, blood protein markers that are repeatedly measurable can be extremely useful in daily clinical practice. Herein, we summarize the molecular mechanism of psoriasis, and we describe the functions and induction mechanisms of these biomarker candidates.

Keywords: inflammatory skin disease; Th17 cells; adipokines; glycoproteins; fatty acid-binding protein

1. Introduction

Psoriasis is a recurrent, persistent inflammatory skin disorder characterized by rough, reddish plaques on frequently chafed body parts, such as the extensor sites of the extremities [1,2]. Individuals with this condition suffer from subjective symptoms, such as itching and pain, but also from skin lesions, especially on exposed areas, such as the scalp, face, hands, and nails, which can have a prominent impact on the patients' quality of life [3–6]. In fact, it has been suggested that the manifestation of psoriasis-related symptoms can trigger stigmatization, leading to social discrimination and alienation [7–9]. Psoriasis often coexists with varied comorbidities represented by psoriatic arthritis (PsA), uveitis, psychiatric disorders, metabolic disorders, and cardiovascular diseases [2,10–13]. Psoriasis is therefore considered to be part of systemic disorders characterized by skin lesions. The process that amplifies localized psoriatic molecular reactions into a systemic inflammatory response is called "psoriatic march" [14].

While severe psoriatic symptoms are often resistant to conventional treatment, recent advances in molecular-targeted therapies have enabled sufficient treatment and control in most cases. The clinical effects of these therapies allow for markedly reduced skin lesions, related symptoms, and comorbidities but also a deep understanding of the molecular mechanism of psoriatic diseases in which the interleukin (IL)-23/IL-17 axis based on Th17-cell-mediating cytokine network plays an essential role [11,15].

Biomarkers are indicators of normal physiological processes, pathogenic reactions, and responses to pathogen/treatment exposure or intervention, including therapeutic interventions [16]. Biomarkers can have molecular biology, histology, radiological images, or other physiologic characteristics [16]. A reliable indicator that reflects sufficient remission of disease activity is indispensable for establishing standardized therapeutic strategies. To date, several biomarker candidates have been proposed to reflect improvement in psoriasis during treatment. Consequently, this review describes the molecular pathogenesis of psoriasis and changes in biomarkers that occur along its disease activity, focusing on blood-protein markers that can be repeatedly measured in daily clinical practice.

2. Molecular Pathogenesis of Psoriasis

As shown by the remarkable efficacy of molecular-targeted therapies, the IL-23/IL-17 axis, which depends mainly on Th17-cell function, is considered the most essential mechanism of psoriasis (Figure 1) [1,2,10,15,17]. Molecules regulated in the downstream of Th17 cytokines are identified as biomarker candidates (Table 1). In the initial stage, a complex of antimicrobial peptides (AMP), such as LL-37, and self-nucleotides derived from damaged keratinocytes via toll-like receptors (TLRs), potentiate the function of plasmacytoid dendritic cells (pDCs) to produce substantive interferon (IFN)-α, which activates myeloid (conventional) DCs [18–20]. These activated DCs release tumor necrosis factor (TNF) and IL-23 that synergistically propel the immune response process. TNF stimulates DCs in an autocrine manner but inhibits the function of pDCs [1,2,10,15,17]. A paradoxical reaction during treatment using TNF inhibitors can depend on pDC activation by cancelling TNF-mediated inhibition [21].

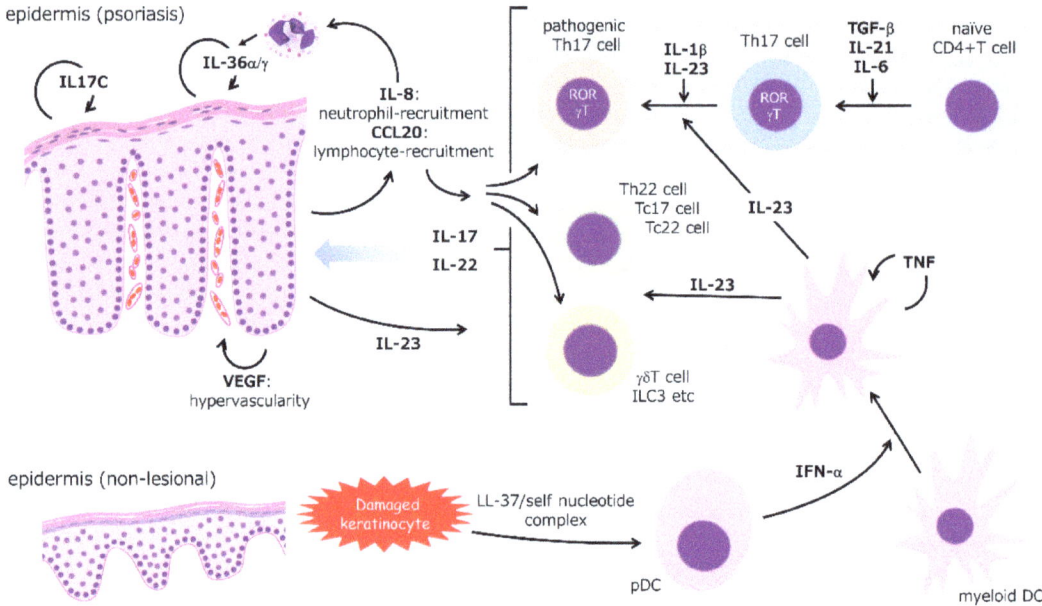

Figure 1. Summarized molecular mechanism of psoriasis. IFN-α released from activated pDCs stimulates myeloid DCs to produce TNF and IL-23. TNF activates DCs in an autocrine manner and enhances the inflammatory responses of various immunocytes. Naïve CD4-positive T cells differentiate into Th17 cells in the presence of the transforming growth factor (TGF)-β, IL-21, and IL-6. The pathogenicity of Th17 cells is potentiated by IL-23. IL-17 and IL-22 are produced by Th17 and other cells with more innate characteristics (e.g., innate lymphoid cell (ILC)-3 and gamma delta T cells). IL-17 and Il-22 induce epidermal hyperproliferation. IL-17 and TNF synergistically accelerate the production of inflammatory cytokines and chemokines from the epidermal keratinocytes, resulting in a vicious circle of inflammatory reactions.

Table 1. Summary of blood-protein biomarkers reflecting the severity of psoriasis.

Group	Biomarkers	Cellular Source	Findings
blood cell counts	NLR	-	increase especially in cases with arthritis
	PLR	-	
cytokines	IL-17A	Th17, Tc17, ILC3, etc.	relation with atherosclerosis, fatty liver, and insulin resistance
	IL-17F	Th17, Tc17, ILC3, colon epithelial cells, etc.	much higher serum IL-17F levels than IL-17A levels
	IL-22	Th17, Th22, Tc22, ILC3, etc.	vascular protective effect; relation with liver fibrosis
	IL-19	monocytes, macrophages, keratinocytes, fibroblasts, etc.	vascular protective effect
	IL-36γ	epidermis	relatively specific to skin lesions
chemokines	Fractalkine	APCs, ECs, and epidermis	close correlation with atherosclerosis
	TARC	DCs, ECs, epidermis, and fibroblasts	a biomarker for AD; possible relation to deeper remission during anti-IL-17 therapy; correlation with severity of GPP
adipokines	Resistin	macrophages, monocytes, and adipocytes	close correlation with atherosclerosis
	Adiponectin	adipocytes	negatively correlated with atherosclerosis
AMPs	β-defensin 2	epidermis	relatively specific to skin lesion; correlation with atherosclerosis
	S100A7	epidermis	
protease inhibitors	SCCA2	epidermis	also increase in AD
	Elafin	Epidermis and immune cells	correlation with CRP and ESR
glycoproteins	LRG	hepatocytes, neutrophils, ECs, and macrophages	correlation with CRP and arthritis
	YKL-40	neutrophils, macrophages, fibroblasts, ECs, and smooth muscle cells	correlation with tumor progression, metabolic diseases, and arthritis
FABPs	FABP-4	adipocytes	increase in cardiovascular diseases; the expression in T_{RM} infiltrating into psoriatic epidermis
	i-FABP	intestine epithelial cells	correlation with disruption of intestine barrier

AMP, antimicrobial peptide; FABP, fatty acid-binding protein; NLR, neutrophils/lymphocytes ratio; PLR, platelets/lymphocytes ratio; TARC, thymus and activation-regulated chemokine; LRG, leucin-rich alpha-2 glycoprotein; APCs, antigen presenting cells; ECs, endothelial cells; DCs, dendritic cells; AD, atopic dermatitis; GPP, generalized pustular psoriasis.

2.1. IL-23

IL-12, IL-23, IL-27, and IL-35 form the IL-12 cytokine family [22] in which subunits and specific receptors are shared [22,23]. For instance, IL-12 and IL-23 share the p40 subunit, but IL-23 specifically possesses the p19 subunit. IL-12 and IL-23 signals are transmitted by pairs of IL-12 receptor β1 (IL-12Rβ1)/IL-12Rβ2 and IL-12Rβ1/IL-23R, respectively. In a psoriatic lesion, both p40 and p19-expressions but also the expression of p40 and p19 subunits increases as opposed to the p35 subunit, which is another component of IL-12, suggesting a more definitive role of IL-23 in the molecular mechanism of psoriasis [24]. IL-12 and IL-23 work differently on T-cell diversity. IL-12 mainly leads to the induction of Th1 cells, whereas IL-23 mainly enhances Th17 cell pathogenicity characterized by IL-17 production [22,23]. IL-23 expression also increases epidermal keratinocytes by TLR-4 stimulation, which can participate in the pathogenesis of interleukin-36 receptor antagonist (DITRA) deficiency [25]. IL-23 stimulates DCs to induce IL-22 release from Th cells [26]. IL-23 expression in keratinocytes is epigenetically regulated, and the mechanism can contribute to the patho-mechanism of psoriasis [27]. IL-23 also potentiates FoxP3-positive regulatory T cells (Treg) to produce IL-17 [28,29]. While DCs are the main source of TNF, TNF is also produced by other cells, such as Th1, Th17, macrophages, neutrophils, mast cells, endothelial cells, and epidermal keratinocytes [11,20,30,31]. TNF induces proinflammatory responses via various signaling pathways, such as nuclear factor (NF)-κB and MAP-kinase signaling, through TNF receptors, which is broadly expressed by various cell types [32]. Consequently, TNF activates DCs and accelerates the inflammatory reactions that involve various immunocytes [10,32]. While IL-23 can fortify the pathogenicity of Th17 cells, it is not required for the differentiation of Th17 cells from naïve CD4+ T cells. In contrast, TGF-β, IL-21, and IL-6 are indispensable for Th17 differentiation, [33,34].

2.2. IL-17

IL-17 consists of IL-17A, IL-17B, IL-17C, IL-17D, IL-17E, and IL-17F homodimers or a IL-17A and IL-17F heterodimer. Ligand-specific IL-17 receptors (IL-17R) transmit IL-17 signaling, whereas IL-17A signaling employs IL-17RA, IL-17RC, and IL-17RD [35–38]. IL-17 receptors share a similar expression of fibroblast growth factor and IL-17R (SEFIR) domain, an intracellular domain essential for recruiting Act-1, a protein that activates NF-κB and MAPK pathways [35–37]. IL-17 is indispensable for host defense against cutaneous and mucosal infection by *Staphylococcus aureus* and *Candida albicans* [35–37,39] and for upholding the intestinal epithelial barrier [40,41]. IL-17A is the most investigated subtype in both physiological and disease conditions, including psoriasis [36], and it is produced by Th17, Tc17, tissue-resident memory T (T_{RM}), innate lymphoid cell (ILC)-3, invariant natural killer T cells (iNKT), gamma delta T cells, and mucosal associated invariant T (MAIT) cells [42]. Free fatty-acid-nourished, CD8-positive T_{RM} is present even in the healed epidermis following psoriasis, and IL-17 released from T_{RM} contributes to lesion recurrence [43,44]. Moreover, IL-17 and IL-22 released from Th17 and other innate cells, such as ILC-3 and gamma delta T cells, induce hyperproliferation of epidermis and accelerate the production of inflammatory cytokines and chemokines, such as IL-8 (CXCL-8), IL-17C, and vascular endothelial growth factor, in the epidermis [1,2,10,17]. According to a study investigating cytokine profile in small and large psoriatic plaques, IL-17 signaling is consistently accelerated in lesional skin; however, suppressed regulation of inflammatory reaction and upregulated TNF signaling are simultaneously observed even in non-lesional skin of patients with large psoriatic plaques. Consequently, this suggests that synergistic effect of IL-17 and TNF signaling induce a systemic inflammatory reaction [45]. These factors play crucial roles in the formation of the psoriatic phenotype and the vicious inflammatory circle of a psoriatic lesion. While the role of IL-17 is broadly shared in other psoriatic diseases, such as PsA [15] and pustular psoriasis [46], the significance of IL-17 inhibition remains unclear in terms of treating palmoplantar pustulosis [47,48].

2.3. CCL20/CCR6 Axis

C-C motif chemokine ligand (CCL) 20, a well-known macrophage inflammatory protein (MIP)-3a or liver activation-regulated chemokine, is a member of the CC-chemokine family and plays a significant role in inflammatory and homeostatic conditions [49,50]. Although a constitutively strong expression is observed in the liver, lung, appendix, and tonsils, this expression can be induced in various cells, such as immune, endothelial, and epithelial cells [50]. CCL20 recruits immunocytes expressing the specific receptor CCR6, and CCR6 expression is observed in DCs, T cells, and B cells [50]. The interaction between CCL20 and CCR6 is an indispensable pathogenic mechanism of autoimmune disorders, including psoriasis, and it is considered a distinct therapeutic target [51]. Th17 cytokines and TNF independently and synergistically induce CCL20 expression in epidermal keratinocytes [52,53]. CCL20 expression is significantly upregulated in scratched keratinocyte sheet, suggesting the contribution of CCL20 in the Koebner phenomenon [54]. Deletion of CCR6 or the dominant-negative form of CCL20 ameliorates skin symptoms in psoriasis model mice [55–57], thus suggesting the indispensable role of the CCL20/CCR6 axis in the pathogenesis of psoriasis [58,59].

2.4. Adipose Tissue

Adipokines and proinflammatory cytokines derived from white adipose tissue (WAT) can enhance and influence the Th17-mediated inflammatory response (Figure 2). Psoriasis is frequently concurrent with obesity and overweight [60,61], which are closely related metabolic abnormalities, and weight reduction interventions are necessary to reduce the severity of skin lesions and comorbidities [62–68]. Similar to obesity, the expression of proinflammatory adipokines, such as TNF, IL-6, leptin, resistin, and chemerin, is upregulated in psoriasis, whereas the expression of anti-inflammatory adipokines, such as adiponectin and omentin, is suppressed [60,69–72]. Although they are possibly more closely associated with systemic inflammation, oxidative stress, and cardiovascular risk [73,74], visceral adipose tissue and subcutaneous adipose tissue have similar cytokine profiles [73]. In obese WAT, macrophage infiltration into the stromal vascular fraction of WAT via monocyte chemoattractantprotein (MCP)-1/CCR2 pathway is a key mechanism of obesity-induced adipose inflammation [75]. Adipose tissue macrophages (ATMs), which resemble M1-macrophages, can be activated via TLR4 stimulation by lipopolysaccharide and saturated fatty acids (SFAs) [76] and release proinflammatory cytokines, such as TNF and IL-6 [77]. SFAs, pathogen-associated molecular patterns (PAMPs), and danger-associated molecular patterns (DAMPs) also activate NLRP3 inflammasomes in ATMs, resulting in enhanced production of IL-1 and IL-18 [78]. WAT also acts as a reservoir of T_{RM} cells that is characterized by high turnover rates and active metabolism, as measured by lipid uptake and mitochondrial respiration [79,80]. The numbers of CD8+ T_{RM} cells can be present in psoriatic skin for long periods, taking in free fatty acids via fatty acid-binding protein (FABP)-4/5 for the regional longevity [44]. These cells play a crucial role in the recurrence of clinically healed psoriasis [43].

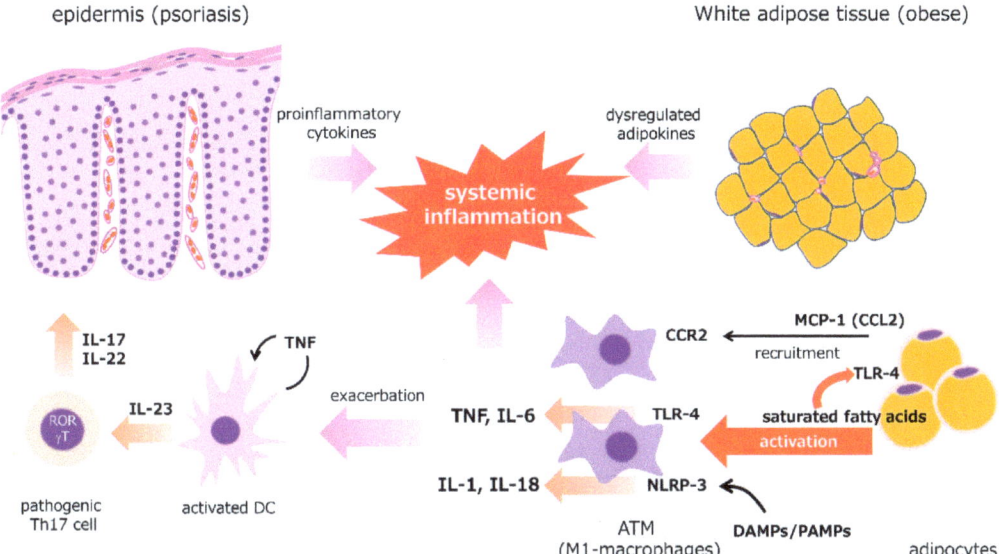

Figure 2. Close correlation between psoriasis and adipose tissue. Adipokines and proinflammatory cytokines derived from white adipose tissue (WAT) enhance and influence the Th17-mediated inflammatory response. In psoriasis and obesity, balance between proinflammatory adipokines and anti-inflammatory adipokines is dysregulated. In obese WAT, macrophages infiltrate the stromal vascular fraction of WAT via the monocyte chemoattractantprotein-1 (MCP-1)/CCR2 pathway. Adipose tissue macrophages (ATMs) activated via TLR4 stimulation by saturated fatty acids (SFAs) release proinflammatory cytokines, such as TNF and IL-6. SFAs, pathogen-associated molecular patterns (PAMPs), and danger-associated molecular patterns (DAMPs) also activate NLRP3 inflammasomes in ATMs, resulting in the enhanced production of IL-1 and IL-18. These proinflammatory cytokines synergistically work with Th17-derived cytokines to enhance systemic inflammatory responses.

3. Biomarkers in Psoriasis Treatment

3.1. Peripheral Blood Cell Counts

Neutrophil-to-Lymphocyte Ratio and Platelet-to-Lymphocyte Ratio

Neutrophils and platelets are primarily associated with biophylactic mechanisms against pathogens and hemostasis, respectively. These mechanisms synergistically work at sites of acute injury and inflammation by forming neutrophil extracellular traps. Dysregulated interaction between neutrophils and platelets can be involved in the patho-mechanism of autoimmune disorders, such as systemic lupus erythematosus (SLE), rheumatoid arthritis (RA), systemic vasculitis [81], and psoriasis [82].

Recently, neutrophil-to-lymphocyte ratio (NLR) and platelet-to-lymphocyte ratio (PLR) have been considered as markers of systemic inflammation in internal malignancies [83] and various inflammatory conditions, such as SLE and RA [84]. While systemic treatment using biologics can reduce NLR and PLR and improve psoriatic skin and arthropathic symptoms [85,86], it is not always correlated with the severity of psoriasis skin lesions as evaluated by the Psoriasis Area and Severity Index (PASI), suggesting that the NLR and PLR are better at reflecting systemic inflammation [87].

3.2. Cytokines and Chemokines

3.2.1. IL-17

As mentioned earlier, IL-17 is a definitive mediator in the patho-mechanism of psoriasis, and it is the most important subtype, as shown by the excellent clinical efficacy of the inhibitors against psoriasis.

Serum IL-17 levels increase as the severity of skin lesions increases, especially in severe psoriatic cases [88], and IL-17A levels are more closely correlated with psoriasis severity compared to IL-17F levels [89]. In contrast, serum IL-23 levels do not increase in psoriatic cases, and changes cannot be detected during successful treatment [90]. IL-17A and IL-17F are targets of IL-17-specific inhibitors but also of other drugs. Tofacitinib, a JAK-inhibitor, and apremilast, a phosphodiesterase inhibitor, decrease serum IL-17A, and IL-17F levels are correlated with the clinical response of skin lesions [91,92]. Serum levels of both subtypes change over the course of treatment and the withdrawal of guselkumab, an IL-23 p19-specific inhibitor [90]. Interestingly, increased serum levels of IL-17F subunit precede skin lesion exacerbation after withdrawal of guselkumab therapy [90], which might depend on the sensitivity of measuring these subunits. While IL-17A and IL-17F are mainly produced by immune cells, such as Th17 and Tc17 cells, the latter is also produced by colon epithelial cells [93], and serum IL-17F levels are significantly higher than serum IL-17A levels [89,90]. IL-17A is also related to the progression of cardiovascular disease, fatty liver, and diabetes [94–96]. Consequently, IL-17A-inhibition can possibly improve non-calcified atherosclerosis of coronary arteries [97].

3.2.2. IL-22

IL-22 is a member of the IL-20 subfamily of cytokines, which belong to the IL-10 family, and it is produced by Th17, Th22, ILC3, Tc22, and gamma delta T cells. However, it plays a crucial role in tissue regeneration, wound healing, and host defenses, especially against fungal infections [98–100]. The signal can be transmitted via a pair of receptors (IL-10 and IL-22) through JAK/STAT pathways [15,99,100]. IL-22 upregulates the proliferation of epidermal keratinocytes and induces acanthosis of epidermis via STAT3 activation in inflammatory dermatoses, such as psoriasis and atopic dermatitis (AD) [101,102]. Serum IL-22 levels increase moderately in psoriasis, in accordance with the skin lesion severity as evaluated by the PASI score [90,103], whereas these levels decrease when implementing an appropriate treatment [90,104]. IL-19, another subfamily of the IL-10 family produced by monocytes, macrophages, keratinocytes, and fibroblasts, is involved in inflammation, angiogenesis, and tissue remodeling [98,105]. Serum IL-19 levels increase in cases of plaque-type psoriasis, and they are very closely correlated with the skin lesion severity as rated by the PASI score [106]. Elevated IL-19 levels in psoriasis can quickly be reduced by ixekizumab or baricitinib treatment. The therapeutic response of psoriasis is predicted by the decrease in the serum IL-19 levels before skin lesions begin to heal [106]. The IL-20 family is also associated with other systemic diseases. IL-19 and IL-22 can be vascular protective cytokines in cardiovascular diseases [107], whereas the synergistic effect of IL-22 and IL-17A can contribute to fibrotic changes in the liver tissue [108].

3.2.3. IL-36

IL-36, an IL-1 family proinflammatory cytokine, consists of IL-36α, IL-36β, and IL-36γ. The IL-36 signal induces an inflammatory response in various tissues [109–112]. IL-36 family of cytokines are produced by immune cells, such as macrophages, DCs, and T cells but also by epithelial tissues, including the epidermis [109,113–115]. Among its subtypes, IL-36α and IL-36γ are significantly expressed in psoriatic epidermis, and the expression can be induced by proinflammatory cytokines that are deeply involved in the molecular patho-mechanism of psoriasis, such as IL-17 and TNF [116]. Furthermore, IL-36 and IL-17A synergistically propel a vicious inflammatory loop [113,114,117]. Serum IL-36γ levels are increased in cases of plaque-type psoriasis, and they are closely correlated with the respective severity; however, the elevated levels can be normalized when adequate treatment is provided [118]. Elevated serum IL-36γ levels constitute a relatively specific diagnostic marker for psoriatic erythroderma that is differentiated from other erythrodermic dermatoses [119].

3.2.4. Fractalkine

Fractalkine (CX3CL1) is a CX3C chemokine expressed in antigen-presenting cells [120], vascular endothelial cells [121], and epidermal keratinocytes [122] in membrane-bound or soluble forms. Fractalkine works as an inflammatory mediator via the specific CX3C chemokine receptor 1 (CX3CR1), and fractalkine expression increases in lesional psoriatic epidermis [122]. This elevated expression contributes to the recruitment of CXCR1-expressing cells, such as natural killer cells, T cells, and monocytes, via the chemotactic effect of the soluble form [123]. Experiments on CX3C-deleted mice revealed that imiquimod could attenuate psoriasis-like inflammation, thus suggesting a key role of the fractalkine/CX3CR1 signaling in the pathogenesis of psoriasis [124]. Serum fractalkine levels increase in cases of psoriasis and AD depending on skin lesion severity [125,126]. Although elevated serum fractalkine levels decrease along with improvement of AD, there are no data on serum fractalkine level changes during psoriasis treatment. Fractalkine is also involved in the molecular mechanism of atherosclerosis [127], and its expression can reflect a systemic inflammatory reaction.

3.2.5. Thymus and Activation-Regulated Chemokine

Thymus and activation-regulated chemokine (TARC)/CCL17 is one of the CC chemokines expressed in the thymus and is produced by various cells, such as dendritic cells (DC), endothelial cells, keratinocytes (KC), bronchial epithelial cells, and fibroblasts [128,129]. The signal is transmitted by the specific receptor CCR4, resulting in lesional infiltration of Th2 cells, basophils, and natural killer cells [129]. TARC is one of the most useful biomarkers for reflecting the current disease activity of AD. TARC expression is slightly upregulated in lesional psoriatic skin, and numbers of CCR4-expressing mononuclear cells infiltrate the lesional skin, suggesting the possible involvement of TARC in the patho-mechanism of psoriasis [130]. While serum TARC levels are lower in psoriasis cases compared to AD cases [131], they tend to increase in more severe cases of psoriasis [132]. Interestingly, the serum TARC level also increases in well-controlled psoriasis cases treated with biologics, especially IL-17 inhibitors [132]. The ILC2 population can possess ILC3-like characteristics when IL-1β and IL-23 are stimulated, both of which are pivotal cytokines in the psoriatic molecular pathogenesis [133]. Details of the induction mechanism of TARC remain unclear, but this process may involve the plasticity of immune cells. In addition, serum levels are higher in cases of generalized pustular psoriasis compared to cases of plaque-type psoriasis, suggesting a relationship with psoriasis severity [134].

3.3. Adipokines

Adipokines (or adipocytokines) are adipose, tissue-derived bioactive proteins that play an essential role in regulating tissue metabolism. Depending on their physiological and pathological effects, adipokines can be classified into proinflammatory and anti-inflammatory groups [135]. In obesity, the balance of adipokines will shift toward a dominant condition of proinflammatory adipokines, and the aberrant secretion contributes to latent systemic inflammation [72,135–137]. These abnormal adipokine states are shared by obesity and psoriatic diseases in which the expression of proinflammatory adipokines leptin, resistin, and chemerin increases, as opposed to the expression of anti-inflammatory adipokines, i.e., adiponectin and omentin, which decreases [69–71,138]. Leptin, which can regulate feeding behaviors by acting on the central nervous system, induces the production of TNF, IL-6, and CC-chemokine from monocytes and macrophages as well as IL-2 and IFN-γ from T cells [135]. Among these adipokines, chemerin, lipocalin-2, resistin, and adiponectin are better biomarker candidates for reflecting psoriasis severity [139].

3.3.1. Resistin

Initially identified in adipose tissue, resitin can be produced in greater quantities by macrophages and monocytes in humans, and its expression is induced by proinflammatory cytokines, such as TNF, IL-1, and IL-6 [135]. Serum resistin levels accurately reflect insulin resistance, and resistin inhibition partially improves the aberrant insulin function [140]. Resistin signaling upregulates the production of proinflammatory cytokines from mononuclear cells, thus forming a vicious inflammatory circle [135]. Plasma resistin levels are correlated with the severity of psoriatic skin lesions, and its levels can decrease as the skin lesions improve following an appropriate treatment approach [141,142]. While serum resistin levels are closely correlated to the PASI score and to the involved body surface area percentage (%BSA) in psoriasis cases before anti-TNF therapy, its levels do not always decrease with the improvement in PASI and %BSA after adalimumab therapy [143]. Serum resistin and leptin levels are also correlated with the intima-media thickness of carotid arteries in psoriasis cases, suggesting their potential contribution to the development of atherosclerosis [144].

3.3.2. Adiponectin

Adiponectin enhances insulin-sensitivity but reduces the TNF-induced dysfunction of endothelial cells and apoptosis of cardiomyocytes [145]. Adiponectin mitigates imiquimod-induced psoriasiform dermatitis via the direct inhibition of IL-17 release from gamma delta T cells [146]. Furthermore, serum adiponectin levels are inversely correlated with skin lesion severity [147,148], and its levels do not always increase with the improvement in skin lesions [142,149]. Serum adiponectin levels exhibit a greater decrease in cases with PsA compared to cases without PsA, suggesting a closer relationship between adiponectin and systemic inflammatory responses [150].

3.4. Antimicrobial Peptides

AMPs are small proteins with approximately 10–50 amino acids that demonstrate biophylactic activity against viral, bacterial, and fungal infections via the disruption of the pathogens' plasma membrane. The main cellular sources for AMPs in the human skin are keratinocytes, mast cells, neutrophils, sebocytes, and eccrine epithelial cells [19,151–153]. AMPs play a critical role in innate immunity, and they are involved in chemotaxis, angiogenesis, and cell proliferation/migration during the host's inflammatory responses [154]. AMP expression is highly upregulated in psoriatic epidermis and is possibly involved in the patho-mechanism of psoriasis [19,154].

3.4.1. Defensin 2

β-defensin 2 (BD-2), a defensin subfamily, is the most investigated molecular biomarker of psoriasis. BD-2 expression is induced by proinflammatory cytokines and microbial products in contrast to the constitutive expression of BD-1 in epithelial cells [155]. TNF, IFN-γ, and IL-17, which are closely involved in the pathogenesis of psoriasis [154], can induce the BD-2 expression in epidermal keratinocytes, and TNF and IL-17A synergistically enhance BD-2-induction [53]. In cases of plaque-type psoriasis, BD-2-protein levels significantly increase both in lesional epidermis and in serum, and serum levels are closely correlated with skin lesion severity as rated by the PASI score [156] and with serum IL-17A levels but not with the IL-17F levels [89]. Several clinical trials have evaluated the efficacy of novel therapeutic options for psoriasis by measuring BD-2 levels [89,157,158]. In moderate to severe psoriasis, elevated serum BD-2 levels decreased and were normalized as the PASI score improved [89,157,158].

3.4.2. S100A

S100 proteins (measuring 10–12 kilodaltons) are low molecular-weight molecules that possess two calcium-binding helix-loop-helix motifs, and they form a family that consists of 25 subtypes [159]. Although S100A7 (psoriasin), S100A8, S100A9, S100A12, and S100A15 (koebnerisin) exhibit antimicrobial activity and are highly expressed in psoriatic epidermis [159,160], S100A7 is the most studied subtype. Proinflammatory cytokines deeply involved in the pathogenesis of psoriasis, such as IL-36, IL-17, and TNF, can independently and synergistically induce S100A7 expression in epidermal keratinocytes, and S100A7 acts as a chemoattractant for lymphocytes, granulocytes, and macrophages, forming an inflammatory loop [161]. Serum S100A7 levels increase in severe psoriatic cases but not in milder ones [162]. Serum S100A7 and S100A15 levels are closely correlated with the intima-media thickness of common carotid arteries [163], suggesting their contribution to the systemic inflammatory response [164].

3.5. Protease Inhibitors

3.5.1. Squamous Cell Carcinoma Antigen

Squamous cell carcinoma antigen (SCCA), which is a recognized serum tumor marker for SCC, is a member of the serpin family of proteins with inhibitory activity against cysteine protease. While SCCA is composed of SCCA1 (SERPINB3) and SCCA2 (SERPINB4), both subtypes are expressed in psoriatic epidermis [165]. SCCA2 expression is significantly upregulated in psoriatic epidermis compared with the normal epidermis in contrast to the constitutive SCCA1 expression in normal and psoriatic epidermis [165]. In psoriasis cases, serum SCCA2 levels are correlated with the PASI score and serum IL-22 levels but not with the IL-17A levels [166]. IL-22, which is involved in the mechanisms of psoriasis and AD, stimulates SCCA1/2 expression in oral SCC-derived cell lines [167] and normal human keratinocytes [166]. IL-17 synergistically acts on the IL-22-mediated induction of SCCA2 in normal keratinocytes [166]. IL-4 and IL-13 signaling can also induce SCCA2 expression in keratinocytes [168]. Thus, serum SCCA2 levels increase in psoriasis but also in other inflammatory dermatoses, such as AD [166,169]. The increased serum SCCA2 levels in psoriasis and AD can be reduced with appropriate treatment [166,169].

3.5.2. Elafin

Elafin, a serine protease inhibitor that is highly expressed in psoriatic epidermis [170–172], is released by epithelial cells and immune cells [173] and plays an essential role in the anti-inflammation mechanism via proteinase inhibition and antimicrobial/immunoregulatory functions [173]. Serum elafin levels increase in psoriasis cases correlate with skin lesion severity and with laboratory findings that reflect inflammation, such as C-reactive protein levels and erythrocyte sedimentation rates [174]. During a cardiovascular event, elafin possibly reduces tissue injury exacerbated by neutrophilic elastase as a result of anti-inflammatory activity [175]. Interestingly, higher elafin expression is associated with a higher likelihood of spontaneous reperfusion, and it is related to a smaller infarct size and more favorable clinical outcomes [176].

3.6. Glycoproteins

3.6.1. Leucin-Rich Alpha-2-Glycoprotein

Leucin-rich alpha-2-glycoprotein (LRG), an approximately 50 kilodalton glycoprotein consisting of abundant amino acid residues with a structure of leucine-rich repeats (LRP), is produced by hepatocytes, neutrophils, endothelial cells, and macrophages following the stimulation of proinflammatory cytokines, such as IL-6, TNF, and IL-1β. LRG is associated with angiogenesis in cooperation with TGF-β signaling [177], and serum LRG levels are a candidate biomarker that reflects cardiovascular risk in cases of kidney diseases [178]. LGR has also been involved in a Th17-differentiation mechanism in a collagen-induced arthritis model [179]. While serum LRG levels increase in cases of psoriasis, depending on the skin lesion severity, its levels are much more closely correlated with serum C-reactive protein levels than with the PASI score [180]. Considering that serum LRG levels are higher in psoriatic cases with arthritis than in cases without arthritis, serum LRG levels might be more reflective of a systemic inflammatory response than of the skin-limited inflammatory level [180].

3.6.2. YKL-40

Chitinase-3 -like 1, also known as YKL-40, is a glycoprotein that contains highly conserved chitin-binding domains without chitinase activity [181–183]. YKL-40 is secreted by various immune cells, such as neutrophils and macrophages, fibroblasts, vascular smooth muscle cells, and endothelial cells [181–183]. YKL-40 expression is upregulated by proinflammatory cytokines, namely IL-6, TNF, IL-13, and IL-18, and is associated with tumor progression, angiogenesis, and various inflammatory responses [181–183]. In psoriatic lesions, YKL-40 expression is detected in infiltrating neutrophils, and serum YKL-40 levels are significantly more elevated in cases of generalized pustular psoriasis compared to cases of plaque-type psoriasis [184]. The levels are moderately correlated with skin lesion severity, and they can be reduced following an appropriate treatment [184,185]. Serum YKL-40 levels are also correlated with arthritis and endothelial dysfunction in cases of psoriasis [186,187], suggesting a close correlation with the systemic inflammatory response.

3.7. Fatty Acid-Binding Protein

The fatty acid-binding protein (FABP) family includes several tissue-specific subtypes of FABP that exhibit prominent affinity with long-chain fatty acid and play a significant role in lipid metabolism [188–190]. Among them, FABP-5 (epidermal FABP, psoriasis-associated-FABP) is highly expressed in psoriatic as opposed to healthy epidermis [191–193], and FABP-5 regulates the differentiation of epidermal keratinocytes [194,195]. There have been numerous studies suggesting a close correlation among blood FABP-4 levels, an adipocyte subtype, and metabolic abnormality related to cardiovascular diseases [188]. FABP-4 and FABP-5 are also specifically expressed in T_{RM} cells compared with other T-cell subtypes, and T_{RM} cells require lipid uptake via FABP-5 and FABP-5 to maintain their longevity in the targeting tissues, such as in psoriatic lesional epidermis [44]. Alteration of the blood fatty acid profile in psoriasis also suggests an essential role for FABP in the pathogenesis of this condition [196]. While FABP-4 does not always relate to psoriasis severity, the serum level increases in psoriasis cases compared with healthy controls and decreases with appropriate treatment [197]. Serum FABP-4 levels are inversely correlated with serum TARC levels, which is possibly related to psoriasis remission [198,199]. Moreover, serum FABP-1 (liver-FABP) levels increase in cases of psoriasis depending on skin lesion severity [200], and FABP-2 (intestinal FABP) potentially reflects the subclinical disruption of the intestinal barrier in severe psoriasis cases [201].

4. Conclusions

The novel and highly efficient therapeutic approaches in psoriasis have enabled the treatment of recalcitrant psoriatic lesions and comorbidities, thus leading to disease remission. The excellent efficacy of molecular-targeted therapies also highlights and reflects the molecular pathogenesis of psoriatic diseases. To refine the underlying therapeutic strategy, useful biomarkers that can reflect disease severity and sufficient remission are indispensable. Further basic and clinical research is required to establish an optimized therapeutic strategy in psoriasis treatment.

Author Contributions: Conceptualization, M.H. and H.N.; data curation, M.H.; writing—original draft preparation, M.H.; writing—review and editing, M.H. and H.N.; project administration, M.H. All authors have read and agreed to the published version of the manuscript.

Funding: This research received no external funding.

Institutional Review Board Statement: Not applicable.

Informed Consent Statement: Not applicable.

Data Availability Statement: Not applicable.

Conflicts of Interest: The authors declare no conflict of interest.

References

1. Nestle, F.O.; Kaplan, D.H.; Barker, J. Psoriasis. *N. Engl. J. Med.* **2009**, *361*, 496–509. [CrossRef]
2. Boehncke, W.H.; Schön, M.P. Psoriasis. *Lancet* **2015**, *386*, 983–994. [CrossRef]
3. Takahashi, H.; Iinuma, S.; Tsuji, H.; Honma, M.; Iizuka, H. Biologics are more potent than other treatment modalities for improvement of quality of life in psoriasis patients. *J. Dermatol.* **2014**, *41*, 686–689. [CrossRef] [PubMed]
4. Imafuku, S.; Kanai, Y.; Murotani, K.; Nomura, T.; Ito, K.; Ohata, C.; Yamazaki, F.; Miyagi, T.; Takahashi, H.; Okubo, Y.; et al. Utility of the Dermatology Life Quality Index at initiation or switching of biologics in real-life Japanese patients with plaque psoriasis: Results from the ProLOGUE study. *J. Dermatol. Sci.* **2021**, *101*, 185–193. [CrossRef] [PubMed]
5. Honma, M.; Cai, Z.; Burge, R.; Zhu, B.; Yotsukura, S.; Torisu-Itakura, H. Relationship Between Rapid Skin Clearance and Quality of Life Benefit: Post Hoc Analysis of Japanese Patients with Moderate-to-Severe Psoriasis Treated with Ixekizumab (UNCOVER-J). *Dermatol. Ther.* **2020**, *10*, 1397–1404. [CrossRef] [PubMed]
6. Meneguin, S.; de Godoy, N.A.; Pollo, C.F.; Miot, H.A.; de Oliveira, C. Quality of life of patients living with psoriasis: A qualitative study. *BMC Dermatol.* **2020**, *20*, 4–9. [CrossRef]
7. Hrehorów, E.; Salomon, J.; Matusiak, L.; Reich, A.; Szepietowski, J.C. Patients with psoriasis feel stigmatized. *Acta Derm. Venereol.* **2012**, *92*, 67–72. [PubMed]
8. Alpsoy, E.; Polat, M.; FettahlıoGlu-Karaman, B.; Karadag, A.S.; Kartal-Durmazlar, P.; YalCın, B.; Emre, S.; Didar-Balcı, D.; Bilgic-Temel, A.; Arca, E.; et al. Internalized stigma in psoriasis: A multicenter study. *J. Dermatol.* **2017**, *44*, 885–891. [CrossRef]
9. Pearl, R.L.; Wan, M.T.; Takeshita, J.; Gelfand, J.M. Stigmatizing attitudes toward persons with psoriasis among laypersons and medical students. *J. Am. Acad. Dermatol.* **2019**, *80*, 1556–1563. [CrossRef]
10. Armstrong, A.W.; Read, C. Pathophysiology, Clinical Presentation, and Treatment of Psoriasis: A Review. *JAMA* **2020**, *323*, 1945–1960. [CrossRef]
11. Ogawa, E.; Sato, Y.; Minagawa, A.; Okuyama, R. Pathogenesis of psoriasis and development of treatment. *J. Dermatol.* **2018**, *45*, 264–272. [CrossRef] [PubMed]
12. Harden, J.L.; Krueger, J.G.; Bowcock, A.M. The immunogenetics of Psoriasis: A comprehensive review. *J. Autoimmun.* **2015**, *64*, 66–73. [CrossRef]
13. Egeberg, A.; Gisondi, P.; Carrascosa, J.M.; Warren, R.B.; Mrowietz, U. The role of the interleukin-23/Th17 pathway in cardiometabolic comorbidity associated with psoriasis. *J. Eur. Acad. Dermatol. Venereol.* **2020**, *34*, 1695–1706. [CrossRef]
14. Boehncke, W.; Boehncke, S.; Tobin, A.; Kirby, B. The 'psoriatic march': A concept of how severe psoriasis may drive cardiovascular comorbidity. *Exp. Dermatol.* **2011**, *20*, 303–307. [CrossRef] [PubMed]
15. Honma, M.; Hayashi, K. Psoriasis: Recent progress in molecular-targeted therapies. *J. Dermatol.* **2021**, *48*, 761–777. [CrossRef]
16. Robb, M.A.; McInnes, P.M.; Califf, R.M. Biomarkers and surrogate endpoints: Developing common terminology and definitions. *JAMA* **2016**, *315*, 1107–1108. [CrossRef]
17. Brembilla, N.C.; Senra, L.; Boehncke, W.H. The IL-17 family of cytokines in psoriasis: IL-17A and beyond. *Front. Immunol.* **2018**, *9*, 1682. [CrossRef] [PubMed]
18. Gilliet, M.; Lande, R. Antimicrobial peptides and self-DNA in autoimmune skin inflammation. *Curr. Opin. Immunol.* **2008**, *20*, 401–407. [CrossRef]

19. Takahashi, T.; Yamasaki, K. Psoriasis and antimicrobial peptides. *Int. J. Mol. Sci.* **2020**, *21*, 6791. [CrossRef] [PubMed]
20. Wang, A.; Bai, Y.P. Dendritic cells: The driver of psoriasis. *J. Dermatol.* **2020**, *47*, 104–113. [CrossRef] [PubMed]
21. Collamer, A.N.; Guerrero, K.T.; Henning, J.S.; Battafarano, D.F. Psoriatic skin lesions induced by tumor necrosis factor antagonist therapy: A literature review and potential mechanisms of action. *Arthritis Rheum.* **2008**, *59*, 996–1001. [CrossRef] [PubMed]
22. Sakkas, L.I.; Mavropoulos, A.; Perricone, C.; Bogdanos, D.P. IL-35: A new immunomodulator in autoimmune rheumatic diseases Treg Breg. *Immunol. Res.* **2018**, *66*, 305–312. [CrossRef]
23. Teng, M.W.L.; Bowman, E.P.; Mcelwee, J.J.; Smyth, M.J.; Casanova, J.; Cooper, A.M.; Cua, D.J. IL-12 and IL-23 cytokines: From discovery to targeted therapies for immune-mediated inflammatory diseases. *Nat. Med.* **2015**, *21*, 719–729. [CrossRef] [PubMed]
24. Lee, E.; Trepicchio, W.L.; Oestreicher, J.L.; Pittman, D.; Wang, F.; Chamian, F.; Dhodapkar, M.; Krueger, J.G. Increased Expression of Interleukin 23 p19 and p40 in Lesional Skin of Patients with Psoriasis Vulgaris. *J. Exp. Med.* **2004**, *199*, 125–130. [CrossRef]
25. Shibata, A.; Sugiura, K.; Furuta, Y.; Mukumoto, Y.; Kaminuma, O.; Akiyama, M. Toll-like receptor 4 antagonist TAK-242 inhibits autoinflammatory symptoms in DITRA. *J. Autoimmun.* **2017**, *80*, 28–38. [CrossRef]
26. Yoon, J.; Leyva Castillo, J.M.; Wang, G.; Galand, C.; Oyoshi, M.K.; Kumar, L.; Hoff, S.; He, R.; Chervonsky, A.; Oppenheim, J.J.; et al. IL-23 induced in keratinocytes by endogenous TLR4 ligands polarizes dendritic cells to drive IL-22 responses to skin immunization. *J. Exp. Med.* **2016**, *213*, 2147–2166. [CrossRef]
27. Li, H.; Yao, Q.; Mariscal, A.G.; Wu, X.; Hülse, J.; Pedersen, E.; Helin, K.; Waisman, A.; Vinkel, C.; Thomsen, S.F.; et al. Epigenetic control of IL-23 expression in keratinocytes is important for chronic skin inflammation. *Nat. Commun.* **2018**, *9*, 1420. [CrossRef]
28. Koenen, H.J.P.M.; Smeets, R.L.; Vink, P.M.; Van Rijssen, E.; Boots, A.M.H.; Joosten, I. Human CD25 high Foxp3 pos regulatory T cells differentiate into IL-17—Producing cells. *Blood* **2008**, *112*, 2340–2353. [CrossRef]
29. Bovenschen, H.J.; Van De Kerkhof, P.C.; Van Erp, P.E.; Woestenenk, R.; Joosten, I.; Koenen, H.J.P.M. Foxp3 regulatory T cells of psoriasis patients easily differentiate into IL-17A-producing cells and are found in lesional skin. *J. Investig. Dermatol.* **2011**, *131*, 1853–1860. [CrossRef] [PubMed]
30. Mylonas, A.; Conrad, C. Psoriasis: Classical vs. Paradoxical. the yin-yang of TNF and Type i interferon. *Front. Immunol.* **2018**, *9*, 2746. [CrossRef] [PubMed]
31. Krueger, G.; Callis, K. Potential of Tumor Necrosis Factor Inhibitors in Psoriasis and Psoriatic Arthritis. *Arch. Dermatol.* **2004**, *140*, 218–225. [CrossRef]
32. Kalliolias, G.D.; Ivashkiv, L.B.; Program, T.D. TNF biology, pathogenic mechanisms and emerging therapeutic strategies. *Nat. Rev. Rheumatol.* **2016**, *12*, 49–62. [CrossRef] [PubMed]
33. Yasuda, K.; Takeuchi, Y.; Hirota, K. The pathogenicity of Th17 cells in autoimmune diseases. *Semin. Immunopathol.* **2019**, *41*, 283–297. [CrossRef] [PubMed]
34. Schmitt, N.; Ueno, H. Regulation of human helper T cell subset differentiation by cytokines. *Curr. Opin. Immunol.* **2015**, *34*, 130–136. [CrossRef]
35. Amatya, N.; Garg, A.V.; Gaffen, S.L. IL-17 Signaling: The Yin and the Yang. *Trends Immunol.* **2017**, *38*, 310–322. [CrossRef] [PubMed]
36. McGeachy, M.J.; Cua, D.J.; Gaffen, S.L. The IL-17 Family of Cytokines in Health and Disease. *Immunity* **2019**, *50*, 892–906. [CrossRef]
37. Monin, L.; Gaffen, S.L. Interleukin 17 Family Cytokines: Signaling and Therapeutic Implications. *Cold Spring Harb. Perspect. Biol.* **2018**, *10*, a028522. [CrossRef] [PubMed]
38. Su, Y.; Huang, J.; Zhao, X.; Lu, H.; Wang, W.; Yang, X.O.; Shi, Y.; Wang, X.; Lai, Y.; Dong, C. Interleukin-17 receptor D constitutes an alternative receptor for interleukin-17A important in psoriasis-like skin inflammation. *Sci. Immunol.* **2019**, *4*, eaau9657. [CrossRef]
39. Matsuzaki, G.; Umemura, M. Interleukin-17 family cytokines in protective immunity against infections: Role of hematopoietic cell-derived and non-hematopoietic cell-derived interleukin-17s. *Microbiol. Immunol.* **2018**, *62*, 1–13. [CrossRef]
40. Lee, J.S.; Tato, C.M.; Joyce-Shaikh, B.; Gulan, F.; Cayatte, C.; Chen, Y.; Blumenschein, W.M.; Judo, M.; Ayanoglu, G.; McClanahan, T.K.; et al. Interleukin-23-Independent IL-17 Production Regulates Intestinal Epithelial Permeability. *Immunity* **2015**, *43*, 727–738. [CrossRef]
41. Maxwell, J.R.; Zhang, Y.; Brown, W.A.; Smith, C.L.; Byrne, F.R.; Fiorino, M.; Stevens, E.; Bigler, J.; Davis, J.A.; Rottman, J.B.; et al. Differential Roles for Interleukin-23 and Interleukin-17 in Intestinal Immunoregulation. *Immunity* **2015**, *43*, 739–750. [CrossRef]
42. McGonagle, D.G.; McInnes, I.B.; Kirkham, B.W.; Sherlock, J.; Moots, R. The role of IL-17A in axial spondyloarthritis and psoriatic arthritis: Recent advances and controversies. *Ann. Rheum. Dis.* **2019**, *78*, 1167–1178. [CrossRef]
43. Cheuk, S.; Wiken, M.; Blomqvist, L.; Nylen, S.; Talme, T.; Stahle, M.; Eidsmo, L.; Wikén, M.; Blomqvist, L.; Nylén, S.; et al. Epidermal Th22 and Tc17 Cells Form a Localized Disease Memory in Clinically Healed Psoriasis. *J. Immunol.* **2014**, *192*, 3111–3120. [CrossRef]
44. Pan, Y.; Tian, T.; Park, C.O.; Lofftus, S.Y.; Mei, S.; Liu, X.; Luo, C.; O'Malley, J.T.; Gehad, A.; Teague, J.E.; et al. Survival of tissue-resident memory T cells requires exogenous lipid uptake and metabolism. *Nature* **2017**, *543*, 252–256. [CrossRef]
45. Kim, J.; Oh, C.H.; Jeon, J.; Baek, Y.; Ahn, J.; Kim, D.J.; Lee, H.S.; Correa, J.; Sua, M.; Lowes, M.A.; et al. Molecular phenotyping small (Asian) versus large (Western) plaque psoriasis shows common activation of IL-17 pathway genes but different regulatory gene sets. *J. Investig. Dermatol.* **2016**, *136*, 161–172. [CrossRef]

46. Imafuku, S.; Honma, M.; Okubo, Y.; Komine, M.; Ohtsuki, M.; Morita, A.; Seko, N.; Kawashima, N.; Ito, S.; Shima, T.; et al. Efficacy and safety of secukinumab in patients with generalized pustular psoriasis: A 52-week analysis from phase III open-label multicenter Japanese study. *J. Dermatol.* **2016**, *43*, 1011–1017. [CrossRef] [PubMed]
47. Mrowietz, U.; Bachelez, H.; Burden, A.D.; Rissler, M.; Sieder, C.; Orsenigo, R.; Chaouche-Teyara, K. Secukinumab for moderate-to-severe palmoplantar pustular psoriasis: Results of the 2PRECISE study. *J. Am. Acad. Dermatol.* **2019**, *80*, 1344–1352. [CrossRef] [PubMed]
48. Honma, M.; Nozaki, H.; Hayashi, K.; Iinuma, S.; Ishida-Yamamoto, A. Palmoplantar pustulosis emerged on a case of generalized pustular psoriasis successfully treated by secukinumab. *J. Dermatol.* **2019**, *46*, e468–e469. [CrossRef] [PubMed]
49. Zlotnik, A.; Yoshie, O. The Chemokine Superfamily Revisited. *Immunity* **2012**, *36*, 705–716. [CrossRef] [PubMed]
50. Schutyser, E.; Struyf, S.; Van Damme, J. The CC chemokine CCL20 and its receptor CCR6. *Cytokine Growth Factor Rev.* **2003**, *14*, 409–426. [CrossRef]
51. Meitei, H.T.; Jadhav, N.; Lal, G. CCR6-CCL20 axis as a therapeutic target for autoimmune diseases. *Autoimmun. Rev.* **2021**, *20*, 102846. [CrossRef]
52. Harper, E.G.; Guo, C.; Rizzo, H.; Lillis, J.V.; Kurtz, S.E.; Skorcheva, I.; Purdy, D.; Fitch, E.; Iordanov, M.; Blauvelt, A. Th17 cytokines stimulate CCL20 expression in keratinocytes in vitro and in vivo: Implications for psoriasis pathogenesis. *J. Investig. Dermatol.* **2009**, *129*, 2175–2183. [CrossRef]
53. Chiricozzi, A.; Guttman-Yassky, E.; Suárez-Fariñas, M.; Nograles, K.E.; Tian, S.; Cardinale, I.; Chimenti, S.; Krueger, J.G. Integrative responses to IL-17 and TNF-α in human keratinocytes account for key inflammatory pathogenic circuits in psoriasis. *J. Investig. Dermatol.* **2011**, *131*, 677–687. [CrossRef]
54. Furue, K.; Ito, T.; Tanaka, Y.; Yumine, A.; Hashimoto-Hachiya, A.; Takemura, M.; Murata, M.; Yamamura, K.; Tsuji, G.; Furue, M. Cyto/chemokine profile of in vitro scratched keratinocyte model: Implications of significant upregulation of CCL20, CXCL8 and IL36G in Koebner phenomenon. *J. Dermatol. Sci.* **2019**, *94*, 244–251. [CrossRef]
55. Mabuchi, T.; Singh, T.P.; Takekoshi, T.; Jia, G.F.; Wu, X.; Kao, M.C.; Weiss, I.; Farber, J.M.; Hwang, S.T. CCR6 is required for epidermal trafficking of γδ-T cells in an IL-23-Induced model of psoriasiform dermatitis. *J. Investig. Dermatol.* **2013**, *133*, 164–171. [CrossRef]
56. Hedrick, M.N.; Lonsdorf, A.S.; Shirakawa, A.K.; Lee, C.C.R.; Liao, F.; Singh, S.P.; Zhang, H.H.; Grinberg, A.; Love, P.E.; Hwang, S.T.; et al. CCR6 is required for IL-23-induced psoriasis-like inflammation in mice. *J. Clin. Investig.* **2009**, *119*, 2317–2329. [CrossRef]
57. Getschman, A.E.; Imai, Y.; Larsen, O.; Peterson, F.C.; Wu, X.; Rosenkilde, M.M.; Hwang, S.T.; Volkman, B.F. Protein engineering of the chemokine CCL20 prevents psoriasiform dermatitis in an IL-23–dependent murine model. *Proc. Natl. Acad. Sci. USA* **2017**, *114*, 12460–12465. [CrossRef]
58. Furue, K.; Ito, T.; Tsuji, G.; Nakahara, T.; Furue, M. The CCL20 and CCR6 axis in psoriasis. *Scand. J. Immunol.* **2020**, *91*, e12846. [CrossRef]
59. Mabuchi, T.; Chang, T.W.; Quinter, S.; Hwang, S.T. Chemokine receptors in the pathogenesis and therapy of psoriasis. *J. Dermatol. Sci.* **2012**, *65*, 4–11. [CrossRef]
60. Jensen, P.; Skov, L. Psoriasis and Obesity. *Dermatology* **2017**, *232*, 633–639. [CrossRef]
61. Huang, Y.H.; Yang, L.C.; Hui, R.Y.; Chang, Y.C.; Yang, Y.W.; Yang, C.H.; Chen, Y.H.; Chung, W.H.; Kuan, Y.Z.; Chiu, C.S. Relationships between obesity and the clinical severity of psoriasis in Taiwan. *J. Eur. Acad. Dermatol. Venereol.* **2010**, *24*, 1035–1039. [CrossRef] [PubMed]
62. Naldi, L.; Conti, A.; Cazzaniga, S.; Patrizi, A.; Pazzaglia, M.; Lanzoni, A.; Veneziano, L.; Pellacani, G.; Miglietta, R.; Padalino, C.; et al. Diet and physical exercise in psoriasis: A randomized controlled trial. *Br. J. Dermatol.* **2014**, *170*, 634–642. [CrossRef] [PubMed]
63. Jensen, P.; Christensen, R.; Zachariae, C.; Geiker, N.R.W.; Schaadt, B.K.; Stender, S.; Hansen, P.R.; Astrup, A.; Skov, L. Long-term effects of weight reduction on the severity of psoriasis in a cohort derived from a randomized trial: A prospective observational follow-up study. *Am. J. Clin. Nutr.* **2016**, *104*, 259–265. [CrossRef]
64. Mahil, S.K.; McSweeney, S.M.; Kloczko, E.; McGowan, B.; Barker, J.N.; Smith, C.H. Does weight loss reduce the severity and incidence of psoriasis or psoriatic arthritis? A Critically Appraised Topic. *Br. J. Dermatol.* **2019**, *181*, 946–953. [CrossRef] [PubMed]
65. Castaldo, G.; Rastrelli, L.; Galdo, G.; Molettieri, P.; Rotondi Aufiero, F.; Cereda, E. Aggressive weight-loss program with a ketogenic induction phase for the treatment of chronic plaque psoriasis: A proof-of-concept, single-arm, open-label clinical trial. *Nutrition* **2020**, *74*, 110757. [CrossRef] [PubMed]
66. Jensen, P.; Zachariae, C.; Christensen, R.; Geiker, N.R.W.; Schaadt, B.K.; Stender, S.; Hansen, P.R.; Astrup, A.; Skov, L. Effect of weight loss on the severity of psoriasis: A randomized clinical study. *JAMA Dermatol.* **2013**, *149*, 795–801. [CrossRef]
67. Debbaneh, M.; Millsop, J.W.; Bhatia, B.K.; Koo, J.; Liao, W. Diet and psoriasis, part I: Impact of weight loss interventions. *J. Am. Acad. Dermatol.* **2014**, *71*, 133–140. [CrossRef]
68. Sako, E.Y.; Famenini, S.; Wu, J.J. Bariatric surgery and psoriasis. *J. Am. Acad. Dermatol.* **2014**, *70*, 774–779. [CrossRef]
69. Coimbra, S.; Catarino, C.; Santos-Silva, A. The triad psoriasis–obesity–adipokine profile. *J. Eur. Acad. Dermatol. Venereol.* **2016**, *30*, 1876–1885. [CrossRef]

70. Gerdes, S.; Rostami-Yazdi, M.; Mrowietz, U. Adipokines and psoriasis. *Exp. Dermatol.* **2011**, *20*, 81–87. [CrossRef]
71. Wong, Y.; Nakamizo, S.; Tan, K.J.; Kabashima, K. An update on the role of adipose tissues in psoriasis. *Front. Immunol.* **2019**, *10*, 1507. [CrossRef]
72. Fantuzzi, G. Adipose tissue, adipokines, and inflammation. *J. Allergy Clin. Immunol.* **2005**, *115*, 911–919. [CrossRef]
73. Pou, K.M.; Massaro, J.M.; Hoffmann, U.; Vasan, R.S.; Maurovich-Horvat, P.; Larson, M.G.; Keaney, J.F.; Meigs, J.B.; Lipinska, I.; Kathiresan, S.; et al. Visceral and subcutaneous adipose tissue volumes are cross-sectionally related to markers of inflammation and oxidative stress: The Framingham Heart Study. *Circulation* **2007**, *116*, 1234–1241. [CrossRef] [PubMed]
74. Alexopoulos, N.; Katritsis, D.; Raggi, P. Visceral adipose tissue as a source of inflammation and promoter of atherosclerosis. *Atherosclerosis* **2014**, *233*, 104–112. [CrossRef]
75. Carvalheira, J.B.C.; Qiu, Y.; Chawla, A. Blood spotlight on leukocytes and obesity. *Blood* **2013**, *122*, 3263–3267. [CrossRef] [PubMed]
76. Rocha, D.M.; Caldas, A.P.; Oliveira, L.L.; Bressan, J.; Hermsdorff, H.H. Saturated fatty acids trigger TLR4-mediated inflammatory response. *Atherosclerosis* **2016**, *244*, 211–215. [CrossRef]
77. Kunz, M.; Simon, J.C.; Saalbach, A. Psoriasis: Obesity and Fatty Acids. *Front. Immunol.* **2019**, *10*, 1807. [CrossRef]
78. Barra, N.G.; Henriksbo, B.D.; Anhê, F.F.; Schertzer, J.D. The NLRP3 inflammasome regulates adipose tissue metabolism. *Biochem. J.* **2020**, *477*, 1089–1107. [CrossRef] [PubMed]
79. Cheuk, S.; Eidsmo, L. The Skinny on Fat T_{RM} Cells. *Immunity* **2017**, *47*, 1012–1014. [CrossRef]
80. Han, S.J.; Glatman Zaretsky, A.; Andrade-Oliveira, V.; Collins, N.; Dzutsev, A.; Shaik, J.; Morais da Fonseca, D.; Harrison, O.J.; Tamoutounour, S.; Byrd, A.L.; et al. White Adipose Tissue Is a Reservoir for Memory T Cells and Promotes Protective Memory Responses to Infection. *Immunity* **2017**, *47*, 1154–1168. [CrossRef]
81. Ramirez, G.A.; Manfredi, A.A.; Maugeri, N. Misunderstandings between platelets and neutrophils build in chronic inflammation. *Front. Immunol.* **2019**, *10*, 2491. [CrossRef] [PubMed]
82. Chiang, C.C.; Cheng, W.J.; Korinek, M.; Lin, C.Y.; Hwang, T.L. Neutrophils in Psoriasis. *Front. Immunol.* **2019**, *10*, 2376. [CrossRef] [PubMed]
83. Sylman, J.L.; Mitrugno, A.; Atallah, M.; Tormoen, G.W.; Shatzel, J.J.; Yunga, S.T.; Wagner, T.H.; Leppert, J.T.; Mallick, P.; McCarty, O.J.T. The predictive value of inflammation-related peripheral blood measurements in cancer staging and prognosis. *Front. Oncol.* **2018**, *8*, 78. [CrossRef] [PubMed]
84. Hao, X.; Li, D.; Wu, D.; Zhang, N. The Relationship between Hematological Indices and Autoimmune Rheumatic Diseases (ARDs), a Meta-Analysis. *Sci. Rep.* **2017**, *7*, 10833. [CrossRef]
85. Asahina, A.; Kubo, N.; Umezawa, Y.; Honda, H.; Yanaba, K. Neutrophil-lymphocyte ratio, platelet-lymphocyte ratio and mean platelet volume in Japanese patients with psoriasis and psoriatic arthritis: Response to therapy with biologics. *J. Dermatol.* **2017**, *44*, 1112–1121. [CrossRef]
86. Najar Nobari, N.; Shahidi Dadras, M.; Nasiri, S.; Abdollahimajd, F.; Gheisari, M. Neutrophil/platelet to lymphocyte ratio in monitoring of response to TNF-α inhibitors in psoriatic patients. *Dermatol. Ther.* **2020**, *33*, e13457. [CrossRef]
87. Paliogiannis, P.; Satta, R.; Deligia, G.; Farina, G.; Bassu, S.; Mangoni, A.A.; Carru, C.; Zinellu, A. Associations between the neutrophil-to-lymphocyte and the platelet-to-lymphocyte ratios and the presence and severity of psoriasis: A systematic review and meta-analysis. *Clin. Exp. Med.* **2019**, *19*, 37–45. [CrossRef]
88. Yilmaz, S.B.; Cicek, N.; Coskun, M.; Yegin, O.; Alpsoy, E. Serum and tissue levels of IL-17 in different clinical subtypes of psoriasis. *Arch. Dermatol. Res.* **2012**, *304*, 465–469. [CrossRef]
89. Kolbinger, F.; Loesche, C.; Valentin, M.A.; Jiang, X.; Cheng, Y.; Jarvis, P.; Peters, T.; Calonder, C.; Bruin, G.; Polus, F.; et al. β-Defensin 2 is a responsive biomarker of IL-17A–driven skin pathology in patients with psoriasis. *J. Allergy Clin. Immunol.* **2017**, *139*, 923–932. [CrossRef]
90. Gordon, K.B.; Armstrong, A.W.; Foley, P.; Song, M.; Shen, Y.K.; Li, S.; Muñoz-Elías, E.J.; Branigan, P.; Liu, X.; Reich, K. Guselkumab Efficacy after Withdrawal Is Associated with Suppression of Serum IL-23-Regulated IL-17 and IL-22 in Psoriasis: VOYAGE 2 Study. *J. Investig. Dermatol.* **2019**, *139*, 2437–2446. [CrossRef]
91. Fitz, L.; Zhang, W.; Soderstrom, C.; Fraser, S.; Lee, J.; Quazi, A.; Wolk, R.; Mebus, C.A.; Valdez, H.; Berstein, G. Association between serum interleukin-17A and clinical response to tofacitinib and etanercept in moderate to severe psoriasis. *Clin. Exp. Dermatol.* **2018**, *43*, 790–797. [CrossRef] [PubMed]
92. Garcet, S.; Nograles, K.; Correa da Rosa, J.; Schafer, P.H.; Krueger, J.G. Synergistic cytokine effects as apremilast response predictors in patients with psoriasis. *J. Allergy Clin. Immunol.* **2018**, *142*, 1010–1013. [CrossRef] [PubMed]
93. Ishigame, H.; Kakuta, S.; Nagai, T.; Kadoki, M.; Nambu, A.; Komiyama, Y.; Fujikado, N.; Tanahashi, Y.; Akitsu, A.; Kotaki, H.; et al. Differential Roles of Interleukin-17A and -17F in Host Defense against Mucoepithelial Bacterial Infection and Allergic Responses. *Immunity* **2009**, *30*, 108–119. [CrossRef]
94. Gomes, A.L.; Teijeiro, A.; Burén, S.; Tummala, K.S.; Yilmaz, M.; Waisman, A.; Theurillat, J.P.; Perna, C.; Djouder, N. Metabolic Inflammation-Associated IL-17A Causes Non-alcoholic Steatohepatitis and Hepatocellular Carcinoma. *Cancer Cell* **2016**, *30*, 161–175. [CrossRef]

95. Von Stebut, E.; Boehncke, W.H.; Ghoreschi, K.; Gori, T.; Kaya, Z.; Thaci, D.; Schäffler, A. IL-17A in Psoriasis and Beyond: Cardiovascular and Metabolic Implications. *Front. Immunol.* **2020**, *10*, 3096. [CrossRef]
96. Ikumi, K.; Odanaka, M.; Shime, H.; Imai, M.; Osaga, S.; Taguchi, O.; Nishida, E.; Hemmi, H.; Kaisho, T.; Morita, A.; et al. Hyperglycemia Is Associated with Psoriatic Inflammation in Both Humans and Mice. *J. Investig. Dermatol.* **2019**, *139*, 1329–1338. [CrossRef] [PubMed]
97. Elnabawi, Y.A.; Dey, A.K.; Goyal, A.; Groenendyk, J.W.; Chung, J.H.; Belur, A.D.; Rodante, J.; Harrington, C.L.; Teague, H.L.; Baumer, Y.; et al. Coronary artery plaque characteristics and treatment with biologic therapy in severe psoriasis: Results from a prospective observational study. *Cardiovasc. Res.* **2019**, *115*, 721–728. [CrossRef]
98. Rutz, S.; Wang, X.; Ouyang, W. The IL-20 subfamily of cytokines-from host defence to tissue homeostasis. *Nat. Rev. Immunol.* **2014**, *14*, 783–795. [CrossRef]
99. Ouyang, W.; O'Garra, A. IL-10 Family Cytokines IL-10 and IL-22: From Basic Science to Clinical Translation. *Immunity* **2019**, *50*, 871–891. [CrossRef]
100. Eyerich, K.; Dimartino, V.; Cavani, A. IL-17 and IL-22 in immunity: Driving protection and pathology. *Eur. J. Immunol.* **2017**, *47*, 607–614. [CrossRef]
101. Honma, M.; Minami-Hori, M.; Takahashi, H.; Iizuka, H. Podoplanin expression in wound and hyperproliferative psoriatic epidermis: Regulation by TGF-β and STAT-3 activating cytokines, IFN-γ, IL-6, and IL-22. *J. Dermatol. Sci.* **2012**, *65*, 134–140. [CrossRef]
102. Guttman-Yassky, E.; Krueger, J.G. Atopic dermatitis and psoriasis: Two different immune diseases or one spectrum? *Curr. Opin. Immunol.* **2017**, *48*, 68–73. [CrossRef]
103. Shimauchi, T.; Hirakawa, S.; Suzuki, T.; Yasuma, A.; Majima, Y.; Tatsuno, K.; Yagi, H.; Ito, T.; Tokura, Y. Serum interleukin-22 and vascular endothelial growth factor serve as sensitive biomarkers but not as predictors of therapeutic response to biologics in patients with psoriasis. *J. Dermatol.* **2013**, *40*, 805–812. [CrossRef]
104. Philipp, S.; Menter, A.; Nikkels, A.F.; Barber, K.; Landells, I.; Eichenfield, L.F.; Song, M.; Randazzo, B.; Li, S.; Hsu, M.C.; et al. Ustekinumab for the treatment of moderate-to-severe plaque psoriasis in paediatric patients (≥6 to <12 years of age): Efficacy, safety, pharmacokinetic and biomarker results from the open-label CADMUS Jr study. *Br. J. Dermatol.* **2020**, *183*, 664–672. [CrossRef]
105. Kragstrup, T.W.; Andersen, T.; Heftdal, L.D.; Hvid, M.; Gerwien, J.; Sivakumar, P.; Taylor, P.C.; Senolt, L.; Deleuran, B. The IL-20 cytokine family in rheumatoid arthritis and spondyloarthritis. *Front. Immunol.* **2018**, *9*, 2226. [CrossRef]
106. Konrad, R.J.; Higgs, R.E.; Rodgers, G.H.; Ming, W.; Qian, Y.W.; Bivi, N.; Mack, J.K.; Siegel, R.W.; Nickoloff, B.J. Assessment and Clinical Relevance of Serum IL-19 Levels in Psoriasis and Atopic Dermatitis Using a Sensitive and Specific Novel Immunoassay. *Sci. Rep.* **2019**, *9*, 5211. [CrossRef] [PubMed]
107. Autieri, M.V. IL-19 and other IL-20 family member cytokines in vascular inflammatory diseases. *Front. Immunol.* **2018**, *9*, 700. [CrossRef] [PubMed]
108. Fabre, T.; Molina, M.F.; Soucy, G.; Goulet, J.P.; Willems, B.; Villeneuve, J.P.; Bilodeau, M.; Shoukry, N.H. Type 3 cytokines IL-17A and IL-22 drive TGF—dependent liver fibrosis. *Sci. Immunol.* **2018**, *3*, eaar7754. [CrossRef] [PubMed]
109. Walsh, P.T.; Fallon, P.G. The emergence of the IL-36 cytokine family as novel targets for inflammatory diseases. *Ann. N. Y. Acad. Sci.* **2016**, *1417*, 23–34. [CrossRef] [PubMed]
110. Yi, G.; Ybe, J.A.; Saha, S.S.; Caviness, G.; Raymond, E.; Ganesan, R.; Mbow, M.L.; Kao, C.C. Structural and functional attributes of the interleukin-36 receptor. *J. Biol. Chem.* **2016**, *291*, 16597–16609. [CrossRef]
111. Fields, J.K.; Günther, S.; Sundberg, E.J. Structural basis of IL-1 family cytokine signaling. *Front. Immunol.* **2019**, *10*, 1412. [CrossRef]
112. Han, Y.; Huard, A.; Mora, J.; da Silva, P.; Brüne, B.; Weigert, A. IL-36 family cytokines in protective versus destructive inflammation. *Cell. Signal.* **2020**, *75*, 109773. [CrossRef] [PubMed]
113. Furue, K.; Yamamura, K.; Tsuji, G.; Mitoma, C.; Uchi, H.; Nakahara, T.; Kido-Nakahara, M.; Kadono, T.; Furue, M. Highlighting interleukin-36 signalling in plaque psoriasis and pustular psoriasis. *Acta Derm. Venereol.* **2018**, *98*, 5–13. [CrossRef]
114. Mercurio, L.; Id, C.M.F.; Capriotti, L.; Scarponi, C.; Facchiano, F.; Morelli, M.; Rossi, S.; Pagnanelli, G.; Id, C.A.; Cavani, A.; et al. Interleukin (IL)-17/IL-36 axis participates to the crosstalk between endothelial cells and keratinocytes during inflammatory skin responses. *PLoS ONE* **2020**, *15*, e0222969. [CrossRef]
115. Buhl, A.L.; Wenzel, J. Interleukin-36 in infectious and inflammatory skin diseases. *Front. Immunol.* **2019**, *10*, 1162. [CrossRef]
116. Madonna, S.; Girolomoni, G.; Dinarello, C.A.; Albanesi, C. The significance of Il-36 hyperactivation and Il-36R targeting in psoriasis. *Int. J. Mol. Sci.* **2019**, *20*, 3318. [CrossRef]
117. Pfaff, C.M.; Marquardt, Y.; Fietkau, K.; Baron, J.M.; Lüscher, B. The psoriasis-associated IL-17A induces and cooperates with IL-36 cytokines to control keratinocyte differentiation and function. *Sci. Rep.* **2017**, *7*, 15631. [CrossRef] [PubMed]
118. D'Erme, A.M.; Wilsmann-Theis, D.; Wagenpfeil, J.; Hölzel, M.; Ferring-Schmitt, S.; Sternberg, S.; Wittmann, M.; Peters, B.; Bosio, A.; Bieber, T.; et al. IL-36γ (IL 1F9) Is a Biomarker for Psoriasis Skin Lesions. *J. Investig. Dermatol.* **2015**, *135*, 1025–1032. [CrossRef]
119. Braegelmann, J.; D'Erme, A.M.; Akmal, S.; Maier, J.; Braegelmann, C.; Wenzel, J. Interleukin-36γ (IL-1F9) identifies psoriasis among patients with erythroderma. *Acta Derm. Venereol.* **2016**, *96*, 386–387. [CrossRef]
120. Raychaudhuri, S.P.; Jiang, W.Y.; Farber, E.M. Cellular localization of fractalkine at sites of inflammation: Antigen-presenting cells in psoriasis express high levels of fractalkine. *Br. J. Dermatol.* **2001**, *144*, 1105–1113. [CrossRef]

121. Fraticelli, P.; Sironi, M.; Bianchi, G.; D'Ambrosio, D.; Albanesi, C.; Stoppacciaro, A.; Chieppa, M.; Allavena, P.; Ruco, L.; Girolomoni, G.; et al. Fractalkine (CX3CL1) as an amplification circuit of polarized Th1 responses. *J. Clin. Investig.* **2001**, *107*, 1173–1181. [CrossRef]
122. Sugaya, M.; Nakamura, K.; Mitsui, H.; Takekoshi, T.; Saeki, H.; Tamaki, K. Human keratinocytes express fractalkine/CX3CL1. *J. Dermatol. Sci.* **2003**, *31*, 179–187. [CrossRef]
123. Plant, D.; Young, H.S.; Watson, R.E.B.; Worthington, J.; Griffiths, C.E.M. The CX3CL1-CX3CR1 system and psoriasis. *Exp. Dermatol.* **2006**, *15*, 900–903. [CrossRef]
124. Morimura, S.; Oka, T.; Sugaya, M.; Sato, S. CX3CR1 deficiency attenuates imiquimod-induced psoriasis-like skin inflammation with decreased M1 macrophages. *J. Dermatol. Sci.* **2016**, *82*, 175–188. [CrossRef]
125. Congjun, J.; Yanmei, Z.; Huiling, J.; Zhen, Y.; Shuo, L. Elevated local and serum CX3CL1(Fractalkine) Expression and its association with disease severity in patients with psoriasis. *Ann. Clin. Lab. Sci.* **2015**, *45*, 556–561.
126. Echigo, T.; Hasegawa, M.; Shimada, Y.; Takehara, K.; Sato, S. Expression of fractalkine and its receptor, CX3CR1, in atopic dermatitis: Possible contribution to skin inflammation. *J. Allergy Clin. Immunol.* **2004**, *113*, 940–948. [CrossRef]
127. Teupser, D.; Pavlides, S.; Tan, M.; Gutierrez-Ramos, J.C.; Kolbeck, R.; Breslow, J.L. Major reduction of antherosclerosis in fractalkine (CX3CL1)-deficient mice is at the brachiocephalic artery, not the aortic root. *Proc. Natl. Acad. Sci. USA* **2004**, *101*, 17795–17800. [CrossRef]
128. Hughes, C.E.; Nibbs, R.J.B. A guide to chemokines and their receptors. *FEBS J.* **2018**, *285*, 2944–2971. [CrossRef]
129. Saeki, H.; Tamaki, K. Thymus and activation regulated chemokine (TARC)/CCL17 and skin diseases. *J. Dermatol. Sci.* **2006**, *43*, 75–84. [CrossRef]
130. Rottman, J.B.; Smith, T.L.; Ganley, K.G.; Kikuchi, T.; Krueger, J.G. Potential role of the chemokine receptors CXCR3, CCR4, and the integrin $\alpha E\beta 7$ in the pathogenesis of psoriasis vulgaris. *Lab. Investig.* **2001**, *81*, 335–347. [CrossRef]
131. Kakinuma, T.; Nakamura, K.; Wakugawa, M.; Mitsui, H.; Tada, Y.; Saeki, H.; Torii, H.; Asahina, A.; Onai, N.; Matsushima, K.; et al. Thymus and activation-regulated chemokine in atopic dermatitis: Serum thymus and activation-regulated chemokine level is closely related with disease activity. *J. Allergy Clin. Immunol.* **2001**, *107*, 535–541. [CrossRef] [PubMed]
132. Shibuya, T.; Honma, M.; Iinuma, S.; Iwasaki, T.; Takahashi, H.; Ishida-Yamamoto, A. Alteration of serum thymus and activation-regulated chemokine level during biologic therapy for psoriasis: Possibility as a marker reflecting favorable response to anti-interleukin-17A agents. *J. Dermatol.* **2018**, *45*, 710–714. [CrossRef] [PubMed]
133. Bernink, J.H.; Ohne, Y.; Teunissen, M.B.M.; Wang, J.; Wu, J.; Krabbendam, L.; Guntermann, C.; Volckmann, R.; Koster, J.; van Tol, S.; et al. c-Kit-positive ILC2s exhibit an ILC3-like signature that may contribute to IL-17-mediated pathologies. *Nat. Immunol.* **2019**, *20*, 992–1003. [CrossRef] [PubMed]
134. Kawasaki, Y.; Kamata, M.; Shimizu, T.; Nagata, M.; Fukaya, S.; Hayashi, K.; Fukuyasu, A.; Tanaka, T.; Ishikawa, T.; Ohnishi, T.; et al. Thymus and activation-regulated chemokine (TARC) in patients with psoriasis: Increased serum TARC levels in patients with generalized pustular psoriasis. *J. Dermatol.* **2020**, *47*, 1149–1156. [CrossRef]
135. Ouchi, N.; Parker, J.L.; Lugus, J.J.; Walsh, K. Adipokines in inflammation and metabolic disease. *Nat. Rev. Immunol.* **2011**, *11*, 85–97. [CrossRef]
136. Fasshauer, M.; Blüher, M. Adipokines in health and disease. *Trends Pharmacol. Sci.* **2015**, *36*, 461–470. [CrossRef]
137. Francisco, V.; Ruiz-Fernández, C.; Pino, J.; Mera, A.; González-Gay, M.A.; Gómez, R.; Lago, F.; Mobasheri, A.; Gualillo, O. Adipokines: Linking metabolic syndrome, the immune system, and arthritic diseases. *Biochem. Pharmacol.* **2019**, *165*, 196–206. [CrossRef]
138. Versini, M.; Jeandel, P.Y.; Rosenthal, E.; Shoenfeld, Y. Obesity in autoimmune diseases: Not a passive bystander. *Autoimmun. Rev.* **2014**, *13*, 981–1000. [CrossRef]
139. Bai, F.; Zheng, W.; Dong, Y.; Wang, J.; Garstka, M.A.; Li, R.; An, J.; Ma, H. Serum levels of adipokines and cytokines in psoriasis patients: A systematic review and meta-analysis. *Oncotarget* **2018**, *9*, 1266–1278. [CrossRef]
140. Steppan, C.M.; Lazar, M.A.; Lazar, M.A. Resistin and obesity-associated insulin resistance. *Trends Endocrinol. Metab.* **2002**, *13*, 18–23. [CrossRef]
141. Takahashi, H.; Tsuji, H.; Honma, M.; Ishida-Yamamoto, A.; Iizuka, H. Increased plasma resistin and decreased omentin levels in Japanese patients with psoriasis. *Arch. Dermatol. Res.* **2013**, *305*, 113–116. [CrossRef]
142. Kyriakou, A.; Patsatsi, A.; Sotiriadis, D.; Goulis, D.G. Effects of treatment for psoriasis on circulating levels of leptin, adiponectin and resistin: A systematic review and meta-analysis. *Br. J. Dermatol.* **2018**, *179*, 273–281. [CrossRef]
143. Pina, T.; Genre, F.; Lopez-Mejias, R.; Armesto, S.; Ubilla, B.; Mijares, V.; Dierssen-Sotos, T.; Gonzalez-Lopez, M.A.; Gonzalez-Vela, M.C.; Blanco, R.; et al. Relationship of Leptin with adiposity and inflammation and Resistin with disease severity in Psoriatic patients undergoing anti-TNF-alpha therapy. *J. Eur. Acad. Dermatol. Venereol.* **2015**, *29*, 1995–2001. [CrossRef]
144. Robati, R.M.; Partovi-Kia, M.; Haghighatkhah, H.R.; Younespour, S.; Abdollahimajd, F. Increased serum leptin and resistin levels and increased carotid intima-media wall thickness in patients with psoriasis: Is psoriasis associated with atherosclerosis? *J. Am. Acad. Dermatol.* **2014**, *71*, 642–648. [CrossRef] [PubMed]
145. Goldstein, B.J.; Scalia, R.G.; Ma, X.L. Protective vascular and myocardial effects of adiponectin. *Nat. Clin. Pract. Cardiovasc. Med.* **2009**, *6*, 27–35. [CrossRef] [PubMed]

146. Shibata, S.; Tada, Y.; Hau, C.S.; Mitsui, A.; Kamata, M.; Asano, Y.; Sugaya, M.; Kadono, T.; Masamoto, Y.; Kurokawa, M.; et al. Adiponectin regulates psoriasiform skin inflammation by suppressing IL-17 production from γδ-T cells. *Nat. Commun.* **2015**, *6*, 7687. [CrossRef] [PubMed]
147. Coimbra, S.; Oliveira, H.; Reis, F.; Belo, L.; Rocha, S.; Quintanilha, A.; Figueiredo, A.; Teixeira, F.; Castro, E.; Rocha-Pereira, P.; et al. Circulating adipokine levels in Portuguese patients with psoriasis vulgaris according to body mass index, severity and therapy. *J. Eur. Acad. Dermatol. Venereol.* **2010**, *24*, 1386–1394. [CrossRef]
148. Boehncke, S.; Salgo, R.; Garbaraviciene, J.; Beschmann, H.; Hardt, K.; Diehl, S.; Fichtlscherer, S.; Thaçi, D.; Boehncke, W.H. Effective continuous systemic therapy of severe plaque-type psoriasis is accompanied by amelioration of biomarkers of cardiovascular risk: Results of a prospective longitudinal observational study. *J. Eur. Acad. Dermatol. Venereol.* **2011**, *25*, 1187–1193. [CrossRef]
149. Gerdes, S.; Pinter, A.; Biermann, M.; Papavassilis, C.; Reinhardt, M. Adiponectin levels in a large pooled plaque psoriasis study population. *J. Dermatolog. Treat.* **2020**, *31*, 531–534. [CrossRef]
150. Johnson, C.M.; Fitch, K.; Merola, J.F.; Han, J.; Qureshi, A.A.; Li, W.Q. Plasma levels of tumour necrosis factor-α and adiponectin can differentiate patients with psoriatic arthritis from those with psoriasis. *Br. J. Dermatol.* **2019**, *181*, 379–380. [CrossRef]
151. Nakatsuji, T.; Gallo, R.L. Antimicrobial Peptides: Old Molecules with New Ideas. *J. Investig. Dermatol.* **2011**, *132*, 887–895. [CrossRef] [PubMed]
152. Lazzaro, B.P.; Zasloff, M.; Rolff, J. Antimicrobial peptides: Application informed by evolution. *Science* **2020**, *368*, eaau5480. [CrossRef]
153. Magana, M.; Pushpanathan, M.; Santos, A.L.; Leanse, L.; Fernandez, M.; Ioannidis, A.; Giulianotti, M.A.; Apidianakis, Y.; Bradfute, S.; Ferguson, A.L.; et al. The value of antimicrobial peptides in the age of resistance. *Lancet Infect. Dis.* **2020**, *20*, e216–e230. [CrossRef]
154. Lai, Y.; Gallo, R.L. AMPed up immunity: How antimicrobial peptides have multiple roles in immune defense. *Trends Immunol.* **2009**, *30*, 131–141. [CrossRef]
155. Ali, R.S.; Falconer, A.; Ikram, M.; Bissett, C.E.; Cerio, R.; Quinn, A.G. Expression of the peptide antibiotics human β defensin-1 and human β defensin-2 in normal human skin. *J. Investig. Dermatol.* **2001**, *117*, 106–111. [PubMed]
156. Jansen, P.A.M.; Rodijk-Olthuis, D.; Hollox, E.J.; Kamsteeg, M.; Tjabringa, G.S.; de Jongh, G.J.; van Vlijmen-Willems, I.M.J.J.; Bergboer, J.G.M.; van Rossum, M.M.; de Jong, E.M.G.J.; et al. β-Defensin-2 protein is a serum biomarker for disease activity in psoriasis and reaches biologically relevant concentrations in lesional skin. *PLoS ONE* **2009**, *4*, e4725. [CrossRef]
157. Morita, A.; Tani, Y.; Matsumoto, K.; Yamaguchi, M.; Teshima, R.; Ohtsuki, M. Assessment of serum biomarkers in patients with plaque psoriasis on secukinumab. *J. Dermatol.* **2020**, *47*, 452–457. [CrossRef] [PubMed]
158. Jin, T.; Sun, Z.; Chen, X.; Wang, Y.; Li, R.; Ji, S.; Zhao, Y. Serum Human Beta-Defensin-2 Is a Possible Biomarker for Monitoring Response to JAK Inhibitor in Psoriasis Patients. *Dermatology* **2017**, *233*, 164–169. [CrossRef]
159. Gonzalez, L.L.; Garrie, K.; Turner, M.D. Role of S100 proteins in health and disease. *Biochim. Biophys. Acta Mol. Cell Res.* **2020**, *1867*, 118677. [CrossRef]
160. Büchau, A.S.; Gallo, R.L. Innate immunity and antimicrobial defense systems in psoriasis. *Clin. Dermatol.* **2007**, *25*, 616–624. [CrossRef]
161. D'Amico, F.; Skarmoutsou, E.; Granata, M.; Trovato, C.; Rossi, G.A.; Mazzarino, M.C. S100A7: A rAMPing up AMP molecule in psoriasis. *Cytokine Growth Factor Rev.* **2016**, *32*, 97–104. [CrossRef]
162. Maurelli, M.; Gisondi, P.; Danese, E.; Gelati, M.; Papagrigoraki, A.; del Giglio, M.; Lippi, G.; Girolomoni, G. Psoriasin (S100A7) is increased in the serum of patients with moderate-to-severe psoriasis. *Br. J. Dermatol.* **2020**, *182*, 1502–1503. [CrossRef] [PubMed]
163. Awad, S.M.; Attallah, D.A.; Salama, R.H.; Mahran, A.M.; Abu El-Hamed, E. Serum levels of psoriasin (S100A7) and koebnerisin (S100A15) as potential markers of atherosclerosis in patients with psoriasis. *Clin. Exp. Dermatol.* **2018**, *43*, 262–267. [CrossRef] [PubMed]
164. Batycka-Baran, A.; Hattinger, E.; Zwicker, S.; Summer, B.; Zack Howard, O.M.; Thomas, P.; Szepietowski, J.C.; Ruzicka, T.; Prinz, J.C.; Wolf, R. Leukocyte-derived koebnerisin (S100A15) and psoriasin (S100A7) are systemic mediators of inflammation in psoriasis. *J. Dermatol. Sci.* **2015**, *79*, 214–221. [CrossRef]
165. Takeda, A.; Higuchi, D.; Takahashi, T.; Ogo, M.; Baciu, P.; Goetinck, P.F.; Hibino, T. Overexpression of serpin squamous cell carcinoma antigens in psoriatic skin. *J. Investig. Dermatol.* **2002**, *118*, 147–154. [CrossRef]
166. Watanabe, Y.; Yamaguchi, Y.; Komitsu, N.; Ohta, S.; Azuma, Y.; Izuhara, K.; Aihara, M. Elevation of serum squamous cell carcinoma antigen 2 in patients with psoriasis: Associations with disease severity and response to the treatment. *Br. J. Dermatol.* **2016**, *174*, 1327–1336. [CrossRef] [PubMed]
167. Naher, L.; Kiyoshima, T.; Kobayashi, I.; Wada, H.; Nagata, K.; Fujiwara, H.; Ookuma, Y.F.; Ozeki, S.; Nakamura, S.; Sakai, H. STAT3 signal transduction through interleukin-22 in oral squamous cell carcinoma. *Int. J. Oncol.* **2012**, *41*, 1577–1586. [CrossRef]
168. Mitsuishi, K.; Nakamura, T.; Sakata, Y.; Yuyama, N.; Arima, K.; Sugita, Y.; Suto, H.; Izuhara, K.; Ogawa, H. The squamous cell carcinoma antigens as relevant biomarkers of atopic dermatitis. *Clin. Exp. Allergy* **2005**, *35*, 1327–1333. [CrossRef]
169. Okawa, T.; Yamaguchi, Y.; Kou, K.; Ono, J.; Azuma, Y.; Komitsu, N.; Inoue, Y.; Kohno, M.; Matsukura, S.; Kambara, T.; et al. Serum levels of squamous cell carcinoma antigens 1 and 2 reflect disease severity and clinical type of atopic dermatitis in adult patients. *Allergol. Int.* **2018**, *67*, 124–130. [CrossRef]

170. Iizuka, H.; Takahashi, H.; Honma, M.; Ishida-Yamamoto, A. Unique keratinization process in psoriasis: Late differentiation markers are abolished because of the premature cell death. *J. Dermatol.* **2004**, *31*, 271–276. [CrossRef]
171. Nakane, H.; Ishida-Yamamoto, A.; Takahashi, H.; Iizuka, H. Elafin, a secretory protein, is cross-linked into the cornified cell envelopes from the inside of psoriatic keratinocytes. *J. Investig. Dermatol.* **2002**, *119*, 50–55. [CrossRef]
172. Nonomura, K.; Yamanishi, K.; Yasuno, H.; Nara, K.; Hirose, S. Up-regulation of elafin/SKALP gene expression in psoriatic epidermis. *J. Investig. Dermatol.* **1994**, *103*, 88–91. [CrossRef] [PubMed]
173. Sallenave, J.M. Secretory leukocyte protease inhibitor and elafin/trappin-2: Versatile mucosal antimicrobials and regulators of immunity. *Am. J. Respir. Cell Mol. Biol.* **2010**, *42*, 635–643. [CrossRef] [PubMed]
174. Elgharib, I.; Khashaba, S.A.; Elsaid, H.H.; Sharaf, M.M. Serum elafin as a potential inflammatory marker in psoriasis. *Int. J. Dermatol.* **2019**, *58*, 205–209. [CrossRef] [PubMed]
175. Alam, S.R.; Newby, D.E.; Henriksen, P.A. Role of the endogenous elastase inhibitor, elafin, in cardiovascular injury: From epithelium to endothelium. *Biochem. Pharmacol.* **2012**, *83*, 695–704. [CrossRef]
176. Shavadia, J.S.; Granger, C.B.; Alemayehu, W.; Westerhout, C.M.; Povsic, T.J.; Brener, S.J.; van Diepen, S.; Defilippi, C.; Armstrong, P.W. High-throughput targeted proteomics discovery approach and spontaneous reperfusion in ST-segment elevation myocardial infarction. *Am. Heart J.* **2020**, *220*, 137–144. [CrossRef]
177. Wang, X.; Abraham, S.; McKenzie, J.A.G.; Jeffs, N.; Swire, M.; Tripathi, V.B.; Luhmann, U.F.O.; Lange, C.A.K.; Zhai, Z.; Arthur, H.M.; et al. LRG1 promotes angiogenesis by modulating endothelial TGF-β signalling. *Nature* **2013**, *499*, 306–311. [CrossRef]
178. Yang, F.J.; Hsieh, C.Y.; Shu, K.H.; Chen, I.Y.; Pan, S.Y.; Chuang, Y.F.; Chiu, Y.L.; Yang, W.S. Plasma Leucine-Rich α-2-Glycoprotein 1 Predicts Cardiovascular Disease Risk in End-Stage Renal Disease. *Sci. Rep.* **2020**, *10*, 5988. [CrossRef]
179. Urushima, H.; Fujimoto, M.; Mishima, T.; Ohkawara, T.; Honda, H.; Lee, H.; Kawahata, H.; Serada, S.; Naka, T. Leucine-rich alpha 2 glycoprotein promotes Th17 differentiation and collagen-induced arthritis in mice through enhancement of TGF-β-Smad2 signaling in naïve helper T cells. *Arthritis Res. Ther.* **2017**, *19*, 137. [CrossRef]
180. Nakajima, H.; Serada, S.; Fujimoto, M.; Naka, T.; Sano, S. Leucine-rich α-2 glycoprotein is an innovative biomarker for psoriasis. *J. Dermatol. Sci.* **2017**, *86*, 170–174. [CrossRef]
181. Libreros, S.; Iragavarapu-Charyulu, V. YKL-40/CHI3L1 drives inflammation on the road of tumor progression. *J. Leukoc. Biol.* **2015**, *98*, 931–936. [CrossRef]
182. Prakash, M.; Bodas, M.; Prakash, D.; Nawani, N.; Khetmalas, M.; Mandal, A.; Eriksson, C. Diverse pathological implications of YKL-40: Answers may lie in "outside-in" signaling. *Cell. Signal.* **2013**, *25*, 1567–1573. [CrossRef] [PubMed]
183. Deng, Y.; Li, G.; Chang, D.; Su, X. YKL-40 as a novel biomarker in cardio-metabolic disorders and inflammatory diseases. *Clin. Chim. Acta* **2020**, *511*, 40–46. [CrossRef] [PubMed]
184. Imai, Y.; Tsuda, T.; Aochi, S.; Futatsugi-Yumikura, S.; Sakaguchi, Y.; Nakagawa, N.; Iwatsuki, K.; Yamanishi, K. YKL-40 (chitinase 3-like-1) as a biomarker for psoriasis vulgaris and pustular psoriasis. *J. Dermatol. Sci.* **2011**, *64*, 75–77. [CrossRef] [PubMed]
185. Khashaba, S.A.; Attwa, E.; Said, N.; Ahmed, S.; Khattab, F. Serum YKL-40 and IL 17 in Psoriasis: Reliability as prognostic markers for disease severity and responsiveness to treatment. *Dermatol. Ther.* **2021**, *34*, e14606. [CrossRef] [PubMed]
186. Ahmed, S.F.; Attia, E.A.S.; Saad, A.A.; Sharara, M.; Fawzy, H.; El Nahrery, E.M.A. Serum YKL-40 in psoriasis with and without arthritis; Correlation with disease activity and high-resolution power Doppler ultrasonographic joint findings. *J. Eur. Acad. Dermatol. Venereol.* **2015**, *29*, 682–688. [CrossRef]
187. Erfan, G.; Guzel, S.; Alpsoy, S.; Rifaioglu, E.N.; Kaya, S.; Kucukyalcın, V.; Topcu, B.; Kulac, M. Serum YKL-40: A potential biomarker for psoriasis or endothelial dysfunction in psoriasis? *Mol. Cell. Biochem.* **2015**, *400*, 207–212. [CrossRef]
188. Hotamisligil, G.S.; Bernlohr, D.A. Metabolic functions of FABPs—Mechanisms and therapeutic implications. *Nat. Rev. Endocrinol.* **2015**, *11*, 592–605. [CrossRef] [PubMed]
189. Storch, J.; Thumser, A.E. Tissue-specific functions in the fatty acid-binding protein family. *J. Biol. Chem.* **2010**, *285*, 32679–32683. [CrossRef] [PubMed]
190. Smathers, R.L.; Petersen, D.R. The human fatty acid-binding protein family: Evolutionary divergences and functions. *Hum. Genom.* **2011**, *5*, 170–191. [CrossRef]
191. Watanabe, R.; Fujii, H.; Yamamoto, A.; Hashimoto, T.; Kameda, K.; Ito, M.; Ono, T. Immunohistochemical distribution of cutaneous fatty acid-binding protein in human skin. *J. Dermatol. Sci.* **1997**, *16*, 17–22. [CrossRef]
192. Kuijpers, A.L.A.; Bergers, M.; Siegenthaler, G.; Zeeuwen, P.L.J.M.; Van De Kerkhof, P.C.M.; Schalkwijk, J. Skin-derived antileukoproteinase (SKALP) and epidermal fatty acid-binding protein (E-FABP): Two novel markers of the psoriatic phenotype that respond differentially to topical steroid. *Acta Derm. Venereol.* **1997**, *77*, 14–19. [PubMed]
193. Madsen, P.; Rasmussen, H.H.; Leffers, H.; Honoré, B.; Celis, J.E. Molecular cloning and expression of a novel keratinocyte protein (psoriasis-associated fatty acid-binding protein [PA-FABP]) that is highly upregulated in psoriatic skin and that shares similarity to fatty acid-binding proteins. *J. Investig. Dermatol.* **1992**, *99*, 299–305. [CrossRef]
194. Ogawa, E.; Owada, Y.; Ikawa, S.; Adachi, Y.; Egawa, T.; Nemoto, K.; Suzuki, K.; Hishinuma, T.; Kawashima, H.; Kondo, H.; et al. Epidermal FABP (FABP5) regulates keratinocyte differentiation by 13(S)-HODE-mediated activation of the NF-B signaling pathway. *J. Investig. Dermatol.* **2011**, *131*, 604–612. [CrossRef] [PubMed]
195. Dallaglio, K.; Marconi, A.; Truzzi, F.; Lotti, R.; Palazzo, E.; Petracchi, T.; Saltari, A.; Coppini, M.; Pincelli, C. E-FABP induces differentiation in normal human keratinocytes and modulates the differentiation process in psoriatic keratinocytes in vitro. *Exp. Dermatol.* **2013**, *22*, 255–261. [CrossRef] [PubMed]

196. Myśliwiec, H.; Baran, A.; Harasim-Symbor, E.; Myśliwiec, P.; Milewska, A.J.; Chabowski, A.; Flisiak, I. Serum fatty acid profile in psoriasis and its comorbidity. *Arch. Dermatol. Res.* **2017**, *309*, 371–380. [CrossRef]
197. Baran, A.; Świderska, M.; Bacharewicz-Szczerbicka, J.; Myśliwiec, H.; Flisiak, I. Serum Fatty Acid-Binding Protein 4 is Increased in Patients with Psoriasis. *Lipids* **2017**, *52*, 51–60. [CrossRef] [PubMed]
198. Honma, M.; Shibuya, T.; Iinuma, S.; Ishida-Yamamoto, A. Serum fatty acid-binding protein 4 level is inversely correlated with serum thymus and activation-regulated chemokine level in psoriatic patients achieving clear skin by biologics. *J. Dermatol.* **2019**, *46*, e116–e117. [CrossRef]
199. Shibuya, T.; Honma, M.; Iinuma, S.; Iwasaki, T.; Ishida-Yamamoto, A. Persistent pruritus in psoriatic patients during administration of biologics. *J. Dermatol.* **2018**, *45*, e223. [CrossRef]
200. Baran, A.; Kiluk, P.; Maciaszek, M.; Świderska, M.; Flisiak, I. Liver fatty acid-binding protein might be a predictive marker of clinical response to systemic treatment in psoriasis. *Arch. Dermatol. Res.* **2019**, *311*, 389–397. [CrossRef]
201. Sikora, M.; Stec, A.; Chrabaszcz, M.; Waskiel-Burnat, A.; Zaremba, M.; Olszewska, M.; Rudnicka, L. Intestinal Fatty Acid Binding Protein, a Biomarker of Intestinal Barrier, is Associated with Severity of Psoriasis. *J. Clin. Med.* **2019**, *8*, 1021. [CrossRef] [PubMed]

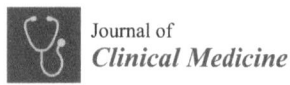

Review

Skin-Resident Memory T Cells: Pathogenesis and Implication for the Treatment of Psoriasis

Trung T. Vu [1,2], Hanako Koguchi-Yoshioka [2,3] and Rei Watanabe [2,3,*]

[1] Department of Cutaneous Immunology, Immunology Frontier Research Center, Osaka University, Osaka 565-0871, Japan; trungvu0406@derma.med.osaka-u.ac.jp
[2] Department of Dermatology, Course of Integrated Medicine, Graduate School of Medicine/Faculty of Medicine, Osaka University, Osaka 565-0871, Japan; stain_way@yahoo.co.jp
[3] Department of Integrative Medicine for Allergic and Immunological Diseases, Course of Integrated Medicine, Graduate School of Medicine/Faculty of Medicine, Osaka University, Osaka 565-0871, Japan
* Correspondence: rwatanabe@derma.med.osaka-u.ac.jp

Abstract: Tissue-resident memory T cells (T_{RM}) stay in the peripheral tissues for long periods of time, do not recirculate, and provide the first line of adaptive immune response in the residing tissues. Although T_{RM} originate from circulating T cells, T_{RM} are physiologically distinct from circulating T cells with the expression of tissue-residency markers, such as CD69 and CD103, and the characteristic profile of transcription factors. Besides defense against pathogens, the functional skew of skin T_{RM} is indicated in chronic skin inflammatory diseases. In psoriasis, IL-17A-producing $CD8^+$ T_{RM} are regarded as one of the pathogenic populations in skin. Although no licensed drugs that directly and specifically inhibit the activity of skin T_{RM} are available to date, psoriatic skin T_{RM} are affected in the current treatments of psoriasis. Targeting skin T_{RM} or using T_{RM} as a potential index for disease severity can be an attractive strategy in psoriasis.

Keywords: skin-resident memory T cells; human; psoriasis; cytokines; autoantigens; treatment

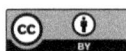

1. Introduction

Once the immune system encounters antigens, memory T cells are generated from the naïve T cells and facilitate a prompt response to the re-exposure of the same antigens. Two populations of memory T cells have been defined from human blood circulation: effector memory T cells (T_{EM}) and central memory T cells (T_{CM}) [1]. T_{EM} are also dominant in peripheral non-lymphoid tissues and T_{CM} have an affinity for secondary lymphoid organs [2,3]. Furthermore, research on murine infectious disease models has revealed that a subpopulation of T_{EM} found in peripheral tissues remain in the same tissues for long periods without recirculation after cure of infection [4–6]. These findings led to the establishment of the new population of memory T cells, tissue-resident memory T cells (T_{RM}).

T_{RM} are superior to their circulating memory counterparts in their ability to provide the local adaptive cellular defense [7–11]. They can respond to the local antigen re-exposure without the recruitment of circulating T cells to the tissue [12]. In addition, recent studies suggest T_{RM} also contribute to systemic immune responses upon subsequent exposure to specific antigens by proliferating and baring circulating populations, such as T_{CM} and T_{EM} [13,14].

The existence and functional activities of T_{RM} were initially investigated in barrier tissues, such as the gut [6,15], skin [4,5,12,16,17], respiratory tract [18,19], and reproductive tract [20,21], in the context of local defense against pathogens in infectious diseases. However, their roles are now recognized in various conditions, including cancer immunity, tissue-specific autoimmune diseases, and chronic inflammatory diseases both in barrier and non-barrier tissues [22].

Skin T_{RM} are among the intensively studied T_{RM} populations not only in murine models but also in humans. The human skin contains an estimate of 20 billion T cells, doubling those in the circulation [23], and over half of these T cells show the T_{RM} phenotype [24]. Besides infectious diseases, the involvement of skin T_{RM} has been reported in allergic contact hypersensitivity [25]; fixed drug eruption [26]; cutaneous malignancies, including malignant melanoma [27,28] and cutaneous T-cell lymphoma [24,29]; and chronic inflammatory diseases, such as vitiligo, alopecia, and psoriasis [30,31].

In this review, we provide an overview of the general characteristics of T_{RM}. Then, narrowing our focus to skin T_{RM} in humans, we summarize the involvement of skin T_{RM} in cutaneous disorders, especially psoriasis. We also mention the possibility of engaging T_{RM} as a disease index and treatment target in psoriasis. Since $CD8^+$ T_{RM} are the best-characterized population, we focus on $CD8^+$ T_{RM} and describe this population as T_{RM} in this review unless otherwise mentioned.

2. The Characteristics of T_{RM}

T cells in the neonatal murine skin are predominant with dendritic epidermal T cells (DETCS) with restricted antigenic specificity [32], and neonatal human skin holds only a few T cells [24]. Thus, T_{RM} are assumed to develop from circulating T cells according to repeated antigen exposure. In the local inflammation caused by specific antigens, the robustly expanded effector T cells emerge in the circulation and the affected tissues, and both T_{CM} and T_{RM} are assumed to arise from a part of these effector T cells [25,33].

The general characteristics of T_{RM} across the tissues include the loss of migration and the gain of retention. The development and maintenance of these characteristics in T_{RM} are driven by complex factors, such as cytokine and chemokine receptors, the other cell-surface molecules being responsible for tissue homing and retention, and transcription factors (Figure 1).

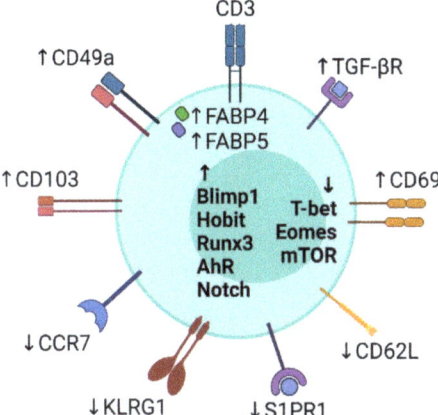

Figure 1. A. Surface markers, intracellular molecules, and transcription factors of T_{RM}. The expression levels of these molecules on T_{RM} are shown by upward arrows (increased expressions) and downward arrows (decreased expressions). Created with BioRender.com (accessed on 21 August 2021).

2.1. Cell Surface Molecules

While homing molecules including chemokine receptors are diverse depending on the target peripheral tissues, the molecules related to tissue retention seem to be shared among various tissues. In general, T_{RM} lack the expression of the secondary lymphoid homing molecules CC-chemokine receptor 7 (CCR7) and L-selectin, which are expressed on T_{CM} and naïve T cells [1]. The tissue retention molecules CD69 and CD103 (αE integrin) are widely recognized as the markers for T_{RM}. CD103 is a ligand of E-cadherin that is expressed on epithelial cells [34], and CD69 interferes with sphingosine-1-phosphate (S1P) receptor-1, which allows the cells to exit from peripheral tissues by sensing the density of S1P [35]. CD69 also reportedly regulates the uptake of L-tryptophan and the intracellular quantity of L-tryptophan-derived activator of the aryl hydrocarbon receptor (AhR) [36], which is reportedly involved in the persistence of T_{RM} [32]. These functions would explain at least partially the importance of these molecules in tissue retention. However, their expression varies, possibly depending on the tissues and the causes of T_{RM} development. T_{RM} lacking CD103 expression have been described in some peripheral tissues and secondary lymphoid organs [37,38] and CD103$^+$ T_{RM} can be found in the dermis and adult central nervous system where E-cadherin is absent, implying that binding to E-cadherin is not required for the persistence of T_{RM} in peripheral tissues [24,39]. Although CD69 is expressed on the majority of T_{RM} in various peripheral tissues, T_{RM} negative for CD69 expression are also noted [33]. We thus have to take into account that these two molecules are not able to cover T_{RM} universally.

2.2. Transcription Factors

Transcriptional regulation is also presumably common among T_{RM} in various tissues. For instance, the expression of AhR is increased in skin T_{RM} as compared with naïve T cells and splenic T cells, possibly favoring the maintenance of skin T_{RM} [32]. Rapamycin inhibits the formation of T_{RM} in the intestinal and vaginal mucosa, highlighting a positive link of mammalian target of rapamycin and the downstream transcription factors with the formation of T_{RM} [40]. The maintenance of lung T_{RM} may be related to Notch signaling, including the upregulation of the downstream transcription factor RBPJ [41]. The augmented uptake of exogenous lipids accompanied by the upregulation of fatty acid binding proteins (FABPs) 4 and 5 is one of the characteristic processes involved in the generation and maintenance of skin T_{RM} [42]. Hypoxia-inducible factor-1α, which is a transcription factor in the downstream of FABP5 signaling, reportedly promotes the residency and anti-tumor function of tumor-infiltrating T cells in the murine malignancy model [43]. The downregulation of T-box transcription factors T-bet and EOMES [44] and the upregulation of Blimp-1, Hobit [45], and Runx3 [46,47] have also been reported to be involved in the differentiation and/or maintenance of T_{RM}.

2.3. Skin-Homing Molecules

In addition to the shared characteristics of various T_{RM}, skin T_{RM} are shown to have their own homing molecules. As one of skin's homing molecules, cutaneous lymphocyte-associated antigen (CLA) binds to E-selectin and P-selectin and allows the cells to migrate into skin [23]. The chemokine receptors CCR4, CCR8, CCR10, CXCR3, and CXCR6 are also regarded as important skin-homing and/or retention molecules for at least some skin T cells [16,48–52].

2.4. Fate Decision of T_{RM}

How the fate of T_{RM} differentiation is decided remains an unsolved question. T_{RM} reportedly derive from circulating T cells lacking high expression of the killer cell lectin-like receptor subfamily G member 1 (KLRG1), which is regarded as a terminal differentiation marker [16,47]. Another report demonstrates that the effector T cells with enriched expression of T_{RM}-associated genes, such as *Itgae* (CD103), *Itga1* (CD49a), *Cd101*, *Ahr*, and *Fabp5*, already exist as memory precursor cells and preferentially differentiate into T_{RM} [53], suggesting that the fate of T_{RM} is at least partially decided in the early stage of adoptive immune memory formation. On the other hand, the time-course single-cell RNA-sequencing analysis in a murine model with lymphocytic-choriomeningitis-virus infection revealed that the transcriptional characteristics of T_{RM} can be detected from gut-infiltrating T cells at the earliest 4 days after infection, and the characteristics are distinct from those found in splenic T cells [54], implying that the T_{RM} differentiation program is initiated after the cells enter the specific peripheral tissues. Further elucidation of the T_{RM} differentiation mechanism will require further research.

3. Human Skin T_{RM}

In general, human T_{RM} and murine T_{RM} share core transcriptional, phenotypic, and functional profiles, including the almost global expression of CD69 and dominant CD103 expression in CD8 fractions [45,55–57]. In patients with cutaneous T-cell lymphoma (CTCL), the treatment with alemtuzumab, which depletes circulating T cells and spares the T_{RM}, does not result in serious infection [58], implying the role of skin T_{RM} in protective immunity. The T_{RM} phenotype of the malignant cells in CTCL is related to the clinical manifestation of well-demarcated lesions, suggesting that the sessile property of T_{RM} also exists in humans [24]. In vitro experiments suggest skin T_{RM} maintain the production of IL-17A and IFN-γ in reaction with pathogen challenges through aging [59]. Using transcriptomic and functional data, human T_{RM} are found to abolish their senescent phenotype and survive for over 10 years in specific circumstances [46], replicating the longevity of T_{RM} in humans.

However, T_{RM} in humans are presumably more diverse and widely distributed. For instance, CD4$^+$ T_{RM} are found in both the epidermis and dermis in humans, although murine skin CD4$^+$ T_{RM} are predominantly found in dermis [17,24,60,61]. T_{RM} are also found in secondary lymphoid organs, such as the spleen, lymph nodes, and tonsils in humans [55,56].

The factors that may cause the difference between human skin T_{RM} properties and those observed in laboratory mice may include the following: (1) the thick epidermis with abundant niche for T_{RM} [24,62]; (2) the low density of hair follicles that express cytokines important for T_{RM} migration and survival, including IL-7 and IL-15 [63,64]; (3) the frequent exposure to foreign antigens; (4) the small population of $\gamma\delta$T cells with the lack of DETC in the human epidermis [65] (however, we do not know whether the recently identified $\alpha\beta\gamma\delta$T cell population in fetal skin can replace DETC) [66]. The longer survival period of human T_{RM} compared to murine life span [46] may also cause difficulty in adapting the findings in murine models to human biology.

The involvement of skin T_{RM} is highlighted in chronic inflammatory disorders and cutaneous malignancies. In the lesional skin of alopecia areata, T_{RM} with the ability to produce granzyme B are dominant and related to disease prognosis, implying their involvement in the pathogenesis [67]. Intraepidermal IFN-γ-producing T_{RM} are enriched in the cured sites of fixed drug eruption [26], suggesting the contribution of this fraction to the reproducible property. In patients with atopic dermatitis, cutaneous T_{RM} with the production of IL-4 and IL-13 are also indicated to be involved in the disease pathogenesis [68]. Dermal T_{RM} are increased with the production potential of perforin, granzyme B, and IFN-γ in vitiligo [30,69], which are presumably specific for melanocyte antigens. In malignant melanoma, skin T_{RM} provide protection against tumor regrowth and are involved in vitiligo formation, suggestive of their specific reactivity against melanoma antigens [70]. Better understanding of cutaneous T_{RM} will pave the way for novel management and treatment of skin diseases.

The methodologies for evaluating skin T_{RM} are summarized in Table 1. In the translational research field, one of the most popular methods for analyzing T_{RM} is fluorescence-activated cell sorting (FACS) analysis. However, conducting this method from biopsied skin specimens is not practical in the daily clinical settings considering the burden for both patients and clinicians. Immunohistochemistry (IHC) and/or immunofluorescence (IF) for T_{RM}-related molecules, such as CD3, CD8, CD69, and CD103, on the residual biopsy specimens carried out for diagnosis is probably more feasible to date. To establish non-invasive methods for predicting the activities of skin T_{RM}, such as analyzing tape-stripped or surface-swabbed samples, will require further research.

4. Skin T_{RM} in the Pathogenesis of Psoriasis

Psoriasis, hereafter referred to as plaque psoriasis, is an immune-mediated chronic inflammatory skin disorder characterized by well-demarcated persistent scaly indurated erythematous plaques. The contributions of environment [71], hereditary predisposition [72], and autoantigens [73] are implied to be involved in disease development. Circulating T cells were previously regarded as responsible for the lesion formation in psoriasis. However, the inhibition of E-selectin, which is required for T-cell migration from the blood stream to skin, was noted to be ineffective [74]. Another blocking strategy of T-cell migration by the biologics targeting CD11a also did not show dramatic efficacy [75]. However, in a humanized murine model where psoriatic nonlesional skin specimens are grafted to immunodeficient mice [76], the healthy-appearing nonlesional skin grafts spontaneously develop psoriatic disease, suggesting that the cells residing in the nonlesional skin are sufficient for the development of psoriatic disease. These results have led to the theory that T_{RM} may play a crucial role in the pathogenesis of psoriasis.

The fate of skin T_{RM} is affected by the skin microenvironment, and in psoriasis, this is also the case. Several skin-constituting factors have been reported to support the development and persistence of IL-17A-producing T_{RM} in psoriasis. Keratinocytes in disease-naïve sites of psoriasis upregulate the expression of chemokines, such as CCL20 upon stimulation by skin commensal fungi [77]. Since CCL20 is a ligand for CCR6, which is a signature molecule of IL-17A-producing T cells, the activated keratinocytes in the disease-naïve sites of psoriasis are to recruit IL-17A-producing T cells to the disease-naïve sites, leading to the accumulation of IL-17A-producing T_{RM} [77]. In turn, IL-17A from T_{RM} stimulates keratinocytes to express CCL20, further accelerating the recruitment of CCR6$^+$ cells [78]. In the resolved skin, the continuous production of IL-23 and IL-15 from Langerhans cells presumably support the maintenance of IL-17A-producing T_{RM} in the epidermis [79]. The reduced repertoire of IL-17A-producing T cells in the resolved skin, which has been observed in different psoriatic patients, implies the existence of common antigens that drive the accumulation of psoriatic T_{RM} [80]. Several potential autoantigens have been reported in psoriasis (Figure 2). For example, cationic antimicrobial peptide LL-37 produced by various cells including keratinocytes binds self-DNA and triggers the activation of plasmacytoid dendritic cells (pDC) and TNF/iNOS-producing dendritic cells (TIP-DC) [81,82]. A disintegrin-like and metalloprotease domain containing thrombospondin type 1 motif-like 5 (ADAMTSL5) in complex with HLA-C*06:02 on the surface of melanocytes confers epidermal CD8$^+$ T-cell response [83]. Neo-lipid antigens generated by phospholipase A2 group 4D (PLA2G4D) from mast cells and keratinocytes trigger the CD1a-reactive T cells to produce IL-17A and IL-22 [84]. Keratin 17, a human epidermal keratin that shares a sequential homology with streptococcal M protein, is recognized by HLA-Cw*0602-restricted IFN-γ-producing CD8$^+$ T cells [85,86]. Taken together, these results suggest the synchronizing roles of the skin microenvironment in the development and persistence of pathogenic cutaneous T_{RM}.

In the lesional skin of patients with psoriasis, T_{RM} consist of both CD4 and CD8 fractions, which synchronize the elevated immune response by the increased expression of inflammatory cytokines, such as IL-17A, IL-22, and IFN-γ [62,80,87,88]. While IL-17A-producing CD4$^+$ T_{RM} also exist in healthy skin, the enrichment of CD8$^+$ T_{RM} producing IL-17A in the epidermis is one of the characteristics of psoriasis [87,88]. In disease-naïve skin that has never experienced disease formation, IL-17A production is augmented by T_{RM} [77], and the increase in IL-17A-producing CD8$^+$ T_{RM} at the dispense of IFN-γ-producing T_{RM} occurs according to disease duration [88].

IFN-γ-producing T_{RM} are also dominant in the epidermis and express the complex of CD49a–CD29, also known as very late antigen 1 (VLA-1) or α1β1 integrin [76]. CD49a$^+$ T_{RM} are involved in the pathogenesis of psoriasis. The number of epidermal CD8$^+$CD49a$^+$ T_{RM} correlates with the severity of the disease [89], and an experimental blockade of CD49a in mice transplanted with psoriatic skin reduces the disease formation [76]. However, since the blockade of whole CD8$^+$ T cells almost completely prevents disease development in the similar psoriatic skin-engrafted murine model [90], CD49a$^+$ T_{RM} with IFN-γ production are not likely the key population for disease development, while the CD8$^+$ T cell population likely includes a critical fraction for disease pathogenesis. In fact, CD8$^+$ T_{RM} without the expression of CD49a are defined as an IL-17A-producing T_{RM} subset [30].

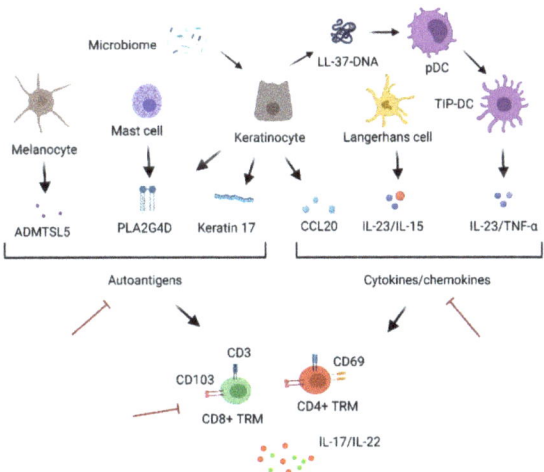

Figure 2. Development of T_{RM} in psoriasis. T_{RM} are activated by either autoantigens or cytokines/chemokines. Autoantigens include ADMTSL5 on the surface of melanocytes, PLAG4D from mast cells and keratinocytes, and keratin 17 from keratinocytes. Antimicrobial peptide LL-37, also from keratinocytes, binds to self-DNA to activate pDC and TIP-DC, leading to the production of IL-23/TNF-α. IL-23/15 from Langerhans cells and CCL20 from keratinocytes also activate T_{RM}. These stimulated T_{RM} produce proinflammatory cytokines, such as IL-17A and IL-22, the hallmarks of psoriasis. The development of pathogenic T_{RM} can be inhibited by stopping pathways related to T_{RM} activation or directly inhibiting the activity of T_{RM} (red inhibition icon). Created with BioRender.com (assessed on 21 August 2021).

Successful treatment with an IL-17A-targeting biologics results in a decreased number of IL-17A-producing T_{RM} in resolved skin, but the frequency of these cells is not altered within the remaining T cells [91]. Another study on residual psoriasis after the use of biologics revealed a decrease in keratinocyte proliferation. However, the percentage of IL-17A-producing $CD103^+$ T_{RM} was not significantly reduced after the treatments [92]. Similarly, a new normal in the persistence of IL-17A-producing T_{RM} with CCR6 and IL-23R expression in the resolved skin has been established [62,80]. IL-17A-producing $CD8^+$ T_{RM} and IL-22-producing $CD4^+$ T_{RM} remain in the psoriatic epidermis for as long as six years after starting the successful TNF-α-targeting treatment [62]. Taken together, these findings highlight the essential standing point of IL-17A-producing T_{RM} as one of the pathogenic populations of skin T_{RM} in psoriasis.

5. Targeting Skin T_{RM} in the Management of Psoriasis

Regardless of the persistence of this population by various treatments in psoriasis, many of the current and upcoming therapeutics in clinical practice presumably exert an indirect influence on cutaneous IL-17A-producing T_{RM}. Since the remission period after successful treatments inversely correlates with the relative IL-17 signaling of the resolved skin compared to IL-10 and IFN-γ signaling [93], the relative reduction, if not elimination, of IL-17A-producing T_{RM} may be of help in controlling psoriatic disease activity.

Biologics targeting the IL-17 pathway reportedly reduce IL-17 signaling and the amount of T cells in the lesion [94]. Furthermore, the biologics targeting IL-23 decrease this fraction from the lesion more strongly compared to those targeting IL-17A [95]. Ultraviolet irradiation leads to the diminishment of IL-17A-producing T cells in skin [96], and this T-cell fraction includes T_{RM}. Topical vitamin D analogues and corticosteroids reportedly reduce the lesional IL-17A-producing T_{RM}, possibly including pathogenic T_{RM} [97,98]. Retinoic acid prevents Th17 differentiation and possibly promotes the properties of regulatory T cells [99,100]. As the oral phosphodiesterase 4 inhibitor (PDE4i) diminishes the proinflammatory cytokine production from circulating T cells [101], the function of both topical and systemic PDE4i could be revisited from the perspective of skin T_{RM}. An AhR agonist modulates the Th17 property of T cells, and the efficacy of its topical form possibly affects IL-17A-producing T cells in skin, including T_{RM} [102].

Proof-of-concept approaches that directly and exclusively target pathogenic populations of T_{RM} should be subjected to further studies. The candidate strategies might include the inhibition of the pathways involved in IL-15 signaling to perturb the survival of pathogenic T_{RM} and the blockade of the pathways processing fatty acids to suppress the lipid metabolism of pathogenic T_{RM}. Targeting the transcription factors specified for differentiation and maintenance of pathogenic T_{RM} is also an attractive strategy. However, although the risk of targeting these populations of T_{RM} is unknown, it may cause the loss of local immune memory against pathogens in the skin. Since the characteristic cell surface molecules and transcription factors found in T_{RM} properties can be overlapped with the sessile properties of other cell types, such as innate lymphoid cells and B cells [103,104], the strategies targeting T_{RM} might also affect the other tissue-sessile immunity. Specific treatment targets for psoriatic dysfunctional T_{RM}, excluding the other T_{RM} and skin-resident immune cells, would be ideal.

6. Conclusions

Extensive studies with rigorous methodologies have broadened our knowledge on T_{RM} in general and those residing in the skin in particular (Table 1). The involvement of skin T_{RM} in the pathogenesis of skin diseases is also being elucidated. Several key points are highlighted below:

- T_{RM} originate from circulating T cells, do not recirculate, and provide the first line of adaptive cellular defense in the residing tissues.
- The functional skew of skin T_{RM} is indicated in chronic skin inflammatory diseases.
- In psoriasis, IL-17-A-producing CD8$^+$ T_{RM} may be among the pathogenic populations in the skin.
- Pathogenic populations of skin T_{RM} can be targeted in the current and future treatments of psoriasis. Skin T_{RM} can also serve as a potential index of the disease.

Further studies on T_{RM} will advance the management of not only psoriasis but other diseases in which this subset of T cells plays a role.

Table 1. Several major findings related to methodologies used in research on humans.

Key Findings	Major Methodologies	
A role of skin T_{RM} in protective immunity in humans	FACS	[58]
Skin T_{RM} with the potential of producing cytokines are infiltrated in the lesion of patients with GVHD	FC, single-cell TCR sequencing, and IF	[46]
Cells residing in nonlesional skin are sufficient, and the recruitment of circulating cells is not necessary for the development of psoriatic disease	Transplantation, FC, quantitative RT-PCR, and IHC	[76]
CD8$^+$ T_{RM} producing IL-17A in the epidermis is one of the characteristics in psoriasis	FC and IHC	[87]
The increase in IL-17A-producing CD8$^+$ T_{RM} during the distribution of IFN-γ-producing T_{RM} occurs according to psoriasis duration	FC and IF	[88]
The successful treatment with IL-17A-targeting biologics results in a decreased number of IL-17A-producing CD8$^+$ T_{RM} in resolved psoriatic skin, but the frequency of these cells is not altered	FC, IHC, and IF	[91]
IL-17A-producing CD8$^+$ T_{RM} and IL-22-producing CD4$^+$ T_{RM} remain in the psoriatic epidermis for as long as six years after starting the successful TNF-α-targeting treatment	FC, quantitative RT-PCR, and IF	[62]

FC: flow cytometry, TCR: T-cell receptor, RT-PCR: reverse transcription polymerase chain reaction, IF: immunofluorescence, IHC: immunohistochemistry.

Author Contributions: Conceptualization, T.T.V., H.K.-Y. and R.W.; writing—original draft preparation, T.T.V.; writing—review and editing T.T.V., H.K.-Y. and R.W.; visualization, T.T.V., H.K.-Y. and R.W.; supervision, R.W. All authors have read and agreed to the published version of the manuscript.

Funding: T.T.V. is funded by Kishimoto Foundation Fellowship.

Conflicts of Interest: R.W. received lecture fees from the companies Abbvie, Eli Lilly, Janssen Pharmaceuticals, Kyowa Kirin, Maruho, and Novartis, and a research grant from the companies Maruho and Janssen Pharmaceuticals. The funders have no role in the writing or in the decision to publish this manuscript.

References

1. Sallusto, F.; Lenig, D.; Förster, R.; Lipp, M.; Lanzavecchia, A. Two subsets of memory T lymphocytes with distinct homing potentials and effector functions. *Nature* **1999**, *401*, 708–712. [CrossRef]
2. Masopust, D.; Vezys, V.; Marzo, A.L.; Lefrançois, L. Preferential Localization of Effector Memory Cells in Nonlymphoid Tissue. *Science* **2001**, *291*, 2413–2417. [CrossRef] [PubMed]
3. Reinhardt, R.L.; Khoruts, A.; Merica, R.; Zell, T.; Jenkins, M.K. Visualizing the generation of memory CD4 T cells in the whole body. *Nature* **2001**, *410*, 101–105. [CrossRef] [PubMed]
4. Gebhardt, T.; Wakim, L.M.; Eidsmo, L.; Reading, P.C.; Heath, W.R.; Carbone, F.R. Memory T cells in nonlymphoid tissue that provide enhanced local immunity during infection with herpes simplex virus. *Nat. Immunol.* **2009**, *10*, 524–530. [CrossRef]
5. Wakim, L.M.; Waithman, J.; van Rooijen, N.; Heath, W.R.; Carbone, F.R. Dendritic Cell-Induced Memory T Cell Activation in Nonlymphoid Tissues. *Science* **2008**, *319*, 198–202. [CrossRef]
6. Masopust, D.; Choo, D.; Vezys, V.; Wherry, E.J.; Duraiswamy, J.; Akondy, R.; Wang, J.; Casey, K.A.; Barber, D.L.; Kawamura, K.S.; et al. Dynamic T cell migration program provides resident memory within intestinal epithelium. *J. Exp. Med.* **2010**, *207*, 553–564. [CrossRef] [PubMed]
7. Khalil, S.; Bardawil, T.; Kurban, M.; Abbas, O. Tissue-resident memory T cells in the skin. *Inflamm. Res.* **2020**, *69*, 245–254. [CrossRef]
8. Watanabe, R. Protective and pathogenic roles of resident memory T cells in human skin disorders. *J. Dermatol. Sci.* **2019**, *95*, 2–7. [CrossRef]
9. Schenkel, J.M.; Masopust, D. Tissue-Resident Memory T Cells. *Immunity* **2014**, *41*, 886–897. [CrossRef]
10. Mueller, S.N.; Mackay, L.K. Tissue-resident memory T cells: Local specialists in immune defence. *Nat. Rev. Immunol.* **2016**, *16*, 79–89. [CrossRef]
11. Carbone, F.R. Tissue-Resident Memory T Cells and Fixed Immune Surveillance in Nonlymphoid Organs. *J. Immunol.* **2015**, *195*, 17–22. [CrossRef]
12. Jiang, X.; Clark, R.A.; Liu, L.; Wagers, A.J.; Fuhlbrigge, R.C.; Kupper, T.S. Skin infection generates non-migratory memory CD8+ TRM cells providing global skin immunity. *Nature* **2012**, *483*, 227–231. [CrossRef] [PubMed]
13. Behr, F.M.; Parga-Vidal, L.; Kragten, N.A.M.; van Dam, T.J.P.; Wesselink, T.H.; Sheridan, B.S.; Arens, R.; van Lier, R.A.W.; Stark, R.; van Gisbergen, K.P.J.M. Tissue-resident memory CD8+ T cells shape local and systemic secondary T cell responses. *Nat. Immunol.* **2020**, *21*, 1070–1081. [CrossRef] [PubMed]
14. Fonseca, R.; Beura, L.K.; Quarnstrom, C.F.; Ghoneim, H.E.; Fan, Y.; Zebley, C.C.; Scott, M.C.; Fares-Frederickson, N.J.; Wijeyesinghe, S.; Thompson, E.A.; et al. Developmental plasticity allows outside-in immune responses by resident memory T cells. *Nat. Immunol.* **2020**, *21*, 412–421. [CrossRef] [PubMed]
15. Masopust, D.; Vezys, V.; Wherry, E.J.; Barber, D.L.; Ahmed, R. Cutting Edge: Gut Microenvironment Promotes Differentiation of a Unique Memory CD8 T Cell Population. *J. Immunol.* **2006**, *176*, 2079–2083. [CrossRef] [PubMed]
16. Mackay, L.K.; Rahimpour, A.; Ma, J.Z.; Collins, N.; Stock, A.T.; Hafon, M.-L.; Vega-Ramos, J.; Lauzurica, P.; Mueller, S.N.; Stefanovic, T.; et al. The developmental pathway for CD103+CD8+ tissue-resident memory T cells of skin. *Nat. Immunol.* **2013**, *14*, 1294–1301. [CrossRef]
17. Gebhardt, T.; Whitney, P.G.; Zaid, A.; Mackay, L.K.; Brooks, A.G.; Heath, W.R.; Carbone, F.R.; Mueller, S.N. Different patterns of peripheral migration by memory CD4+ and CD8+ T cells. *Nature* **2011**, *477*, 216–219. [CrossRef]
18. Teijaro, J.R.; Turner, D.; Pham, Q.; Wherry, E.J.; Lefrançois, L.; Farber, D.L. Cutting Edge: Tissue-Retentive Lung Memory CD4 T Cells Mediate Optimal Protection to Respiratory Virus Infection. *J. Immunol.* **2011**, *187*, 5510–5514. [CrossRef]
19. Anderson, K.G.; Sung, H.; Skon, C.N.; Lefrancois, L.; Deisinger, A.; Vezys, V.; Masopust, D. Cutting Edge: Intravascular Staining Redefines Lung CD8 T Cell Responses. *J. Immunol.* **2012**, *189*, 2702–2706. [CrossRef]
20. Schenkel, J.M.; Fraser, K.A.; Vezys, V.; Masopust, D. Sensing and alarm function of resident memory CD8+ T cells. *Nat. Immunol.* **2013**, *14*, 509–513. [CrossRef]
21. Iijima, N.; Iwasaki, A. A local macrophage chemokine network sustains protective tissue-resident memory CD4 T cells. *Science* **2014**, *346*, 93–98. [CrossRef] [PubMed]
22. Sasson, S.C.; Gordon, C.L.; Christo, S.N.; Klenerman, P.; Mackay, L.K. Local heroes or villains: Tissue-resident memory T cells in human health and disease. *Cell. Mol. Immunol.* **2020**, *17*, 113–122. [CrossRef] [PubMed]

23. Clark, R.A.; Chong, B.; Mirchandani, N.; Brinster, N.K.; Yamanaka, K.; Dowgiert, R.K.; Kupper, T.S. The Vast Majority of CLA+ T Cells Are Resident in Normal Skin. *J. Immunol.* **2006**, *176*, 4431–4439. [CrossRef]
24. Watanabe, R.; Gehad, A.; Yang, C.; Scott, L.L.; Teague, J.E.; Schlapbach, C.; Elco, C.P.; Huang, V.; Matos, T.R.; Kupper, T.S.; et al. Human skin is protected by four functionally and phenotypically discrete populations of resident and recirculating memory T cells. *Sci. Transl. Med.* **2015**, *7*, 279ra39. [CrossRef]
25. Gaide, O.; Emerson, R.O.; Jiang, X.; Gulati, N.; Nizza, S.; Desmarais, C.; Robins, H.; Krueger, J.G.; Clark, R.A.; Kupper, T.S. Common clonal origin of central and resident memory T cells following skin immunization. *Nat. Med.* **2015**, *21*, 647–653. [CrossRef] [PubMed]
26. Mizukawa, Y.; Yamazaki, Y.; Teraki, Y.; Hayakawa, J.; Hayakawa, K.; Nuriya, H.; Kohara, M.; Shiohara, T. Direct Evidence for Interferon-γ Production by Effector-Memory-Type Intraepidermal T Cells Residing at an Effector Site of Immunopathology in Fixed Drug Eruption. *Am. J. Pathol.* **2002**, *161*, 1337–1347. [CrossRef]
27. Amsen, D.; van Gisbergen, K.P.J.M.; Hombrink, P.; van Lier, R.A.W. Tissue-resident memory T cells at the center of immunity to solid tumors. *Nat. Immunol.* **2018**, *19*, 538–546. [CrossRef]
28. Edwards, J.; Wilmott, J.S.; Madore, J.; Gide, T.N.; Quek, C.; Tasker, A.; Ferguson, A.; Chen, J.; Hewavisenti, R.; Hersey, P.; et al. CD103+ Tumor-Resident CD8+ T Cells Are Associated with Improved Survival in Immunotherapy-Naïve Melanoma Patients and Expand Significantly During Anti–PD-1 Treatment. *Clin. Cancer Res.* **2018**, *24*, 3036–3045. [CrossRef]
29. Vieyra-Garcia, P.; Crouch, J.D.; O'Malley, J.T.; Seger, E.W.; Yang, C.H.; Teague, J.E.; Vromans, A.M.; Gehad, A.; Win, T.S.; Yu, Z.; et al. Benign T cells drive clinical skin inflammation in cutaneous T cell lymphoma. *JCI Insight* **2019**, *4*, e124233. [CrossRef]
30. Cheuk, S.; Schlums, H.; Gallais Sérézal, I.; Martini, E.; Chiang, S.C.; Marquardt, N.; Gibbs, A.; Detlofsson, E.; Introini, A.; Forkel, M.; et al. CD49a Expression Defines Tissue-Resident CD8+ T Cells Poised for Cytotoxic Function in Human Skin. *Immunity* **2017**, *46*, 287–300. [CrossRef]
31. Xing, L.; Dai, Z.; Jabbari, A.; Cerise, J.E.; Higgins, C.A.; Gong, W.; de Jong, A.; Harel, S.; DeStefano, G.M.; Rothman, L.; et al. Alopecia areata is driven by cytotoxic T lymphocytes and is reversed by JAK inhibition. *Nat. Med.* **2014**, *20*, 1043–1049. [CrossRef]
32. Zaid, A.; Mackay, L.K.; Rahimpour, A.; Braun, A.; Veldhoen, M.; Carbone, F.R.; Manton, J.H.; Heath, W.R.; Mueller, S.N. Persistence of skin-resident memory T cells within an epidermal niche. *Proc. Natl. Acad. Sci. USA* **2014**, *111*, 5307–5312. [CrossRef] [PubMed]
33. Steinert, E.M.; Schenkel, J.M.; Fraser, K.A.; Beura, L.K.; Manlove, L.S.; Igyártó, B.Z.; Southern, P.J.; Masopust, D. Quantifying Memory CD8 T Cells Reveals Regionalization of Immunosurveillance. *Cell* **2015**, *161*, 737–749. [CrossRef] [PubMed]
34. Cepek, K.L.; Shaw, S.K.; Parker, C.M.; Russell, G.J.; Morrow, J.S.; Rimm, D.L.; Brenner, M.B. Adhesion between epithelial cells and T lymphocytes mediated by E-cadherin and the αEβ7 integrin. *Nature* **1994**, *372*, 190–193. [CrossRef]
35. Mackay, L.K.; Braun, A.; Macleod, B.L.; Collins, N.; Tebartz, C.; Bedoui, S.; Carbone, F.R.; Gebhardt, T. Cutting Edge: CD69 Interference with Sphingosine-1-Phosphate Receptor Function Regulates Peripheral T Cell Retention. *J. Immunol.* **2015**, *194*, 2059–2063. [CrossRef]
36. Cibrian, D.; Saiz, M.L.; De La Fuente, H.; Sánchez-Díaz, R.; Moreno-Gonzalo, O.; Jorge, I.; Ferrarini, A.; Vázquez, J.; Punzón, C.; Fresno, M.; et al. CD69 controls the uptake of L-tryptophan through LAT1-CD98 and AhR-dependent secretion of IL-22 in psoriasis. *Nat. Immunol.* **2016**, *17*, 985–996. [CrossRef] [PubMed]
37. Bergsbaken, T.; Bevan, M.J. Proinflammatory microenvironments within the intestine regulate the differentiation of tissue-resident CD8+ T cells responding to infection. *Nat. Immunol.* **2015**, *16*, 406–414. [CrossRef]
38. Schenkel, J.M.; Fraser, K.A.; Masopust, D. Cutting Edge: Resident Memory CD8 T Cells Occupy Frontline Niches in Secondary Lymphoid Organs. *J. Immunol.* **2014**, *192*, 2961–2964. [CrossRef] [PubMed]
39. Wakim, L.M.; Woodward-Davis, A.; Bevan, M.J. Memory T cells persisting within the brain after local infection show functional adaptations to their tissue of residence. *Proc. Natl. Acad. Sci. USA* **2010**, *107*, 17872–17879. [CrossRef]
40. Sowell, R.T.; Rogozinska, M.; Nelson, C.E.; Vezys, V.; Marzo, A.L. Cutting Edge: Generation of Effector Cells That Localize to Mucosal Tissues and Form Resident Memory CD8 T Cells Is Controlled by mTOR. *J. Immunol.* **2014**, *193*, 2067–2071. [CrossRef]
41. Hombrink, P.; Helbig, C.; Backer, R.A.; Piet, B.; Oja, A.E.; Stark, R.; Brasser, G.; Jongejan, A.; Jonkers, R.E.; Nota, B.; et al. Programs for the persistence, vigilance and control of human CD8+ lung-resident memory T cells. *Nat. Immunol.* **2016**, *17*, 1467–1478. [CrossRef]
42. Pan, Y.; Tian, T.; Park, C.O.; Lofttus, S.Y.; Mei, S.; Liu, X.; Luo, C.; O'Malley, J.T.; Gehad, A.; Teague, J.E.; et al. Survival of tissue-resident memory T cells requires exogenous lipid uptake and metabolism. *Nature* **2017**, *543*, 252–256. [CrossRef] [PubMed]
43. Liikanen, I.; Lauhan, C.; Quon, S.; Omilusik, K.; Phan, A.T.; Bartrolí, L.B.; Ferry, A.; Goulding, J.; Chen, J.; Scott-Browne, J.P.; et al. Hypoxia-inducible factor activity promotes antitumor effector function and tissue residency by CD8+ T cells. *J. Clin. Investig.* **2021**, *131*, e143729. [CrossRef]
44. Mackay, L.K.; Wynne-Jones, E.; Freestone, D.; Pellicci, D.G.; Mielke, L.A.; Newman, D.M.; Braun, A.; Masson, F.; Kallies, A.; Belz, G.T.; et al. T-box Transcription Factors Combine with the Cytokines TGF-β and IL-15 to Control Tissue-Resident Memory T Cell Fate. *Immunity* **2015**, *43*, 1101–1111. [CrossRef] [PubMed]
45. Mackay, L.K.; Minnich, M.; Kragten, N.A.M.; Liao, Y.; Nota, B.; Seillet, C.; Zaid, A.; Man, K.; Preston, S.; Freestone, D.; et al. Hobit and Blimp1 instruct a universal transcriptional program of tissue residency in lymphocytes. *Science* **2016**, *352*, 459–463. [CrossRef] [PubMed]

46. Strobl, J.; Pandey, R.V.; Krausgruber, T.; Bayer, N.; Kleissl, L.; Reininger, B.; Vieyra-Garcia, P.; Wolf, P.; Jentus, M.-M.; Mitterbauer, M.; et al. Long-term skin-resident memory T cells proliferate in situ and are involved in human graft-versus-host disease (GVHD). *Sci. Transl. Med.* **2020**, *12*, eabb7028. [CrossRef] [PubMed]
47. Milner, J.J.; Toma, C.; Yu, B.; Zhang, K.; Omilusik, K.; Phan, A.T.; Wang, D.; Getzler, A.J.; Nguyen, T.; Crotty, S.; et al. Runx3 programs CD8$^+$ T cell residency in non-lymphoid tissues and tumours. *Nature* **2017**, *552*, 253–257. [CrossRef]
48. Campbell, J.J.; Haraldsen, G.; Pan, J.; Rottman, J.; Qin, S.; Ponath, P.; Andrew, D.P.; Warnke, R.; Ruffing, N.; Kassam, N.; et al. The chemokine receptor CCR4 in vascular recognition by cutaneous but not intestinal memory T cells. *Nature* **1999**, *400*, 776–780. [CrossRef]
49. Homey, B.; Alenius, H.; Müller, A.; Soto, H.; Bowman, E.P.; Yuan, W.; McEvoy, L.; Lauerma, A.I.; Assmann, T.; Bünemann, E.; et al. CCL27–CCR10 interactions regulate T cell–mediated skin inflammation. *Nat. Med.* **2002**, *8*, 157–165. [CrossRef]
50. McCully, M.L.; Ladell, K.; Hakobyan, S.; Mansel, R.E.; Price, D.A.; Moser, B. Epidermis instructs skin homing receptor expression in human T cells. *Blood* **2012**, *120*, 4591–4598. [CrossRef]
51. Xia, M.; Hu, S.; Fu, Y.; Jin, W.; Yi, Q.; Matsui, Y.; Yang, J.; McDowell, M.A.; Sarkar, S.; Kalia, V.; et al. CCR10 regulates balanced maintenance and function of resident regulatory and effector T cells to promote immune homeostasis in the skin. *J. Allergy Clin. Immunol.* **2014**, *134*, 634–644. [CrossRef] [PubMed]
52. Zaid, A.; Hor, J.L.; Christo, S.N.; Groom, J.R.; Heath, W.R.; Mackay, L.K.; Mueller, S.N. Chemokine Receptor–Dependent Control of Skin Tissue–Resident Memory T Cell Formation. *J. Immunol.* **2017**, *199*, 2451–2459. [CrossRef]
53. Kok, L.; Dijkgraaf, F.E.; Urbanus, J.; Bresser, K.; Vredevoogd, D.W.; Cardoso, R.F.; Perié, L.; Beltman, J.B.; Schumacher, T.N. A committed tissue-resident memory T cell precursor within the circulating CD8$^+$ effector T cell pool. *J. Exp. Med.* **2020**, *217*, e20191711. [CrossRef]
54. Kurd, N.S.; He, Z.; Louis, T.L.; Milner, J.J.; Omilusik, K.D.; Jin, W.; Tsai, M.S.; Widjaja, C.E.; Kanbar, J.N.; Olvera, J.G.; et al. Early precursors and molecular determinants of tissue-resident memory CD8$^+$ T lymphocytes revealed by single-cell RNA sequencing. *Sci. Immunol.* **2020**, *5*, eaaz6894. [CrossRef]
55. Sathaliyawala, T.; Kubota, M.; Yudanin, N.; Turner, D.; Camp, P.; Thome, J.J.C.; Bickham, K.L.; Lerner, H.; Goldstein, M.; Sykes, M.; et al. Distribution and Compartmentalization of Human Circulating and Tissue-Resident Memory T Cell Subsets. *Immunity* **2013**, *38*, 187–197. [CrossRef]
56. Kumar, B.V.; Ma, W.; Miron, M.; Granot, T.; Guyer, R.S.; Carpenter, D.J.; Senda, T.; Sun, X.; Ho, S.-H.; Lerner, H.; et al. Human Tissue-Resident Memory T Cells Are Defined by Core Transcriptional and Functional Signatures in Lymphoid and Mucosal Sites. *Cell Rep.* **2017**, *20*, 2921–2934. [CrossRef]
57. Wong, M.T.; Ong, D.E.H.; Lim, F.S.H.; Teng, K.W.W.; McGovern, N.; Narayanan, S.; Ho, W.Q.; Cerny, D.; Tan, H.K.K.; Anicete, R.; et al. A High-Dimensional Atlas of Human T Cell Diversity Reveals Tissue-Specific Trafficking and Cytokine Signatures. *Immunity* **2016**, *45*, 442–456. [CrossRef]
58. Clark, R.A.; Watanabe, R.; Teague, J.E.; Schlapbach, C.; Tawa, M.C.; Adams, N.; Dorosario, A.A.; Chaney, K.S.; Cutler, C.S.; LeBoeuf, N.R.; et al. Skin Effector Memory T Cells Do Not Recirculate and Provide Immune Protection in Alemtuzumab-Treated CTCL Patients. *Sci. Transl. Med.* **2012**, *4*, 117ra7. [CrossRef]
59. Koguchi-Yoshioka, H.; Hoffer, E.; Cheuk, S.; Matsumura, Y.; Vo, S.; Kjellman, P.; Grema, L.; Ishitsuka, Y.; Nakamura, Y.; Okiyama, N.; et al. Skin T cells maintain their diversity and functionality in the elderly. *Commun. Biol.* **2021**, *4*, 13. [CrossRef]
60. Park, C.O.; Fu, X.; Jiang, X.; Pan, Y.; Teague, J.E.; Collins, N.; Tian, T.; O'Malley, J.T.; Emerson, R.O.; Kim, J.H.; et al. Staged development of long-lived T-cell receptor αβ TH17 resident memory T-cell population to Candida albicans after skin infection. *J. Allergy Clin. Immunol.* **2018**, *142*, 647–662. [CrossRef] [PubMed]
61. Collins, N.; Jiang, X.; Zaid, A.; Macleod, B.L.; Li, J.; Park, C.O.; Haque, A.; Bedoui, S.; Heath, W.R.; Mueller, S.N.; et al. Skin CD4$^+$ memory T cells exhibit combined cluster-mediated retention and equilibration with the circulation. *Nat. Commun.* **2016**, *7*, 11514. [CrossRef] [PubMed]
62. Cheuk, S.; Wikén, M.; Blomqvist, L.; Nylén, S.; Talme, T.; Ståhle, M.; Eidsmo, L. Epidermal Th22 and Tc17 Cells Form a Localized Disease Memory in Clinically Healed Psoriasis. *J. Immunol.* **2014**, *192*, 3111–3120. [CrossRef]
63. Adachi, T.; Kobayashi, T.; Sugihara, E.; Yamada, T.; Ikuta, K.; Pittaluga, S.; Saya, H.; Amagai, M.; Nagao, K. Hair follicle–derived IL-7 and IL-15 mediate skin-resident memory T cell homeostasis and lymphoma. *Nat. Med.* **2015**, *21*, 1272–1279. [CrossRef] [PubMed]
64. Tokura, Y.; Phadungsaksawasdi, P.; Kurihara, K.; Fujiyama, T.; Honda, T. Pathophysiology of Skin Resident Memory T Cells. *Front. Immunol.* **2021**, *11*, 3789. [CrossRef] [PubMed]
65. Adams, E.J.; Gu, S.; Luoma, A.M. Human gamma delta T cells: Evolution and ligand recognition. *Cell. Immunol.* **2015**, *296*, 31–40. [CrossRef] [PubMed]
66. Reitermaier, R.; Krausgruber, T.; Fortelny, N.; Ayub, T.; Vieyra-Garcia, P.A.; Kienzl, P.; Wolf, P.; Scharrer, A.; Fiala, C.; Kölz, M.; et al. αβγδ T cells play a vital role in fetal human skin development and immunity. *J. Exp. Med.* **2021**, *218*, e20201189. [CrossRef]
67. Koguchi-Yoshioka, H.; Watanabe, R.; Matsumura, Y.; Okiyama, N.; Ishitsuka, Y.; Nakamura, Y.; Fujisawa, Y.; Fujimoto, M. The Possible Linkage of Granzyme B-Producing Skin T Cells with the Disease Prognosis of Alopecia Areata. *J. Investig. Dermatol.* **2021**, *141*, 427–429. [CrossRef] [PubMed]
68. Kim, S.; Park, C.; Shin, J.; Noh, J.; Kim, H.; Kim, J.; Lee, H.; Lee, J.; Kupper, T.S.; Lee, K. Multicytokine-producing tissue resident memory (TRM) cells in atopic dermatitis patient. *J. Investig. Dermatol.* **2016**, *136*, S9. [CrossRef]

69. Boniface, K.; Jacquemin, C.; Darrigade, A.-S.; Dessarthe, B.; Martins, C.; Boukhedouni, N.; Vernisse, C.; Grasseau, A.; Thiolat, D.; Rambert, J.; et al. Vitiligo Skin Is Imprinted with Resident Memory CD8 T Cells Expressing CXCR3. *J. Investig. Dermatol.* **2018**, *138*, 355–364. [CrossRef]
70. Han, J.; Zhao, Y.; Shirai, K.; Molodtsov, A.; Kolling, F.W.; Fisher, J.L.; Zhang, P.; Yan, S.; Searles, T.G.; Bader, J.M.; et al. Resident and circulating memory T cells persist for years in melanoma patients with durable responses to immunotherapy. *Nat. Cancer* **2021**, *2*, 300–311. [CrossRef]
71. Zeng, J.; Luo, S.; Huang, Y.; Lu, Q. Critical role of environmental factors in the pathogenesis of psoriasis. *J. Dermatol.* **2017**, *44*, 863–872. [CrossRef]
72. Li, Q.; Chandran, V.; Tsoi, L.; O'Rielly, D.; Nair, R.P.; Gladman, D.; Elder, J.T.; Rahman, P. Quantifying Differences in Heritability among Psoriatic Arthritis (PsA), Cutaneous Psoriasis (PsC) and Psoriasis vulgaris (PsV). *Sci. Rep.* **2020**, *10*, 4925. [CrossRef]
73. Lande, R.; Botti, E.; Jandus, C.; Dojcinovic, D.; Fanelli, G.; Conrad, C.; Chamilos, G.; Feldmeyer, L.; Marinari, B.; Chon, S.; et al. The antimicrobial peptide LL37 is a T-cell autoantigen in psoriasis. *Nat. Commun.* **2014**, *5*, 5621. [CrossRef]
74. Bhushan, M.; Bleiker, T.O.; Ballsdon, A.E.; Allen, M.H.; Sopwith, M.; Robinson, M.K.; Clarke, C.; Weller, R.P.J.B.; Graham-Brown, R.A.C.; Keefe, M.; et al. Anti-E-selectin is ineffective in the treatment of psoriasis: A randomized trial. *Br. J. Dermatol.* **2002**, *146*, 824–831. [CrossRef]
75. Lebwohl, M.; Tyring, S.K.; Hamilton, T.K.; Toth, D.; Glazer, S.; Tawfik, N.H.; Walicke, P.; Dummer, W.; Wang, X.; Garovoy, M.R.; et al. A Novel Targeted T-Cell Modulator, Efalizumab, for Plaque Psoriasis. *N. Engl. J. Med.* **2003**, *349*, 2004–2013. [CrossRef]
76. Conrad, C.; Boyman, O.; Tonel, G.; Tun-Kyi, A.; Laggner, U.; de Fougerolles, A.; Kotelianski, V.; Gardner, H.; Nestle, F.O. α1β1 integrin is crucial for accumulation of epidermal T cells and the development of psoriasis. *Nat. Med.* **2007**, *13*, 836–842. [CrossRef] [PubMed]
77. Gallais Sérézal, I.; Hoffer, E.; Ignatov, B.; Martini, E.; Zitti, B.; Ehrström, M.; Eidsmo, L. A skewed pool of resident T cells triggers psoriasis-associated tissue responses in never-lesional skin from patients with psoriasis. *J. Allergy Clin. Immunol.* **2019**, *143*, 1444–1454. [CrossRef] [PubMed]
78. Nograles, K.E.; Zaba, L.C.; Guttman-Yassky, E.; Fuentes-Duculan, J.; Suárez-Fariñas, M.; Cardinale, I.; Khatcherian, A.; Gonzalez, J.; Pierson, K.C.; White, T.R.; et al. Th17 cytokines interleukin (IL)-17 and IL-22 modulate distinct inflammatory and keratinocyte-response pathways. *Br. J. Dermatol.* **2008**, *159*, 1092–1102. [CrossRef] [PubMed]
79. Martini, E.; Wikén, M.; Cheuk, S.; Gallais Sérézal, I.; Baharom, F.; Ståhle, M.; Smed-Sörensen, A.; Eidsmo, L. Dynamic Changes in Resident and Infiltrating Epidermal Dendritic Cells in Active and Resolved Psoriasis. *J. Investig. Dermatol.* **2017**, *137*, 865–873. [CrossRef]
80. Matos, T.R.; O'Malley, J.T.; Lowry, E.L.; Hamm, D.; Kirsch, I.R.; Robins, H.S.; Kupper, T.S.; Krueger, J.G.; Clark, R.A. Clinically resolved psoriatic lesions contain psoriasis-specific IL-17–producing αβ T cell clones. *J. Clin. Investig.* **2017**, *127*, 4031–4041. [CrossRef]
81. Lande, R.; Gregorio, J.; Facchinetti, V.; Chatterjee, B.; Wang, Y.-H.; Homey, B.; Cao, W.; Wang, Y.-H.; Su, B.; Nestle, F.O.; et al. Plasmacytoid dendritic cells sense self-DNA coupled with antimicrobial peptide. *Nature* **2007**, *449*, 564–569. [CrossRef] [PubMed]
82. Zaba, L.C.; Krueger, J.G.; Lowes, M.A. Resident and "Inflammatory" Dendritic Cells in Human Skin. *J. Investig. Dermatol.* **2009**, *129*, 302–308. [CrossRef]
83. Arakawa, A.; Siewert, K.; Stöhr, J.; Besgen, P.; Kim, S.-M.; Rühl, G.; Nickel, J.; Vollmer, S.; Thomas, P.; Krebs, S.; et al. Melanocyte antigen triggers autoimmunity in human psoriasis. *J. Exp. Med.* **2015**, *212*, 2203–2212. [CrossRef]
84. Cheung, K.L.; Jarrett, R.; Subramaniam, S.; Salimi, M.; Gutowska-Owsiak, D.; Chen, Y.-L.; Hardman, C.; Xue, L.; Cerundolo, V.; Ogg, G. Psoriatic T cells recognize neolipid antigens generated by mast cell phospholipase delivered by exosomes and presented by CD1a. *J. Exp. Med.* **2016**, *213*, 2399–2412. [CrossRef]
85. Jin, L.; Wang, G. Keratin 17: A Critical Player in the Pathogenesis of Psoriasis. *Med. Res. Rev.* **2014**, *34*, 438–454. [CrossRef]
86. Johnston, A.; Gudjonsson, J.E.; Sigmundsdottir, H.; Love, T.J.; Valdimarsson, H. Peripheral blood T cell responses to keratin peptides that share sequences with streptococcal M proteins are largely restricted to skin-homing CD8$^+$ T cells. *Clin. Exp. Immunol.* **2004**, *138*, 83–93. [CrossRef]
87. Kurihara, K.; Fujiyama, T.; Phadungsaksawasdi, P.; Ito, T.; Tokura, Y. Significance of IL-17A-producing CD8$^+$CD103$^+$ skin resident memory T cells in psoriasis lesion and their possible relationship to clinical course. *J. Dermatol. Sci.* **2019**, *95*, 21–27. [CrossRef] [PubMed]
88. Vo, S.; Watanabe, R.; Koguchi-Yoshioka, H.; Matsumura, Y.; Ishitsuka, Y.; Nakamura, Y.; Okiyama, N.; Fujisawa, Y.; Fujimoto, M. CD8 resident memory T cells with interleukin 17A-producing potential are accumulated in disease-naïve nonlesional sites of psoriasis possibly in correlation with disease duration. *Br. J. Dermatol.* **2019**, *181*, 410–412. [CrossRef]
89. Fenix, K.; Wijesundara, D.K.; Cowin, A.J.; Grubor-Bauk, B.; Kopecki, Z. Immunological memory in imiquimod-induced murine model of psoriasiform dermatitis. *Int. J. Mol. Sci.* **2020**, *21*, 7228. [CrossRef] [PubMed]
90. Di Meglio, P.; Villanova, F.; Navarini, A.A.; Mylonas, A.; Tosi, I.; Nestle, F.O.; Conrad, C. Targeting CD8$^+$ T cells prevents psoriasis development. *J. Allergy Clin. Immunol.* **2016**, *138*, 274–276.e6. [CrossRef] [PubMed]
91. Fujiyama, T.; Umayahara, T.; Kurihara, K.; Shimauchi, T.; Ito, T.; Aoshima, M.; Otobe, E.; Hashizume, H.; Yagi, H.; Tokura, Y. Skin infiltration of pathogenic migratory and resident T cells is decreased by Secukinumab treatment in psoriasis. *J. Investig. Dermatol.* **2020**, *140*, 2073–2076. [CrossRef]

92. Mashiko, S.; Edelmayer, R.M.; Bi, Y.; Olson, L.M.; Wetter, J.B.; Wang, J.; Maari, C.; Saint-Cyr Proulx, E.; Kaimal, V.; Li, X.; et al. Persistence of Inflammatory Phenotype in Residual Psoriatic Plaques in Patients on Effective Biologic Therapy. *J. Investig. Dermatol.* **2020**, *140*, 1015–1025.e4. [CrossRef]
93. Gallais Sérézal, I.; Classon, C.; Cheuk, S.; Barrientos-Somarribas, M.; Wadman, E.; Martini, E.; Chang, D.; Xu Landén, N.; Ehrström, M.; Nylén, S.; et al. Resident T Cells in Resolved Psoriasis Steer Tissue Responses that Stratify Clinical Outcome. *J. Investig. Dermatol.* **2018**, *138*, 1754–1763. [CrossRef]
94. Papp, K.A.; Reich, K.; Paul, C.; Blauvelt, A.; Baran, W.; Bolduc, C.; Toth, D.; Langley, R.G.; Cather, J.; Gottlieb, A.B.; et al. A prospective phase III, randomized, double-blind, placebo-controlled study of brodalumab in patients with moderate-to-severe plaque psoriasis. *Br. J. Dermatol.* **2016**, *175*, 273–286. [CrossRef]
95. Mehta, H.; Mashiko, S.; Angsana, J.; Rubio, M.; Hsieh, Y.-C.M.; Maari, C.; Reich, K.; Blauvelt, A.; Bissonnette, R.; Muñoz-Elías, E.J.; et al. Differential Changes in Inflammatory Mononuclear Phagocyte and T-Cell Profiles within Psoriatic Skin during Treatment with Guselkumab vs. Secukinumab. *J. Investig. Dermatol.* **2021**, *141*, 1707–1718.e9. [CrossRef] [PubMed]
96. Søyland, E.; Heier, I.; Rodríguez-Gallego, C.; Mollnes, T.E.; Johansen, F.-E.; Holven, K.B.; Halvorsen, B.; Aukrust, P.; Jahnsen, F.L.; de la Rosa Carrillo, D.; et al. Sun exposure induces rapid immunological changes in skin and peripheral blood in patients with psoriasis. *Br. J. Dermatol.* **2011**, *164*, 344–355. [CrossRef]
97. Dyring-Andersen, B.; Bonefeld, C.M.; Bzorek, M.; Løvendorf, M.B.; Lauritsen, J.P.H.; Skov, L.; Geisler, C. The Vitamin D Analogue Calcipotriol Reduces the Frequency of $CD8^+IL-17^+$ T Cells in Psoriasis Lesions. *Scand. J. Immunol.* **2015**, *82*, 84–91. [CrossRef]
98. Fujiyama, T.; Ito, T.; Umayahara, T.; Ikeya, S.; Tatsuno, K.; Funakoshi, A.; Hashizume, H.; Tokura, Y. Topical application of a vitamin D3 analogue and corticosteroid to psoriasis plaques decreases skin infiltration of TH17 cells and their ex vivo expansion. *J. Allergy Clin. Immunol.* **2016**, *138*, 517–528. [CrossRef] [PubMed]
99. Gottlieb, S.L.; Hayes, E.; Gilleaudeau, P.; Cardinale, I.; Gottlieb, A.B.; Krueger, J.G. Cellular actions of etretinate in psoriasis: Enhanced epidermal differentiation and reduced cell-mediated inflammation are unexpected outcomes. *J. Cutan. Pathol.* **1996**, *23*, 404–418. [CrossRef]
100. Xiao, S.; Jin, H.; Korn, T.; Liu, S.M.; Oukka, M.; Lim, B.; Kuchroo, V.K. Retinoic Acid Increases Foxp3+ Regulatory T Cells and Inhibits Development of Th17 Cells by Enhancing TGF-β-Driven Smad3 Signaling and Inhibiting IL-6 and IL-23 Receptor Expression. *J. Immunol.* **2008**, *181*, 2277–2284. [CrossRef] [PubMed]
101. Gottlieb, A.B.; Matheson, R.T.; Menter, A.; Leonardi, C.L.; Day, R.M.; Hu, C.; Schafer, P.H. Efficacy, tolerability, and pharmacodynamics of apremilast in recalcitrant plaque psoriasis: A phase II open-label study. *J. Drugs Dermatol.* **2013**, *12*, 888–897. [PubMed]
102. Robbins, K.; Bissonnette, R.; Maeda-Chubachi, T.; Ye, L.; Peppers, J.; Gallagher, K.; Kraus, J.E. Phase 2, randomized dose-finding study of tapinarof (GSK2894512 cream) for the treatment of plaque psoriasis. *J. Am. Acad. Dermatol.* **2019**, *80*, 714–721. [CrossRef] [PubMed]
103. Kobayashi, T.; Ricardo-Gonzalez, R.R.; Moro, K. Skin-Resident Innate Lymphoid Cells—Cutaneous Innate Guardians and Regulators. *Trends Immunol.* **2020**, *41*, 100–112. [CrossRef] [PubMed]
104. Weisel, N.M.; Weisel, F.J.; Farber, D.L.; Borghesi, L.A.; Shen, Y.; Ma, W.; Luning Prak, E.T.; Shlomchik, M.J. Comprehensive analyses of B-cell compartments across the human body reveal novel subsets and a gut-resident memory phenotype. *Blood* **2020**, *136*, 2774–2785. [CrossRef] [PubMed]

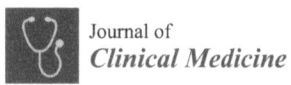

Review

The Defect in Regulatory T Cells in Psoriasis and Therapeutic Approaches

Naoko Kanda [1,*], Toshihiko Hoashi [2] and Hidehisa Saeki [2]

1. Department of Dermatology, Nippon Medical School, Chiba Hokusoh Hospital, Inzai 270-1694, Japan
2. Department of Dermatology, Nippon Medical School, Tokyo 113-8602, Japan; t-hoashi@nms.ac.jp (T.H.); h-saeki@nms.ac.jp (H.S.)
* Correspondence: n-kanda@nms.ac.jp; Tel.: +81-476-99-1111

Abstract: Psoriasis is a chronic inflammatory skin disease characterized by accelerated tumor necrosis factor-α/interleukin (IL)-23/IL-17 axis. Patients with psoriasis manifest functional defects in $CD4^+CD25^+$ forkhead box protein 3 (Foxp3)$^+$ regulatory T cells (Tregs), which suppress the excess immune response and mediate homeostasis. Defects in Tregs contribute to the pathogenesis of psoriasis and may attribute to enhanced inhibition and/or impaired stimulation of Tregs. IL-23 induces the conversion of Tregs into type 17 helper T (Th17) cells. IL-17A reduces transforming growth factor (TGF)-β1 production, Foxp3 expression, and suppresses Treg activity. Short-chain fatty acids (SCFAs), butyrate, propionate, and acetate are microbiota-derived fermentation products that promote Treg development and function by inducing *Foxp3* expression or inducing dendritic cells or intestinal epithelial cells to produce retinoic acids or TGF-β1, respectively. The gut microbiome of patients with psoriasis revealed reduced SCFA-producing bacteria, *Bacteroidetes*, and *Faecallibacterium*, which may contribute to the defect in Tregs. Therapeutic agents currently used, viz., anti-IL-23p19 or anti-IL-17A antibodies, retinoids, vitamin D3, dimethyl fumarate, narrow-band ultraviolet B, or those under development for psoriasis, viz., signal transducer and activator of transcription 3 inhibitors, butyrate, histone deacetylase inhibitors, and probiotics/prebiotics restore the defected Tregs. Thus, restoration of Tregs is a promising therapeutic target for psoriasis.

Keywords: psoriasis; regulatory T cell; forkhead box protein 3; short chain fatty acid; butyrate; interleukin-17A; interleukin-23; dendritic cell; gut microbiome

1. Introduction

Psoriasis is a chronic inflammatory skin disease characterized by accelerated tumor necrosis factor-α (TNF-α)/interleukin-23 (IL-23)/IL-17 axis and hyperproliferation and aberrant differentiation of epidermal keratinocytes (Figure 1) [1–3]. Dendritic cells (DCs) activated by various stimuli secrete TNF-α, which acts on themselves and induces their IL-23 secretion. IL-23 induces type 17 helper T (Th17) cells to proliferate and overproduce IL-17A and IL-22, which act on keratinocytes to promote their proliferation and production of the cytokines TNF-α and IL-17C; antimicrobial peptides or chemokines CXCL1/8 and CCL20 that recruit neutrophils, lymphocytes, and monocytes. Innate immune cells, such as type 3 innate lymphoid cells, γδT cells, or invariant natural killer T cells, also produce IL-17A, and are involved in the pathogenesis of psoriasis.

$CD4^+CD25^+$ forkhead box protein 3 (Foxp3)$^+$ regulatory T cells (Tregs) suppress the excess immunity against various antigens, including self-antigens, and mediate self-tolerance and homeostasis. The transcription factor Foxp3 plays a central role in the development and function of Tregs [4]. In psoriasis, Tregs are functionally defective [5,6] and cannot sufficiently suppress the proliferation or inflammatory cytokine production of Th17 cells (Figure 1). Defects in Tregs may contribute to the development and exacerbation of psoriasis. Although Tregs increase in psoriatic lesional skin compared to healthy skin [7,8], the ratio of Th17 cells to Tregs is higher in the lesions. The results are conflicting regarding

Treg frequency in the blood, with the frequency decreasing, no difference, or increasing in patients with psoriasis compared to that in healthy controls [8].

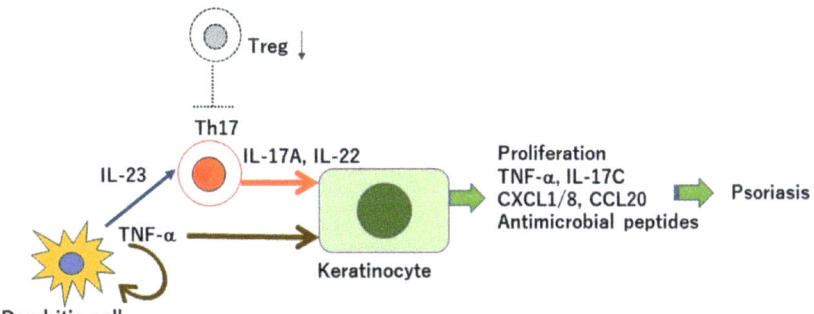

Figure 1. Tumor necrosis factor (TNF)-α/interleukin (IL)-23/IL-17 axis, and the defect in regulatory T cells (Tregs) in the pathogenesis of psoriasis. Dendritic cells secrete TNF-α that induces IL-23 secretion. IL-23 induces type 17 helper T (Th17) cells to produce IL-17A and IL-22, which act on keratinocytes and promote the proliferation and production of cytokines, antimicrobial peptides, or chemokines; thus, inducing inflammation. In psoriasis, Tregs are dysfunctional and cannot sufficiently suppress the activity of Th17 cells.

Natural Tregs are classified into thymus-derived Tregs (tTregs) and peripherally derived Tregs (pTregs). tTregs arise in the thymus and stably express Foxp3. pTregs arise in peripheral sites from conventional T cells in the presence of transforming growth factor (TGF)-β and IL-2 and by binding of self-antigens to the T-cell receptor (TCR) in combination with a co-stimulatory signal CD28. Foxp3 expression in pTregs is less stable than that in tTregs. Tregs can be generated in vitro from conventional T cells in the presence of TGF-β, and this population is known as in vitro-induced Tregs (iTregs). The demethylation level of Treg signature genes and stability of Foxp3 are lower in iTregs than pTregs [9]. In addition to Foxp3$^+$ Tregs, CD4$^+$ type 1 T regulatory (Tr1) cells represent another subset of Tregs defined by the expression of IL-10 and surface marker lymphocyte activation gene 3 and CD49b without Foxp3 and CD25 expression [10]. The relationship between Foxp3$^+$ Tregs and Tr1 cells remains obscure, with both subsets employing common effector pathways, including IL-10, TGF-β, and cytotoxic T lymphocyte antigen 4 (CTLA4) [11].

The suppressive function of Tregs is mediated by multiple mechanisms (Figure 2) [12]; Tregs kill effector T cells or DCs through granzymes [13]; Tregs compete for IL-2 with effector T cells via CD25 and deprive IL-2, thus, inducing apoptosis [14,15]; Tregs release IL-10 and TGF-β, suppressing the proliferation of effector T cells [16,17], and the interaction of CTLA4 with CD80/86 downregulates CD80/86 on DCs and decreases their potency of antigen-presenting cells (APCs) to activate T cells [18]; interactions with Tregs induce the activity of indoleamine 2,3-dioxygenase in DCs, which in turn upregulates heme oxygenase-1 activity in Tregs, and secretion of its product carbon monoxide inhibits the proliferation of effector T cells [19].

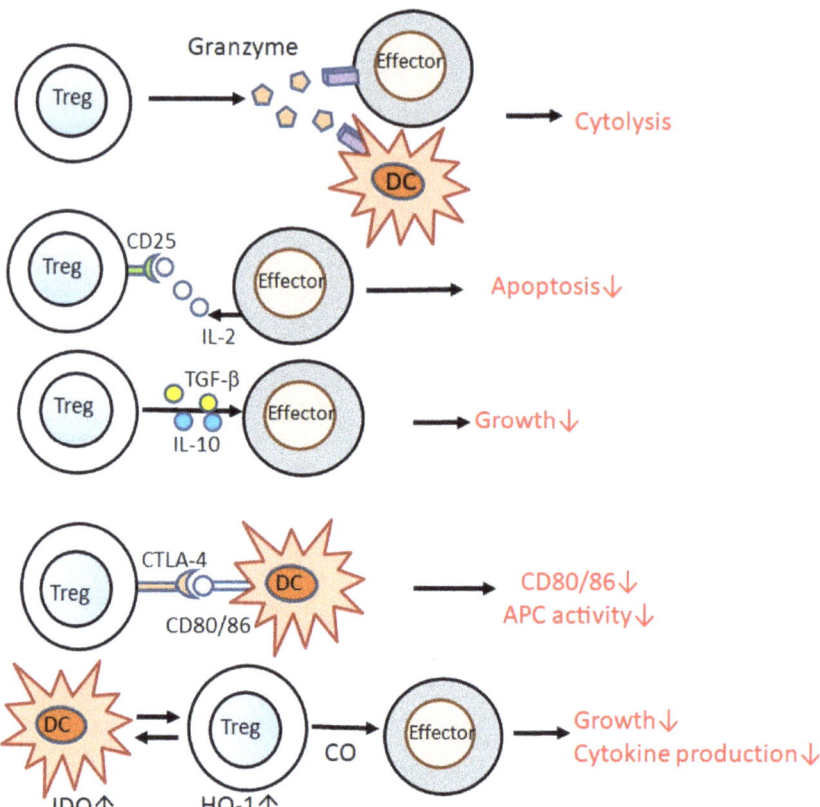

Figure 2. Possible mechanisms for immunosuppression by CD4$^+$CD25$^+$ Forkhead box protein 3 (Foxp3)$^+$ regulatory T cells (Tregs). Tregs kill effector T cells and dendritic cells (DCs) by granzymes; Tregs deprive interleukin (IL)-2 from effector T cells; Tregs secrete IL-10 and transforming growth factor-β (TGF-β), which suppress the proliferation of effector T cells; cytotoxic T-lymphocyte antigen 4 (CTLA4) binding to CD80/86 downregulates CD80/86 and capacity of antigen-presenting cells (APCs) in DCs; interaction with Tregs induces the activity of indoleamine 2,3-dioxygenase (IDO) in DCs, which further activates heme-oxygenase-1 (HO-1) in Tregs, releasing carbon monoxide (CO), which inhibits the activity of effector T cells.

The binding of Foxp3 to target genes induces the expression of *CD25*, *CTLA4*, *GITR*, or *HELIOS* while repressing the expression of *IL-2*, *IFN-γ*, or *RORγt* in Tregs. *Foxp3* expression is mediated by five enhancer elements [4]: 5′-first conserved non-coding sequence (CNS) 0, promoter region, and three further CNS (CNS1–3); these elements are bound by specific transcription factors (Figure 3) [4]. CNS2 is called the Treg-specific demethylation region (TSDR), whose demethylated status confers the stability of Foxp3 expression [6]. In tTregs, CNS2 is fully demethylated and bound by full sets of transcription factors [6]. In pTregs, CNS2 is demethylated with lower stability, whereas in iTregs, this locus is rarely demethylated, making this subset very unstable [6]. *Foxp3* expression is initiated by the binding of self-antigens to TCR in combination with CD28 together with IL-2 and TGF-β [4]. The TCR/CD28 signal activates the binding of nuclear factor of activated T cells (NFAT), activator protein-1, forkhead box-containing protein O subfamily 1 (FOXO1), and nuclear receptor 4a to the promoter, NFAT binding to CNS1, cyclic AMP response element-binding protein binding to CNS2, and c-Rel binding to CNS3 [4]. TGF-β induces Smad2/3 binding to CNS1, whereas IL-2 induces signal transducer and activator of transcription (STAT) 5 binding to the promoter and CNS2 [4].

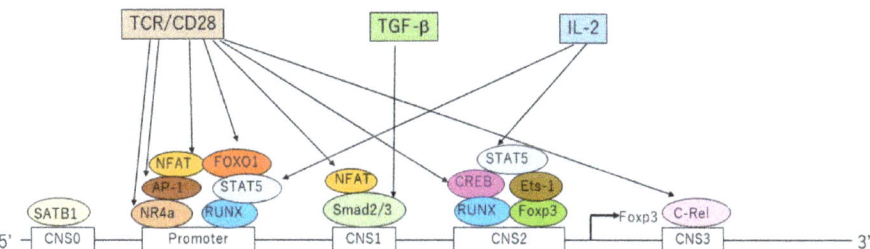

Figure 3. *Forkhead box protein 3 (Foxp3)* gene expression in regulatory T cells. *Foxp3* gene contains five enhancer elements: four conserved non-coding sequences (CNS0–3) and a promoter. *Foxp3* expression is initiated by the binding of self-antigens to the T-cell receptor (TCR) in combination with a co-stimulatory signal, CD28, together with transforming growth factor (TGF)-β and interleukin (IL)-2. These activation signals provoke the recruitment and binding of transcription factors to individual response elements. The TCR/CD28 signal induces the binding of activator protein-1 (AP-1), nuclear factor of activated T cells (NFAT), nuclear receptor 4a (NR4a), forkhead box-containing protein O subfamily 1 (FOXO1), cyclic AMP response element-binding protein (CREB), and c-Rel. TGF-β induces the binding of Smad2/3, and IL-2 induces the binding of signal transducer and activator of transcription 5 (STAT5). SATB1, special AT-rich sequence-binding protein 1; RUNX, runt-related transcription factor.

In this article, we review recent studies regarding the defect of Tregs in psoriasis and the therapeutic agents that restore the defective Tregs. The defect in Tregs in psoriasis may attribute to enhanced inhibition and/or impaired stimulation of the generation and maintenance of Tregs. Restoration of Tregs is necessary for the control of psoriasis, and is a promising therapeutic target.

2. Genetic and Epigenetic Evidence for Defected Tregs in Psoriasis

Gao et al. reported that Chinese patients with psoriasis showed polymorphisms in *Foxp3* [20]. The *Foxp3*-3279 AC and IVS9+459 GG genotypes were associated with an increased risk of psoriasis in a Chinese population, indicating that they may increase the risk for psoriasis by quantitatively and functionally influencing Tregs. Larger population-based studies are needed to confirm the universality of these findings.

Ngalamilka et al. reported that the peripheral blood of patients with psoriasis had significantly higher methylation levels of *Foxp3* TSDR compared to healthy controls [21]. TSDR hypermethylation is associated with chromatin condensation and downregulation of *Foxp3* expression; therefore, the results indicate downregulation of *Foxp3* and reduction of Tregs in psoriasis patients' blood.

3. Downregulation of Tregs by Cytokines or Mediators Which Are Upregulated in Psoriasis

$CD4^+CD25^+Foxp3^+$ Tregs in psoriatic skin lesions can be converted to retinoic acid (RA) receptor-related orphan nuclear receptor γt (RORγt)$^+$IL-17A-producing cells, and the conversion is promoted by IL-23 [22]. IL-23 reduces Foxp3 expression in Tregs [22]. IL-23 is produced by APCs and keratinocytes in psoriatic skin lesions [23], and keratinocyte-derived IL-23 may contribute to the downregulation of Tregs.

IL-17A acts on human Tregs and reduces their suppressive activity on effector T cell proliferation, suppresses Foxp3 and TGF-β expression, and enhances IFN-γ and T-bet expression [24]. These results indicate a downregulatory role of IL-17A in Tregs. However, contradictory results have been reported. IL-17A knockout mice failed to induce Tregs as efficiently as wild-type mice with autoimmune uveitis [25], and blocking IL-17A abolished the $CD4^+CD25^+$ Treg function required for preventing corneal allograft rejection [26]; thus, indicating that IL-17A is required for the induction and/or maintenance of Tregs in the eyes. Either up- or down-regulation by IL-17A in Tregs may depend on the target organs or species, and further studies are needed for clarification.

Yang et al. reported that Tregs from the peripheral blood of patients with psoriasis produced IFN-γ, TNF-α, and IL-17A, together with enhanced phosphorylation of STAT3 and impaired suppressive functions [27]. STAT3 inhibitor Stattic V restrained IFN-γ, TNF-α, and IL-17A expression and restored the suppressive function of Tregs in vitro [27]. IL-6, IL-21, and IL-23 induced the phosphorylation of STAT3 in Tregs in vitro [27]. These findings indicate that IL-6, IL-21, and IL-23 cytokines whose expressions are elevated in psoriatic lesions, may impair the suppressive function of Tregs and induce the conversion of Tregs into Th1/Th17 cells via STAT3 phosphorylation. IL-6 and IL-21 also render effector T cells refractory to Treg-mediated suppression via the STAT3 pathway [28,29].

Akt-induced phosphorylation and inactivation of the transcription factor FOXO1 is another mechanism underlying Treg dysfunction in psoriasis [30]. Circulating Tregs in patients with psoriasis expressed high levels of T-bet and IFN-γ mRNAs, showing a Th1-like phenotype in addition to enhanced phosphorylation of FOXO1 and Akt and cytoplasmic localization of FOXO1. FOXO1 can bind to the promoter of TBX21, which codes T-bet, to inhibit its expression, whereas Akt-induced phosphorylation of FOXO1 induces its cytoplasmic translocation from the nucleus and impairs its transrepressive activity. Serum from patients with psoriasis induced the activation of Akt and phosphorylation and cytoplasmic translocation of FOXO1 in Tregs from healthy controls in vitro, although the Akt-inducing molecules in the serum were not identified.

The expression of microRNA-210 is increased in circulating $CD4^+$ T cells from patients with psoriasis, and this increase may contribute to the reduced Foxp3 mRNA and protein levels in the patients' $CD4^+$ T cells [31]. microRNA-210 binds to the 3'-untranslated region of *Foxp3*, and the overexpression of microRNA-210 inhibits Foxp3 expression in $CD4^+$ T cells from healthy controls, whereas inhibition of microRNA-210 increases Foxp3 expression in $CD4^+$ T cells from patients with psoriasis.

4. Stimulators for Tregs and Their Impairment in Psoriasis

Short-chain fatty acids (SCFAs), such as butyrate, propionate, and acetate, are derived from gut microbial fermentation of dietary fiber, and promote the generation and function of Tregs in the gut and systemically [32]. Skin commensals, such as *Cutibacterium acnes*, also produce SCFAs [33,34], which may stimulate Tregs in the skin. Butyrate acts on DCs and induces the expression of retinaldehyde dehydrogenase, an enzyme that synthesizes RAs [35,36] that promote *Foxp3* expression in pTregs. Butyrate acts as an inhibitor of histone deacetylase (HDAC) and induces histone H3 acetylation on *Foxp3* intronic enhancer, allowing the expression of *Foxp3* in naïve $CD4^+$ T cells, inducing their differentiation into pTregs. SCFAs induce intestinal epithelial cells to produce TGF-β [37], which can contribute to de novo generation of pTregs by inducing *Foxp3* expression via Smad2/3.

Acetate, propionate, and butyrate stimulate the proliferation of tTregs via cell surface GPR43 [38]. Butyrate binds GPR41 on medullary thymic epithelial cells, and promotes the expression of a transcription factor autoimmune regulator (AIRE), which induces the generation of tTregs [39]. Acetate also induces AIRE expression in cortical thymic epithelial cells [40].

It has been reported that the gut microbiome of patients with psoriasis and psoriatic arthritis showed a decrease in SCFA-producing bacteria, including *Bacteroidetes, Prevotella, Akkermansia, Faecalibacterium*, and *Ruminococcus* [41,42]. In particular, a decrease in *Faecalibacterium prausnitzi* and *Akkermansia muciniphila*, which produce butyrate, was noted in patients with psoriasis and psoriatic arthritis [43,44]. The gut microbiome of patients with psoriasis is characterized by an increase in the phylum *Firmicutes* and a decrease in the phylum *Bacteroidetes* [45], which is related to an impaired gut epithelial barrier and reduced butyrate production. Shapiro et al. reported that genes encoding butyrate kinase and phosphate butyryltransferase, enzymes involved in butyrate synthesis, were present in lower proportions in the feces of patients with psoriasis than in the control cohort [46]. The alteration of the gut microbiome in patients with psoriasis may contribute to the defect of Tregs via the reduction of SCFAs.

Vitamin D3, obtained via dietary intake or synthesis in the skin by sun exposure, is metabolized to its active form, 1,25-dihydroxyvitamin D3. 1,25-Dihydroxyvitamin D3 binds to the vitamin D receptor (VDR) that heterodimerizes with the retinoid X receptor (RXR); the heterodimer binds to the vitamin D response element on the *Foxp3* enhancer CNS1 in naïve T cells, leading to *Foxp3* expression and generation of pTregs [4]. It has been reported that serum 25-hydroxyvitamin D3 levels are reduced in patients with psoriasis or psoriatic arthritis compared to controls [47] and that the expression of VDR is decreased in psoriatic skin lesions [48]. The reduced levels of vitamin D3 and/or VDR may be related to defects in Tregs in psoriasis via the reduction of *Foxp3* expression.

5. Therapeutic Approach to Restore the Defect of Tregs in Psoriasis

Restoration of defective Tregs is a promising therapeutic target for psoriasis and psoriatic arthritis. Therapeutic modalities that potentiate Tregs should be selected for a patient population with defective Tregs. For such selection, specific and convenient methods of testing Treg numbers and functions should be developed in the near future.

5.1. Therapeutic Agents Currently Used for Psoriasis

Several biologics or low-molecular-weight agents currently used for psoriasis can restore defective Tregs in psoriasis (Table 1).

Table 1. Therapeutic Agents Restoring Defected Regulatory T Cells (Tregs) in Psoriasis.

Therapeutic Agents	Mechanisms for Restoring Tregs
Currently Used	
Anti-IL-23p19 or anti-IL-12/23p40 antibodies	Reversing conversion from Tregs into Th17 cells
Anti-IL-17A or anti-IL-17RA antibodies	Increasing TGF-β secretion, Foxp3 expression, and suppressive function of Tregs
Topical vitamin D3	Increasing Foxp3 expression through VDR
Retinoids	Increasing Foxp3 expression through RAR
Narrow-band UVB	Increasing RANKL expression in keratinocytes and inducing DCs to expand Tregs
Dimethyl fumarate	Increasing the frequency of Tregs resistant to dimethyl fumarate-induced oxidative stress or increasing SCFA-producing bacteria in the gut
Under development	
SCFAs	Increasing Foxp3 expression via HDAC inhibition, TGF-β production in IEC, RA synthesis in DCs, and proliferation of tTregs
STAT3 inhibitors	Increasing Foxp3 expression via induction of STAT5
Probiotics	Increasing SCFA production in the gut
Prebiotics	Increasing SCFA-producing bacteria in the gut
HDAC inhibitors	Increasing Foxp3 expression and stabilization

IL, interleukin; Th17, type 17 helper T; SCFA, short-chain fatty acid; HDAC, histone deacetylase; STAT, signal transducer and activator of transcription; Foxp3, Forkhead box protein 3; DC, dendritic cell; IEC, intestinal epithelial cell; RANKL, receptor activator of the nuclear factor-κB ligand; RAR, retinoic acid receptor; VDR, vitamin D receptor; TGF, transforming growth factor; tTreg, thymus-derived Treg; UV, ultraviolet.

5.1.1. Biologics

Anti-IL-23p19 antibodies, risankizumab, guselkumab, tralokinumab, or anti-IL-12/23p40 antibody ustekinumab may reverse the IL-23-induced conversion of Tregs into pathogenic Th17 cells and may increase the number and/or suppressive function of Tregs in psoriasis. Anti-IL-23p19 antibody treatment in an imiquimod-induced psoriasis mouse model increased the number of Foxp3$^+$ cells in the lesions, and adoptive transfer of Tregs from anti-IL-23p19 antibody-treated mice improved psoriasis-like dermatitis in the donor mice [49].

Anti-IL-17A antibodies, secukinumab and ixekizumab, or the anti-IL-17RA antibody brodalumab may counteract IL-17A-induced impairment of Tregs. Treatment with secukinumab in patients with psoriasis restored the suppressive function and increased TGF-β production in Tregs, as well as reduced the psoriasis area and severity index (PASI) [24].

5.1.2. Vitamin D3

Topical treatment with maxacalcitol, vitamin D3, in imiquimod-induced psoriasis mice model increased Treg infiltration and IL-10 expression in skin lesions, and adoptive transfer of Tregs from maxacalcitol-treated mice ameliorated psoriasis-like dermatitis in donor mice, indicating a functional suppressive phenotype [50]. Several randomized controlled trials (RCTs) have reported that systemic vitamin D supplementation reduces PASI scores [32,51]. However, the effects have not been verified by a systematic review and meta-analysis of RCTs [52]. More RCTs with larger sample sizes are needed to produce robust results.

5.1.3. Retinoids

Synthetic vitamin A derivatives, retinoids, such as etretinate or acitretin, are absorbed in the small intestine and delivered to the fat, liver, gut, or kidney, where they are metabolized to the active acid form RAs [53]. RA binds to the retinoic acid receptor (RAR), which heterodimerizes with RXR, and the heterodimer binds the RA response element on CNS1 of *Foxp3*, inducing *Foxp3* expression and the generation of pTregs from naïve T cells.

5.1.4. Narrow-Band Ultraviolet (UV) B Therapy

Narrow-band UVB therapy increased Treg number and Foxp3 mRNA levels in peripheral blood mononuclear cells of patients with psoriasis and reduced Th1/Th17 cells [54]. Moreover, narrow-band UVB treatment on keratinocytes upregulates the expression of receptors of activated nuclear factor-κB ligand (RANKL), which interacts with RANK on DCs, promoting DCs to expand the number of Tregs systemically [55,56].

5.1.5. Dimethyl Fumarate (DMF)

The European Medicines Agency approved an oral formulation of DMF for the treatment of moderate-to-severe psoriatic plaque in adults in 2017 [57]. DMF and its active metabolite monomethylfumarate downregulate inflammatory cytokine production in T cells and induce the shift from Th1/Th17 to Th2 by modulation of intracellular glutathione levels and, ultimately, cellular responses to oxidative stress; hence, modulating the activity of the transcription factors nuclear factor-erythroid 2-related factor 2, NF-κB, and hypoxia-inducible factor 1-α or binding to cell surface hydroxyl–carboxylic acid receptor 2 [58].

Oral DMF treatment in Lewis rats increased Foxp3 mRNA levels in the ileum and CD4$^+$CD25$^+$ Tregs in Peyer's patches [59]. The adaptive transfer of these Tregs effectively improved experimental autoimmune neuritis in recipient rats [59]. The upregulation of Tregs by DMF may be mediated by SCFAs as DMF treatment increased the number of SCFAs-producing bacteria, such as *Gemella*, *Roseburia*, *Bacillus*, and *Bacteroides* in the gut [60].

DMF treatment increased Treg frequency and decreased Th17 cells in patients with psoriasis [61]. In vitro DMF treatment induced oxidative stress, which reduced the viability and proliferation of CD4$^+$CD25$^-$ conventional T cells but did not reduce Tregs [62], by virtue of the increased expression of cell surface-reduced thiols [61] or thioredoxin-1 [63], protecting Tregs from oxidative stress. The oxidative effects of DMF may favor Tregs relative to Th17 cells, which may be another mechanism for the anti-psoriatic effects of DMF.

5.1.6. Janus Kinase (JAK) Inhibitors

The JAK family of non-receptor tyrosine kinases transduce signals from a multitude of cytokines [64]. The binding of cytokines to their receptors enables the activation of receptor-associated JAK and JAK-induced phosphorylation of receptors, allowing STAT to bind to receptors and to be phosphorylated by JAKs, leading to the dimerization of STATs, nuclear translocation, and transcription of target genes. JAK inhibitors suppress the JAK/STAT signaling pathways and, thus, block the effects of inflammatory cytokines, such as IL-6, IFN-γ, IL-22, and IL-21, which are involved in the pathogenesis of psoriasis.

The JAK 1/3 inhibitor tofacitinib is approved by the Food and Drug Administration for the treatment of psoriatic arthritis [64]. The JAK1 inhibitor upadacitinib is approved in Japan for psoriatic arthritis. To date, the effects of JAK inhibitors on the number or function of Tregs in patients with psoriasis, or psoriasis mice models, have not been reported. However, tofacitinib increased the number of Tregs and reduced the number of Th17 cells in the liver and spleen of mice with concanavalin A-induced hepatitis [65]. Although the precise mechanism is unknown, it has been reported that the suppressive capacity of Tregs on effector T cells is resistant to the blocking effects of tofacitinib, whereas the function of effector T cells is more sensitive to these effects [66].

5.2. Therapeutic Agents under Development

Therapeutic agents under development that promote the generation and function of Tregs for psoriasis treatment are mentioned in Table 1. Patients resistant to or with insufficient response to current therapy modes, such as systemic immunosuppressive medicine, may include a population with prominent defects in Tregs. For such a population, agents promoting Tregs may complement the therapeutic effects of the current therapy.

5.2.1. SCFAs

Ex vivo treatment of psoriatic lesional skin with sodium butyrate restored the reduced Treg number and IL-10 and Foxp3 expression and normalized the enhanced expression of IL-17A and IL-6 [67]. Topical application of sodium butyrate to imiquimod-induced psoriasis-like dermatitis in mice increased *IL-10* and *Foxp3* transcripts and reduced inflammation and *IL-17A* transcripts [67]. The beneficial effects of sodium butyrate are abolished by the depletion of Tregs [67]. Topical SCFAs may be a promising therapy for psoriasis.

5.2.2. STAT3 Inhibitors

Topical treatment with STA-21, a STAT3 inhibitor, improved human psoriatic skin lesions as well as psoriasis-like dermatitis in K5.Stat3C transgenic mice, indicating a promising role of this agent in the treatment of psoriasis [68]. STA-21 increased the number and function of $CD4^+CD25^+Foxp3^+$ Tregs in IL1-receptor α knockout mice, a model for rheumatoid arthritis [69]. Adoptive transfer of Tregs from STA-21-treated mice markedly suppressed inflammatory arthritis, and in vitro treatment with STA-21 increased Foxp3 mRNA levels in human and murine $CD4^+$ T cells [69]. STA-21 increased the level and phosphorylation of STAT5, a critical transcription factor of *Foxp3* expression, in addition to a reduction in STAT3 levels and phosphorylation [69]. The reciprocal regulation of STAT3 and STAT5 by STA-21 may increase *Foxp3* expression and the suppressive function of Tregs. In vitro treatment of murine splenocytes with STA-21 also increased the frequency of $CD4^+CD25^+Foxp3^+$ Tregs [70]. Stattic V, another STAT3 inhibitor, restored the suppressive function of Tregs in patients with psoriasis [27]. STAT3 inhibitors, including STA-21, may improve psoriasis by potentiating Tregs.

5.2.3. Probiotics/Prebiotics

Probiotics are living microorganisms that confer health benefits to the host when administered in adequate amounts [71]. Most microorganism probiotics belong to the lactic acid-producing genera *Lactobacillus* and *Bifidobacterium*. Oral administration of these genera increased $Foxp3^+$ Treg responses in dextran sulfate sodium-induced colitis [72] or experimental autoimmune encephalomyelitis [73] in mice as well as ameliorated inflammation. Prebiotics are non-digestible fructooligosaccharides, inulins, or galactooligosaccharides that stimulate the growth of beneficial bacteria, such as *Bifidobacterium* [74]. Inulin, a soluble dietary fiber, is fermented by the gut microbiome to generate SCFAs. Oral administration of inulin in rats altered the composition of the gut microbiome and increased the probiotic bacteria *Lactobacillus* and SCFA-producing bacteria *Lachnospiraceae*, *Phascolarctobacterium*, and *Bacteroides* [75]. Female mice fed an inulin-enriched diet during pregnancy and lactation showed an abundance of *Bacteroides* in the gut microbiome and increased plasma SCFA levels, and their offspring had increased frequencies of tTregs and pTregs and increased expression of AIRE in the thymus [39].

Oral administration of *B. infantis* 35624 in patients with psoriasis reduced plasma levels of TNF-α and CRP [76]. Oral administration of *B. longum* CECT 7347, *B. lactis* CECT 8145, and *L. rhamnosus* CECT 8361 in patients with psoriasis resulted in higher PASI 75 compared to the placebo group [77] with an increase in the probiotic bacteria *Collinsella* and *Lactobacillus* in the gut. Feeding a diet rich in fucoidan (a seaweed fiber) in the psoriasis mice model, induced by a *Traf3ip2* mutation, ameliorated symptoms of psoriasis-like dermatitis with increasing *Bacteroides* in the gut [78]. However, whether these probiotic/prebiotic treatments improve the number or function of Tregs has not been examined in patients with psoriasis or mice models and should be further verified. Future studies using synbiotics, probiotics combined with prebiotics, might be promising.

5.2.4. HDAC Inhibitors

The enhancer elements of *Foxp3* are bound by histones, and histone acetylation of these elements allows the gene to be accessible for transcription factors and RNA polymerase, promoting gene expression [4]. HDAC inhibitors enhance histone acetylation of these elements and induce *Foxp3* expression [4]. Foxp3 is also regulated post-transcriptionally. Foxp3 protein associates with histone acetylase and HDAC, and acetylation of this protein increases its stability, whereas its deacetylation makes it susceptible to proteasomal degradation [4]. HDAC inhibitors may, thus, stabilize Foxp3 protein. The pan-HDAC inhibitor trichostatin A acts on human peripheral blood-derived $CD4^+CD25^+Foxp3^+$ Tregs, reversing their conversion into Th17 cells and increasing *Foxp3* expression in healthy controls [79] and in patients with psoriasis [22]. These results indicate a promising role for HDAC inhibitors in psoriasis treatment. However, HDAC inhibitors have not been examined as therapeutic agents other than in oncology. Thus far, 18 HDAC enzymes have been identified; 11 are Zn^{2+}-dependent (HDAC 1–11), and seven require nicotinamide adenine dinucleotide (Sirt 1–7). Among these, Tregs express HDAC 1–11 and Sirt 1–4. Individual HDAC isoforms differentially regulate the transcription and/or stabilization of Foxp3 [4]; thus, specific inhibitors for individual HDACs should be examined for their ability to generate and/or maintain Tregs.

6. Conclusions

Patients with psoriasis are associated with the impaired function of Tregs and disturbed Treg/Th17 balance, which may contribute to the development and exacerbation of this disease. The defect in Tregs in psoriasis may be attributable to enhanced inhibition and/or impaired stimulation of the generation and maintenance of Tregs. Tregs can convert into Th17- or Th1-like phenotypes in patients with psoriasis. Cytokines or mediators that are upregulated in psoriasis, such as IL-23, IL-17A, IL-6, and IL-21, may induce the conversion of Tregs into Th17/Th1 cells. SCFAs stimulate the induction of Tregs via *Foxp3* expression or through their action on DCs or intestinal epithelial cells. The reduction of SCFA-producing bacteria, such as *Bacteroides*, in the gut microbiome of patients with psoriasis, may contribute to the defect in Tregs. Several therapeutic modalities currently used for psoriasis treatment, such as anti-IL-23p19 or anti-IL-17A antibodies, retinoids, topical vitamin D3, DMF, and narrow-band UVB, can restore defective Tregs. Agents that potentiate Tregs, such as STAT3 inhibitors, butyrate, HDAC inhibitors, or probiotics/prebiotics, are under development for the treatment of psoriasis. Restoration of defective Tregs may be a promising therapeutic target for psoriasis.

Author Contributions: N.K. wrote the first draft of the manuscript. T.H. updated the bibliography and figures. H.S. critically revised the manuscript. All authors have read and agreed to the published version of the manuscript.

Funding: This research received no external funding.

Institutional Review Board Statement: Not applicable.

Informed Consent Statement: Not applicable.

Data Availability Statement: Not applicable.

Conflicts of Interest: The authors declare no conflict of interest.

References

1. Takeshita, J.; Grewal, S.; Langan, S.; Mehta, N.N.; Ogdie, A.; Van Voorhees, A.S.; Gelfand, J. Psoriasis and comorbid diseases. *J. Am. Acad. Dermatol.* **2017**, *76*, 377–390. [CrossRef]
2. Furue, K.; Ito, T.; Furue, M. Differential efficacy of biologic treatments targeting the TNF-α/IL-23/IL-17 axis in psoriasis and psoriatic arthritis. *Cytokine* **2018**, *111*, 182–188. [CrossRef] [PubMed]
3. Ogawa, E.; Sato, Y.; Minagawa, A.; Okuyama, R. Pathogenesis of psoriasis and development of treatment. *J. Dermatol.* **2018**, *45*, 264–272. [CrossRef] [PubMed]
4. Von Knethen, A.; Heinicke, U.; Weigert, A.; Zacharowski, K.; Brüne, B. Histone Deacetylation Inhibitors as Modulators of Regulatory T Cells. *Int. J. Mol. Sci.* **2020**, *21*, 2356. [CrossRef] [PubMed]
5. Sugiyama, H.; Gyulai, R.; Toichi, E.; Garaczi, E.; Shimada, S.; Stevens, S.R.; McCormick, T.S.; Cooper, K. Dysfunctional Blood and Target Tissue CD4+CD25high Regulatory T Cells in Psoriasis: Mechanism Underlying Unrestrained Pathogenic Effector T Cell Proliferation. *J. Immunol.* **2005**, *174*, 164–173. [CrossRef] [PubMed]
6. Komine, M. Recent Advances in Psoriasis Research; the Clue to Mysterious Relation to Gut Microbiome. *Int. J. Mol. Sci.* **2020**, *21*, 2582. [CrossRef] [PubMed]
7. Kalekar, L.A.; Rosenblum, M.D. Regulatory T cells in inflammatory skin disease: From mice to humans. *Int. Immunol.* **2019**, *31*, 457–463. [CrossRef]
8. Nussbaum, L.; Chen, Y.; Ogg, G. Role of regulatory T cells in psoriasis pathogenesis and treatment. *Br. J. Dermatol.* **2021**, *184*, 14–24. [CrossRef]
9. Shevach, E.M.; Thornton, A.M. tTregs, pTregs, and iTregs: Similarities and differences. *Immunol. Rev.* **2014**, *259*, 88–102. [CrossRef]
10. Gagliani, N.; Magnani, C.F.; Huber, S.; Gianolini, M.E.; Pala, M.; Licona-Limon, P.; Guo, B.; Herbert, D.R.; Bulfone, A.; Trentini, F.; et al. Coexpression of CD49b and LAG-3 identifies human and mouse T regulatory type 1 cells. *Nat. Med.* **2013**, *19*, 739–746. [CrossRef]
11. Gregori, S.; Goudy, K.S.; Roncarolo, M.G. The Cellular and Molecular Mechanisms of Immuno-Suppression by Human Type 1 Regulatory T Cells. *Front. Immunol.* **2012**, *3*, 30. [CrossRef]
12. Jacek, R.W. The characterization and role of regulatory T cells in immune reactions. *Front. Biosci.* **2008**, *13*, 2266–2274. [CrossRef]
13. Gondek, D.C.; Lu, L.-F.; Quezada, S.; Sakaguchi, S.; Noelle, R.J. Cutting Edge: Contact-Mediated Suppression by CD4+CD25+ Regulatory Cells Involves a Granzyme B-Dependent, Perforin-Independent Mechanism. *J. Immunol.* **2005**, *174*, 1783–1786. [CrossRef] [PubMed]
14. Wang, G.; Khattar, M.; Guo, Z.; Miyahara, Y.; Linkes, S.P.; Sun, Z.; He, X.; Stepkowski, S.M.; Chen, W. IL-2-deprivation and TGF-β are two non-redundant suppressor mechanisms of CD4+CD25+ regulatory T cell which jointly restrain CD4+CD25− cell activation. *Immunol. Lett.* **2010**, *132*, 61–68. [CrossRef]
15. Pandiyan, P.; Zheng, L.; Ishihara, S.; Reed, J.; Lenardo, M.J. CD4+CD25+Foxp3+ regulatory T cells induce cytokine deprivation–mediated apoptosis of effector CD4+ T cells. *Nat. Immunol.* **2007**, *8*, 1353–1362. [CrossRef] [PubMed]
16. Li, M.O.; Flavell, R.A. Contextual Regulation of Inflammation: A Duet by Transforming Growth Factor-β and Interleukin-10. *Immunity* **2008**, *28*, 468–476. [CrossRef] [PubMed]
17. Saraiva, M.; O'Garra, A. The regulation of IL-10 production by immune cells. *Nat. Rev. Immunol.* **2010**, *10*, 170–181. [CrossRef]
18. Wing, K.; Onishi, Y.; Prieto-Martin, P.; Yamaguchi, T.; Miyara, M.; Fehervari, Z.; Nomura, T.; Sakaguchi, S. CTLA-4 Control over Foxp3+ Regulatory T Cell Function. *Science* **2008**, *322*, 271–275. [CrossRef]
19. Brusko, T.M.; Wasserfall, C.H.; Agarwal, A.; Kapturczak, M.H.; Atkinson, M.A. An Integral Role for Heme Oxygenase-1 and Carbon Monoxide in Maintaining Peripheral Tolerance by CD4+CD25+ Regulatory T Cells. *J. Immunol.* **2005**, *174*, 5181–5186. [CrossRef]
20. Gao, L.; Li, K.; Li, F.; Li, H.; Liu, L.; Wang, L.; Zhang, Z.; Gao, T.; Liu, Y. Polymorphisms in the FOXP3 gene in Han Chinese psoriasis patients. *J. Dermatol. Sci.* **2010**, *57*, 51–56. [CrossRef]
21. Ngalamika, O.; Liang, G.; Zhao, M.; Yu, X.; Yang, Y.; Yin, H.; Liu, Y.; Yung, S.; Chan, T.M.; Lu, Q. Peripheral whole blood FOXP3 TSDR methylation: A potential marker in severity assessment of autoimmune diseases and chronic infections. *Immunol. Investig.* **2014**, *44*, 126–136. [CrossRef]
22. Bovenschen, H.J.; van de Kerkhof, P.C.; van Erp, P.E.; Woestenenk, R.; Joosten, I.; Koenen, H.J.P.M. Foxp3+ Regulatory T Cells of Psoriasis Patients Easily Differentiate into IL-17A-Producing Cells and Are Found in Lesional Skin. *J. Investig. Dermatol.* **2011**, *131*, 1853–1860. [CrossRef]
23. Li, H.; Yao, Q.; Mariscal, A.G.; Wu, X.; Hülse, J.; Pedersen, E.; Helin, K.; Waisman, A.; Vinkel, C.; Thomsen, S.F.; et al. Epigenetic control of IL-23 expression in keratinocytes is important for chronic skin inflammation. *Nat. Commun.* **2018**, *9*, 1–18. [CrossRef]
24. Liu, Y.; Zhang, C.; Li, B.; Yu, C.; Bai, X.; Xiao, C.; Wang, L.; Dang, E.; Yang, L.; Wang, G. A novel role of IL-17A in contributing to the impaired suppressive function of Tregs in psoriasis. *J. Dermatol. Sci.* **2021**, *101*, 84–92. [CrossRef]

25. Chong, W.P.; Zhong, Y.; Mattapallil, M.; Chen, J.; Caspi, R.R. Essential role of IL-17A in Tregs induction in autoimmune uveitis. *J. Immunol.* **2019**, *202*, 116.6.
26. Cunnusamy, K.; Chen, P.W.; Niederkorn, J.Y. IL-17A–Dependent CD4+CD25+ Regulatory T Cells Promote Immune Privilege of Corneal Allografts. *J. Immunol.* **2011**, *186*, 6737–6745. [CrossRef]
27. Yang, L.; Li, B.; Dang, E.; Jin, L.; Fan, X.; Wang, G. Impaired function of regulatory T cells in patients with psoriasis is mediated by phosphorylation of STAT3. *J. Dermatol. Sci.* **2016**, *81*, 85–92. [CrossRef]
28. Goodman, W.A.; Levine, A.D.; Massari, J.V.; Sugiyama, H.; McCormick, T.S.; Cooper, K.D. IL-6 Signaling in Psoriasis Prevents Immune Suppression by Regulatory T Cells. *J. Immunol.* **2009**, *183*, 3170–3176. [CrossRef]
29. Peluso, I.; Fantini, M.C.; Fina, D.; Caruso, R.; Boirivant, M.; Macdonald, T.T.; Pallone, F.; Monteleone, G. IL-21 counteracts the regulatory T cell-mediated suppression of human CD4+ T lymphocytes. *J. Immunol.* **2007**, *178*, 732–739. [CrossRef]
30. Li, B.; Lei, J.; Yang, L.; Gao, C.; Dang, E.; Cao, T.; Xue, K.; Zhuang, Y.; Shao, S.; Zhi, D.; et al. Dysregulation of Akt-FOXO1 Pathway Leads to Dysfunction of Regulatory T Cells in Patients with Psoriasis. *J. Investig. Dermatol.* **2019**, *139*, 2098–2107. [CrossRef]
31. Zhao, M.; Wang, L.-T.; Liang, G.-P.; Zhang, P.; Deng, X.-J.; Tang, Q.; Zhai, H.-Y.; Chang, C.C.; Su, Y.-W.; Lu, Q.-J. Up-regulation of microRNA-210 induces immune dysfunction via targeting FOXP3 in CD4+ T cells of psoriasis vulgaris. *Clin. Immunol.* **2014**, *150*, 22–30. [CrossRef]
32. Kanda, N.; Hoashi, T.; Saeki, H. Nutrition and Psoriasis. *Int. J. Mol. Sci.* **2020**, *21*, 5405. [CrossRef]
33. Keshari, S.; Wang, Y.; Herr, D.R.; Wang, S.-M.; Yang, W.-C.; Chuang, T.-H.; Chen, C.-L. Skin *Cutibacterium acnes* Mediates Fermentation to Suppress the Calcium Phosphate-Induced Itching: A Butyric Acid Derivative with Potential for Uremic Pruritus. *J. Clin. Med.* **2020**, *9*, 312. [CrossRef]
34. Rozas, M.; de Ruijter, A.H.; Fabrega, M.; Zorgani, A.; Guell, M.; Paetzold, B.; Brillet, F. From Dysbiosis to Healthy Skin: Major Contributions of *Cutibacterium acnes* to Skin Homeostasis. *Microorganisms* **2021**, *9*, 628. [CrossRef]
35. Isobe, J.; Maeda, S.; Obata, Y.; Iizuka, K.; Nakamura, Y.; Fujimura, Y.; Kimizuka, T.; Hattori, K.; Kim, Y.-G.; Morita, T.; et al. Commensal-bacteria-derived butyrate promotes the T-cell-independent IgA response in the colon. *Int. Immunol.* **2019**, *32*, 243–258. [CrossRef] [PubMed]
36. Kaisar, M.M.M.; Pelgrom, L.; van der Ham, A.; Yazdanbakhsh, M.; Everts, B. Butyrate Conditions Human Dendritic Cells to Prime Type 1 Regulatory T Cells via both Histone Deacetylase Inhibition and G Protein-Coupled Receptor 109A Signaling. *Front. Immunol.* **2017**, *8*, 1429. [CrossRef]
37. Martin-Gallausiaux, C.; Béguet-Crespel, F.; Marinelli, L.; Jamet, A.; LeDue, F.; Blottière, H.M.; Lapaque, N. Butyrate produced by gut commensal bacteria activates TGF-beta1 expression through the transcription factor SP1 in human intestinal epithelial cells. *Sci. Rep.* **2018**, *8*, 1–13. [CrossRef] [PubMed]
38. Smith, P.M.; Howitt, M.R.; Panikov, N.; Michaud, M.; Gallini, C.A.; Bohlooly, Y.M.; Glickman, J.N.; Garrett, W.S. The Microbial Metabolites, Short-Chain Fatty Acids, Regulate Colonic Treg Cell Homeostasis. *Science* **2013**, *341*, 569–573. [CrossRef]
39. Nakajima, A.; Kaga, N.; Nakanishi, Y.; Ohno, H.; Miyamoto, J.; Kimura, I.; Hori, S.; Sasaki, T.; Hiramatsu, K.; Okumura, K.; et al. Maternal High Fiber Diet during Pregnancy and Lactation Influences Regulatory T Cell Differentiation in Offspring in Mice. *J. Immunol.* **2017**, *199*, 3516–3524. [CrossRef]
40. Hu, M.; Eviston, D.; Hsu, P.; Mariño, E.; Chidgey, A.; Santner-Nanan, B.; Wong, K.; Richards, J.L.; Yap, Y.-A.; The BIS Investigator Group; et al. Decreased maternal serum acetate and impaired fetal thymic and regulatory T cell development in preeclampsia. *Nat. Commun.* **2019**, *10*, 1–13. [CrossRef]
41. Olejniczak-Staruch, I.; Ciążyńska, M.; Sobolewska-Sztychny, D.; Narbutt, J.; Skibińska, M.; Lesiak, A. Alterations of the Skin and Gut Microbiome in Psoriasis and Psoriatic Arthritis. *Int. J. Mol. Sci.* **2021**, *22*, 3998. [CrossRef]
42. Scher, J.U.; Ubeda, C.; Artacho, A.; Attur, M.; Isaac, S.; Reddy, S.; Marmon, S.; Neimann, A.; Brusca, S.; Patel, T.; et al. Decreased Bacterial Diversity Characterizes the Altered Gut Microbiota in Patients with Psoriatic Arthritis, Resembling Dysbiosis in Inflammatory Bowel Disease. *Arthritis Rheumatol.* **2015**, *67*, 128–139. [CrossRef]
43. Tan, L.; Zhao, S.; Zhu, W.; Wu, L.; Li, J.; Sheng, M.; Lei, L.; Chen, X.; Peng, C. The Akkermansia muciniphila is a gut microbiota signature in psoriasis. *Exp. Dermatol.* **2018**, *27*, 144–149. [CrossRef]
44. Eppinga, H.; Weiland, C.J.S.; Thio, H.B.; van der Woude, C.J.; Nijsten, T.E.C.; Peppelenbosch, M.P.; Konstantinov, S.R. Similar Depletion of Protective *Faecalibacterium prausnitziiin* Psoriasis and Inflammatory Bowel Disease, but not in Hidradenitis Suppurativa. *J. Crohns Coliti* **2016**, *10*, 1067–1075. [CrossRef]
45. Chen, Y.; Ho, H.J.; Tseng, C.; Lai, Z.; Shieh, J.-J.; Wu, C.-Y. Intestinal microbiota profiling and predicted metabolic dysregulation in psoriasis patients. *Exp. Dermatol.* **2018**, *27*, 1336–1343. [CrossRef]
46. Shapiro, J.; Cohen, N.A.; Shalev, V.; Uzan, A.; Koren, O.; Maharshak, N. Psoriatic patients have a distinct structural and functional fecal microbiota compared with controls. *J. Dermatol.* **2019**, *46*, 595–603. [CrossRef]
47. Umar, M.; Sastry, K.S.; Al Ali, F.; Al-Khulaifi, M.; Wang, E.; Chouchane, A.I. Vitamin D and the Pathophysiology of Inflammatory Skin Diseases. *Ski. Pharmacol. Physiol.* **2018**, *31*, 74–86. [CrossRef]
48. Filoni, A.; Vestita, M.; Congedo, M.; Giudice, G.; Tafuri, S.; Bonamonte, D. Association between psoriasis and vitamin D. *Medicine* **2018**, *97*, e11185. [CrossRef]
49. Shimizu, T.; Kamata, M.; Fukaya, S.; Hayashi, K.; Fukuyasu, A.; Tanaka, T.; Ishikawa, T.; Ohnishi, T.; Tada, Y. Anti-IL-17A and IL-23p19 antibodies but not anti-TNFα antibody induce expansion of regulatory T cells and restoration of their suppressive function in imiquimod-induced psoriasiform dermatitis. *J. Dermatol. Sci.* **2019**, *95*, 90–98. [CrossRef]

50. Hau, C.S.; Shimizu, T.; Tada, Y.; Kamata, M.; Takeoka, S.; Shibata, S.; Mitsui, A.; Asano, Y.; Sugaya, M.; Kadono, T.; et al. The vitamin D3 analog, maxacalcitol, reduces psoriasiform skin inflammation by inducing regulatory T cells and downregulating IL-23 and IL-17 production. *J. Dermatol. Sci.* **2018**, *92*, 117–126. [CrossRef]
51. Perez, A.; Raab, R.; Chen, T.C.; Turner, A.; Holick, M.F. Safety and efficacy of oral calcitriol (1,25-dihydroxyvitamin D3) for the treatment of psoriasis. *Br. J. Dermatol.* **1996**, *134*, 1070–1078. [CrossRef]
52. Theodoridis, X.; Grammatikopoulou, M.G.; Stamouli, E.-M.; Talimtzi, P.; Pagkalidou, E.; Zafiriou, E.; Haidich, A.-B.; Bogdanos, D.P. Effectiveness of oral vitamin D supplementation in lessening disease severity among patients with psoriasis: A systematic review and meta-analysis of randomized controlled trials. *Nutrition* **2021**, *82*, 111024. [CrossRef]
53. Khalil, S.; Bardawil, T.; Stephan, C.; Darwiche, N.; Abbas, O.; Kibbi, A.G.; Nemer, G.; Kurban, M. Retinoids: A journey from the molecular structures and mechanisms of action to clinical uses in dermatology and adverse effects. *J. Dermatol. Treat.* **2017**, *28*, 684–696. [CrossRef]
54. Wang, X.; Wang, G.; Gong, Y.; Liu, Y.; Gu, J.; Chen, W.; Shi, Y. Disruption of Circulating CD4+ T-Lymphocyte Subpopulations in Psoriasis Patients is Ameliorated by Narrow-Band UVB Therapy. *Cell Biophys.* **2014**, *71*, 499–507. [CrossRef] [PubMed]
55. Loser, K.; Mehling, A.; Loeser, S.; Apelt, J.; Kuhn, A.; Grabbe, S.; Schwarz, T.; Penninger, J.; Beissert, S. Epidermal RANKL controls regulatory T-cell numbers via activation of dendritic cells. *Nat. Med.* **2006**, *12*, 1372–1379. [CrossRef] [PubMed]
56. Akiyama, T.; Shinzawa, M.; Akiyama, N. RANKL-RANK interaction in immune regulatory systems. *World J. Orthop.* **2012**, *3*, 142–150. [CrossRef]
57. Mrowietz, U.; Van De Kerkhof, P.; Schoenenberger, A.; Ryzhkova, A.; Pau-Charles, I.; Llamas-Velasco, M.; Daudén, E.; Carrascosa, J.M.; De La Cueva, P.; Salgado-Boquete, L.; et al. Efficacy of dimethyl fumarate treatment for moderate-to-severe plaque psoriasis: Presentation extracts from the 29th EADV virtual congress, 29–31 October 2020. *Expert Rev. Clin. Immunol.* **2021**, *17*, 1–11. [CrossRef]
58. Brück, J.; Dringen, R.; Amasuno, A.; Pau-Charles, I.; Ghoreschi, K. A review of the mechanisms of action of dimethylfumarate in the treatment of psoriasis. *Exp. Dermatol.* **2018**, *27*, 611–624. [CrossRef]
59. Pitarokoili, K.; Bachir, H.; Sgodzai, M.; Grüter, T.; Haupeltshofer, S.; Duscha, A.; Pedreiturria, X.; Motte, J.; Gold, R. Induction of Regulatory Properties in the Intestinal Immune System by Dimethyl Fumarate in Lewis Rat Experimental Autoimmune Neuritis. *Front. Immunol.* **2019**, *10*, 2132. [CrossRef]
60. Ma, N.; Wu, Y.; Xie, F.; Du, K.; Wang, Y.; Shi, L.; Ji, L.; Liu, T.; Ma, X. Dimethyl fumarate reduces the risk of mycotoxins via improving intestinal barrier and microbiota. *Oncotarget* **2017**, *8*, 44625–44638. [CrossRef]
61. Sulaimani, J.; Cluxton, D.; Clowry, J.; Petrasca, A.; Molloy, O.; Moran, B.; Sweeney, C.; Malara, A.; McNicholas, N.; McGuigan, C.; et al. Dimethyl fumarate modulates the Treg–Th17 cell axis in patients with psoriasis. *Br. J. Dermatol.* **2021**, *184*, 495–503. [CrossRef]
62. Mougiakakos, D.; Johansson, C.C.; Kiessling, R. Naturally occurring regulatory T cells show reduced sensitivity toward oxidative stress–induced cell death. *Blood* **2009**, *113*, 3542–3545. [CrossRef] [PubMed]
63. Mougiakakos, D.; Johansson, C.C.; Jitschin, R.; Böttcher, M.; Kiessling, R. Increased thioredoxin-1 production in human naturally occurring regulatory T cells confers enhanced tolerance to oxidative stress. *Blood* **2011**, *117*, 857–861. [CrossRef]
64. Virtanen, A.T.; Haikarainen, T.; Raivola, J.; Silvennoinen, O. Selective JAKinibs: Prospects in Inflammatory and Autoimmune Diseases. *BioDrugs* **2019**, *33*, 15–32. [CrossRef] [PubMed]
65. Wang, H.; Feng, X.; Han, P.; Lei, Y.; Xia, Y.; Tian, D.; Yan, W. The JAK inhibitor tofacitinib ameliorates immune-mediated liver injury in mice. *Mol. Med. Rep.* **2019**, *20*, 4883–4892. [CrossRef]
66. Sewgobind, V.D.K.D.; Quaedackers, M.E.; van der Laan, L.; Kraaijeveld, R.; Korevaar, S.S.; Chan, G.; Weimar, W.; Baan, C.C. The Jak Inhibitor CP-690,550 Preserves the Function of CD4+CD25brightFoxP3+ Regulatory T Cells and Inhibits Effector T Cells. *Arab. Archaeol. Epigr.* **2010**, *10*, 1785–1795. [CrossRef] [PubMed]
67. Schwarz, A.; Philippsen, R.; Schwarz, T. Induction of regulatory T cells and correction of cytokine dysbalance by short chain fatty acids—Implications for the therapy of psoriasis. *J. Investig. Dermatol.* **2020**, *141*, 95.e2–104.e2. [CrossRef] [PubMed]
68. Miyoshi, K.; Takaishi, M.; Nakajima, K.; Ikeda, M.; Kanda, T.; Tarutani, M.; Iiyama, T.; Asao, N.; DiGiovanni, J.; Sano, S. Stat3 as a Therapeutic Target for the Treatment of Psoriasis: A Clinical Feasibility Study with STA-21, a Stat3 Inhibitor. *J. Investig. Dermatol.* **2011**, *131*, 108–117. [CrossRef]
69. Park, J.-S.; Kwok, S.-K.; Lim, M.-A.; Kim, E.-K.; Ryu, J.-G.; Kim, S.-M.; Oh, H.-J.; Ju, J.H.; Park, S.-H.; Kim, H.-Y.; et al. STA-21, a Promising STAT-3 Inhibitor That Reciprocally Regulates Th17 and Treg Cells, Inhibits Osteoclastogenesis in Mice and Humans and Alleviates Autoimmune Inflammation in an Experimental Model of Rheumatoid Arthritis. *Arthritis Rheumatol.* **2014**, *66*, 918–929. [CrossRef]
70. Park, J.-S.; Kim, S.-M.; Hwang, S.-H.; Choi, S.-Y.; Kwon, J.Y.; Kwok, S.-K.; Cho, M.-L.; Park, S.-H. Combinatory treatment using tacrolimus and a STAT3 inhibitor regulate Treg cells and plasma cells. *Int. J. Immunopathol. Pharmacol.* **2018**, *32*, 2058738418778724. [CrossRef]
71. Alzahrani, Y.A.; Alesa, D.I.; Alshamrani, H.M.; Alamssi, D.N.; Alzahrani, N.S.; Almohammadi, M.E. The role of gut microbiome in the pathogenesis of psoriasis and the therapeutic effects of probiotics. *J. Fam. Med. Prim. Care* **2019**, *8*, 3496–3503. [CrossRef] [PubMed]

72. Zheng, B.; Van Bergenhenegouwen, J.; Overbeek, S.; Van De Kant, H.J.G.; Garssen, J.; Folkerts, G.; Vos, P.; Morgan, M.E.; Kraneveld, A.D. Bifidobacterium breve Attenuates Murine Dextran Sodium Sulfate-Induced Colitis and Increases Regulatory T Cell Responses. *PLoS ONE* **2014**, *9*, e95441. [CrossRef]
73. Salehipour, Z.; Haghmorad, D.; Sankian, M.; Rastin, M.; Nosratabadi, R.; Dallal, M.M.S.; Tabasi, N.; Khazaee, M.; Nasiraii, L.R.; Mahmoudi, M. Bifidobacterium animalis in combination with human origin of *Faecalibacterium prausnitziiin* ameliorate neuroinflammation in experimental model of multiple sclerosis by altering CD4+ T cell subset balance. *Biomed. Pharmacother.* **2017**, *95*, 1535–1548. [CrossRef] [PubMed]
74. Kanda, N.; Hoashi, T.; Saeki, H. Nutrition and atopic dermatitis. *J. Nippon. Med Sch.* **2021**, *88*, 171–177. [CrossRef]
75. Zhang, Q.; Yu, H.; Xiao, X.; Hu, L.; Xin, F.; Yu, X. Inulin-type fructan improves diabetic phenotype and gut microbiota profiles in rats. *PeerJ* **2018**, *6*, e4446. [CrossRef] [PubMed]
76. Groeger, D.; O'Mahony, L.; Murphy, E.F.; Bourke, J.F.; Dinan, T.; Kiely, B.; Shanahan, F.; Quigley, E.M. Bifidobacterium infantis35624 modulates host inflammatory processes beyond the gut. *Gut Microbes* **2013**, *4*, 325–339. [CrossRef]
77. Navarro-López, V.; Martínez-Andrés, A.; Ramírez-Boscá, A.; Ruzafa-Costas, B.; Núñez-Delegido, E.; Carrión-Gutiérrez, M.; Prieto-Merino, D.; Codoñer-Cortés, F.; Ramón-Vidal, D.; Genovés-Martínez, S.; et al. Efficacy and Safety of Oral Administration of a Mixture of Probiotic Strains in Patients with Psoriasis: A Randomized Clinical Trial. *Acta Derm. Venereol.* **2019**, *99*, 1078–1084. [CrossRef]
78. Takahashi, M.; Takahashi, K.; Abe, S.; Yamada, K.; Suzuki, M.; Masahisa, M.; Endo, M.; Abe, K.; Inoue, R.; Hoshi, H. Improvement of Psoriasis by Alteration of the Gut Environment by Oral Administration of Fucoidan from Cladosiphon Okamuranus. *Mar. Drugs* **2020**, *18*, 154. [CrossRef]
79. Koenen, H.J.P.M.; Smeets, R.L.; Vink, P.M.; Van Rijssen, E.; Boots, A.M.H.; Joosten, I. Human CD25highFoxp3pos regulatory T cells differentiate into IL-17–producing cells. *Blood* **2008**, *112*, 2340–2352. [CrossRef]

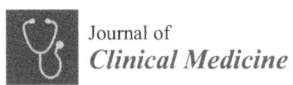

Article

The Antidiabetic Agent Metformin Inhibits IL-23 Production in Murine Bone-Marrow-Derived Dendritic Cells

Tomoyo Matsuda-Taniguchi [1], Masaki Takemura [1], Takeshi Nakahara [1], Akiko Hashimoto-Hachiya [1], Ayako Takai-Yumine [1], Masutaka Furue [1] and Gaku Tsuji [1,2,*]

[1] Department of Dermatology, Graduate School of Medical Sciences, Kyushu University, Fukuoka 812-8582, Japan; taniguchi.tomoyo.735@s.kyushu-u.ac.jp (T.M.-T.); take0917@dermatol.med.kyushu-u.ac.jp (M.T.); nakahara.takeshi.930@m.kyushu-u.ac.jp (T.N.); ahachi@dermatol.med.kyushu-u.ac.jp (A.H.-H.); a-takai@med.kyushu-u.ac.jp (A.T.-Y.); furue@dermatol.med.kyushu-u.ac.jp (M.F.)

[2] Research and Clinical Center for Yusho and Dioxin, Kyushu University Hospital, Fukuoka 812-8582, Japan

* Correspondence: gakku@dermatol.med.kyushu-u.ac.jp; Tel.: +81-92-642-5585

Citation: Matsuda-Taniguchi, T.; Takemura, M.; Nakahara, T.; Hashimoto-Hachiya, A.; Takai-Yumine, A.; Furue, M.; Tsuji, G. The Antidiabetic Agent Metformin Inhibits IL-23 Production in Murine Bone-Marrow-Derived Dendritic Cells. *J. Clin. Med.* **2021**, *10*, 5610. https://doi.org/10.3390/jcm10235610

Academic Editor: Francesco Lacarrubba

Received: 25 October 2021
Accepted: 29 November 2021
Published: 29 November 2021

Publisher's Note: MDPI stays neutral with regard to jurisdictional claims in published maps and institutional affiliations.

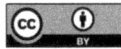

Copyright: © 2021 by the authors. Licensee MDPI, Basel, Switzerland. This article is an open access article distributed under the terms and conditions of the Creative Commons Attribution (CC BY) license (https://creativecommons.org/licenses/by/4.0/).

Abstract: Psoriasis is a chronic inflammatory skin disease, and its immune mechanism has been profoundly elucidated. Biologics targeting interleukin (IL)-23 have prevented the development of psoriasis. As major sources of IL-23, dendritic cells (DCs) play a pivotal role in psoriasis; however, the regulatory mechanism of IL-23 in DCs remains unclear. IL-36γ was reported to reflect the disease activity of psoriasis. Therefore, we hypothesized that IL-36γ may affect IL-23 production in DCs. To reveal the mechanism by which IL-36γ controls IL-23 production in DCs, we analyzed murine bone marrow-derived DCs (BMDCs) stimulated with IL-36γ. IL-36γ stimulation upregulated the mRNA and protein expression of Nfkbiz in BMDCs. Nfkbiz knockdown using siRNA transfection partially inhibited the upregulation of IL-23 mRNA expression induced by IL-36γ stimulation. Since NF-κB signaling regulates Nfkbiz expression and the anti-diabetic agent metformin reportedly modulates NF-κB signaling, we examined the effect of metformin treatment on IL-36γ-induced IL-23 production. Metformin treatment impaired the phosphorylation of NF-κB induced by IL-36γ stimulation with the subsequent downregulation of Nfkbiz, resulting in the inhibition of IL-23 production in BMDCs. These data provided evidence that metformin treatment can inhibit IL-36γ-mediated IL-23 production in BMDCs, which might contribute to the prevention of psoriasis.

Keywords: BMDCs; IL-23; IL-36γ; psoriasis; metformin

1. Introduction

Psoriasis is an immune-mediated inflammatory skin disease affecting 2–4% of the global population [1]. The skin lesions in psoriasis manifest desquamative erythema, which profoundly impairs patients' quality of the life [2]. The pathology of psoriasis is characterized by epidermal hyperproliferation, the intraepidermal accumulation of neutrophils, and the infiltration of dermal inflammatory cells such as T-cells, macrophages, and dendritic cells (DCs) [3]. Among these immune cells, DC counts are increased significantly in psoriatic lesions [4]. Furthermore, autoantigens from keratinocytes activate plasmacytoid DCs (pDCs) in the dermis. pDCs produce type I interferon and tumor necrosis factor-α, which activates classical DCs (cDCs), resulting in interleukin (IL)-23 secretion. IL-23 is mostly produced by cDCs, which correspond to CD1c+ DCs in humans. IL-23 by cDCs promotes Th17 differentiation in mice and humans [5]. In a murine model of psoriasis induced by topical imiquimod (IMQ), DCs were identified as the major source of IMQ-induced IL-23, which is critical for the development of psoriatic skin lesions [6,7]. Several reports have shown that IL-23 derived from DCs is involved in the pathogenesis of psoriasis [8–10]. Therefore, IL-23-producing DCs play a central role in the pathogenesis of psoriasis, which supports clinical evidence that the administration of monoclonal antibodies against IL-23 such as guselkmab, rizankizumab, and tildrakizumab can facilitate the achievement of a Psoriasis Area and Severity Index 90 response at week 16 (67–75%) [11–13]. Whereas IL-23 is a key regulator of IL-17 production, the mechanism of IL-23 production by DCs in psoriasis remains unclear. Recently, serum levels of IL-36γ, a member of the IL-36 family, were identified as a disease activity marker of psoriasis [14]. Meanwhile, IL-36γ is highly expressed in the epidermis in psoriatic lesions [15]. As IL-36γ derived from keratinocytes potentially activates DCs [16], we hypothesized that IL-36γ is involved in IL-23 production in DCs during the pathogenesis of psoriasis. To test this hypothesis, we analyzed murine bone marrow-derived DCs (BMDCs) stimulated with IL-36γ.

Furthermore, we examined whether metformin, an antidiabetic agent, modulates IL-36γ signaling in BMDCs. Metformin is mostly used to treat type 2 diabetes (T2DM), and a high prevalence of T2DM in patients with severe psoriasis has been identified [17]. In clinical studies of patients with psoriasis, long-term treatment with metformin has been shown to reduce the risk of psoriasis [18]. In addition, metformin administration has been shown to improve the severity of psoriasis [19,20]. These clinical results support the likelihood that metformin treatment is effective against both psoriasis and T2DM; however, the molecular mechanism remains unknown.

2. Materials and Methods

2.1. Reagents and Antibodies

Anti-murine NF-κB p65 monoclonal rabbit antibody (Abcam, Cambridge, UK), anti-murine NF-κB p65 (phospho Ser536) polyclonal rabbit antibody (Abcam), anti-murine IκBζ (protein corded by NFKBIZ gene) polyclonal rabbit antibody, and anti-murine β-actin monoclonal mouse antibody (Cell Signaling Technology, Danvers, MA, USA) were used for Western blotting. Dimethyl Sulfoxide (DMSO) was purchased from Nacalai Tesque, Inc. (Kyoto, Japan). Metformin hydrochloride and BAY 11-7082 were obtained from Tokyo Chemical Industry Co., Ltd. (Tokyo, Japan). Murine recombinant IL-36γ was obtained from R&D Systems (Minneapolis, MN, USA).

2.2. Generation of BMDCs and Cell Culture

C57BL/6N female mice were housed in a clean facility until 6 weeks of age by CLEA Japan, Inc. (Fujinomiya, Japan). The animal experiments were conducted in accordance with a protocol reviewed and approved by the animal facility center of Kyushu University (A21-283-0, 2021–2023). Bone marrow cells freshly isolated from the femoral and tibial bones of mice were cultured in RPMI 1640 medium (Merck KGaA, Darmstadt, Germany) containing 1 mmol/L sodium pyruvate (Thermo Fisher Scientific, Waltham, MA, USA), 10 mmol/L 4-(2-hydroxyethyl)-1-piperazineethanesulfonic acid (Thermo Fisher Scientific), 1% Minimum Essential Medium Non-Essential Amino Acids (Thermo Fisher Scientific), 10% FBS (Capricorn Scientific GmbH, Ebsdorfergrund, Germany), 50 nmol/L β-mercaptoethanol (Nacalai Tesque), and antibiotic–antimycotic 100× (100 U/mL penicillin, 100 mg/mL streptomycin, and 0.25 μg/mL amphotericin B; Thermo Fisher Scientific) containing GM-CSF (10 ng/mL) (PeproTech, Cranbury, NJ, USA). On day 3, half of the culture medium and GM-CSF were added. On day 5, non-adherent cells were subcultured, and GM-CSF was added. On day 7, half of the culture medium and GM-CSF were added. On day 9, non-adherent cells were harvested. These cells were purified immunomagnetically via three rounds of positive selection with CD11c (N418) MicroBeads (Miltenyi Biotec, Bergisch Gladbach, Germany). Purified BMDCs were cultured with/without stimulants such as IL-36γ, metformin, and BAY 11-7082 for the indicated times. Culture supernatant was collected after 24 h and analyzed by ELISA. Cells were also collected for quantitative reverse transcription (qRT)-PCR or Western blotting.

2.3. Transfection of Small Interfering RNAs (siRNAs) against Nfkbiz

siRNAs against Nfkbiz and non-targeting siRNA (control siRNA) were obtained from Thermo Fisher Scientific. Cells were incubated in culture medium with a mixture containing 300 nM siRNA for transfection using program DK-100 following the Amaxa® 4D-Nucleofector® Protocol for Immature Mouse Dendritic Cells For 4D-Nucleofector® X Unit (Lonza Group AG, Basel, Switzerland).

2.4. qRT-PCR

Total RNA was extracted using an RNeasy® Mini kit (Qiagen, Venlo, The Netherlands). Reverse transcription was performed using a PrimeScript™ RT reagent kit (Takara Bio, Shiga, Japan). qRT-PCR was conducted on a CFX Connect™ Real-time System (Bio-Rad, Hercules, CA, USA). Gene expression levels of IL-23 and Nfkbiz were determined by qRT-PCR using TaqMan Fast Advanced Master Mix (Thermo Fisher Scientific). Amplification was initiated at 95 °C for 20 s as the first step, followed by 40 cycles of qRT-PCR at 95 °C for 3 s and at 60 °C for 30 s as the second step. mRNA expression was measured in triplicate with normalization by the housekeeping gene Ywhaz, and expression was indicated as the fold change relative to the control group. Primer sequences are listed in Table S1.

2.5. Western Blotting

Cells were incubated for 5 min in cOmplete™ Lysis-M (Roche Diagnostics, Basel, Switzerland). The protein concentration in the lysate was measured using a BCA Protein Assay Kit (Thermo Fisher Scientific). Equal amounts of protein (15 µg) were dissolved in Bolt LDS sample buffer (Thermo Fisher Scientific) and a 10% sample reducing agent (Thermo Fisher Scientific). The lysates were boiled at 70 °C for 10 min and then to electrophoresis in NuPAGE 4–12% Bis-Tris gels (Thermo Fisher Scientific) at 200 V for 25 min. The proteins were then transferred onto polyvinylidene difluoride membranes (Thermo Fisher Scientific), which were blocked with WesternBreeze Blocker/Diluent (Thermo Fisher Scientific). The membranes were then probed with anti-murine NF-κB p65 monoclonal rabbit antibody, anti-murine NF-κB p65 (phospho Ser536) polyclonal rabbit antibody, and anti-murine IκBζ polyclonal rabbit antibody (all from Cell Signaling Technology) overnight at 4 °C. Horseradish peroxidase-conjugated anti-rabbit IgG antibodies (Cell Signaling Technology) served as secondary antibodies. Protein bands were visualized with Chemi-Lumi One Super (Nacalai Tesque) using the ChemiDoc touch imaging system (Bio-Rad). The membranes were then re-blotted with Restore™ PLUS Western Blot Stripping Buffer (Thermo Fisher Scientific) and anti-murine β-actin mouse antibody 30 min at room temperature. Horseradish peroxidase-conjugated anti-mouse IgG antibodies served as secondary antibodies. Protein bands were visualized with SuperSignal™ West Pico PLUS Chemiluminescent Substrate (Thermo Fisher Scientific) using the ChemiDoc touch imaging system (Bio-Rad). Densitometric analysis of the bands was performed using ImageJ software. ImageJ is a public domain, Java-based image processing program developed at the National Institutes of Health (Bethesda, MD, USA). Experiments were repeated three times in separate experiments.

2.6. ELISA

A murine IL-23 ELISA Kit (R&D Systems) was used for ELISA in accordance with the manufacturer's protocol. Optical density was measured using a DTX 800 Multimode Detector (Beckman Coulter, Brea, CA, USA).

2.7. Statistical Analysis

Statistical analysis was performed with GraphPad Prism 5.0 (GraphPad Software, Inc., La Jolla, CA, USA). An unpaired Student's *t*-test was used to analyze the results, and a *p*-value of less than 0.05 was considered statistically significant.

3. Results

3.1. IL-36γ Stimulation Upregulated IL-23 and Nfkbiz Expression in BMDCs

To investigate the mechanism by which IL-36γ regulates IL-23 expression in DCs, we analyzed murine BMDCs stimulated with IL-36γ. qRT-PCR analysis revealed that IL-36γ stimulation (100 ng/mL) for 1, 2, 4, or 6 h upregulated IL-23 mRNA expression with expression peaking at 1 h (Figure 1A). Additionally, IL-36γ stimulation (1, 10, 50, or 100 ng/mL) for 1 h upregulated IL-23 mRNA expression in a concentration-dependent manner (Figure 1B). Furthermore, ELISA of the culture medium of BMDCs stimulated with IL-36γ (1, 10, 50, or 100 ng/mL) for 24 h revealed IL-23 production in a concentration-dependent manner (Figure 1C). We measured IL-23 production by ELISA following stimulation for 1 or 6 h; however, IL-23 was undetectable (data not shown). We believe that 24 h are required for IL-23 secretion to proceed after IL-23 mRNA expression is increased. As NFKBIZ is reported to be a key transcriptional regulator of IL-36-related gene expression in human psoriatic keratinocytes [21,22], we evaluated Nfkbiz expression in addition to IL-23 expression in murine BMDCs. qRT-PCR analysis illustrated that IL-36γ stimulation upregulated Nfkbiz mRNA expression (Figure 1D), which was in a concentration-dependent manner (Figure 1E). Western blotting analysis confirmed that IL-36γ stimulation (100 ng/mL) for 1, 2, 4, or 6 h upregulated IκBζ (protein corded by Nfkbiz gene) protein expression (Figure 1F).

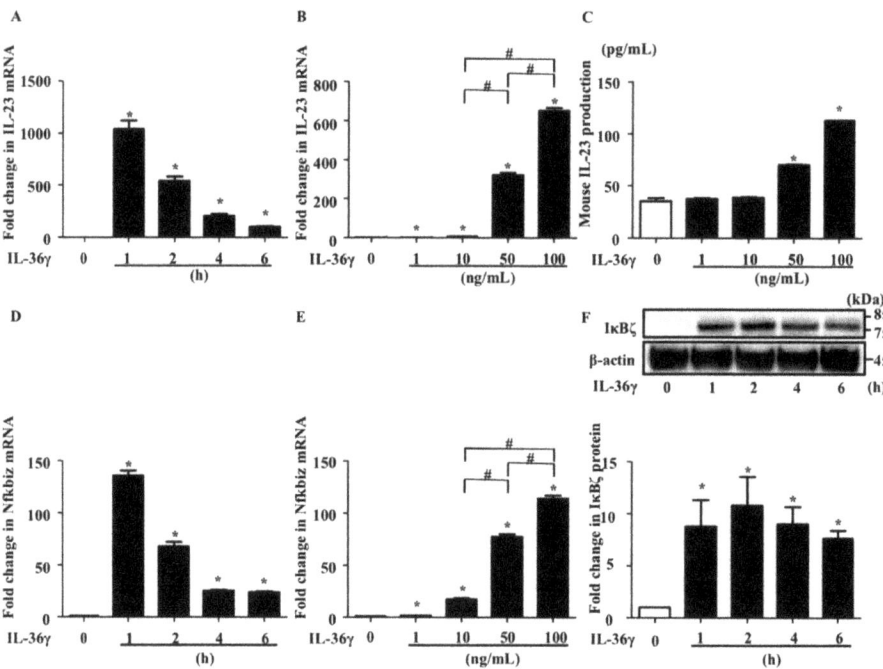

Figure 1. IL-36γ stimulation upregulated IL-23 and Nfkbiz in bone marrow-derived dendtitic cells (BMDCs). (**A,D,F**) BMDCs were stimulated with IL-36γ (100 ng/mL) for 1, 2, 4, or 6 h. (**A,D**) Quantitative reverse transcription (qRT)-PCR. (**F**) Western blotting. IκBζ protein levels are normalized to β-actin protein levels using ImageJ and expressed as fold change. (**B,C,E**) BMDCs were stimulated with IL-36γ (1, 10, 50, or 100 ng/mL) for 1 h. (**B,C**) qRT-PCR. (**E**) BMDCs were stimulated with IL-36γ (100 ng/mL) for 24 h, and IL-23 production in the culture supernatant was measured by ELISA. (**A–D**) Data are expressed as the mean ± standard error of the mean (SEM); $n = 3$/group. * Significant differences between the IL-36γ-stimulated groups and control groups ($p < 0.05$). # Significant differences between the IL-36γ-stimulated groups of each dose ($p < 0.05$). mRNA levels normalized for Ywhaz expression were expressed as the fold change compared to that in the control group. (**C**) Data are expressed as the mean ± SEM; $n = 3$/group; * $p < 0.05$. (**F**) Data are representative of experiments repeated three times with similar results.

3.2. IL-36γ Stimulation Upregulated IL-23 via Nfkbiz in BMDCs

Next, we examined whether Nfkbiz is involved in IL-23 upregulation induced by IL-36γ in murine BMDCs. We transfected BMDCs with either scrambled siRNA (si-control) or siRNA targeting Nfkbiz (si-Nfkbiz) and then stimulated the cells with IL-36γ (10 ng/mL) for 1 h. Although the transfection of si-Nfkbiz alone did not alter mRNA and IκBζ protein expression in BMDCs, it successfully downregulated Nfkbiz mRNA (Figure 2A) and protein expression (Figure 2B) in BMDCs stimulated with IL-36γ. This finding may be related to the partial depletion of the target gene because siRNA transfection is difficult in DCs [23]. Furthermore, we observed that depletion of Nfkbiz via siRNA transfection partially canceled IL-36γ stimulation-induced IL-23 mRNA upregulation (Figure 2C). Although we attempted to measure IL-23 production in the culture supernatant of siRNA-transfected BMDCs using ELISA, we could not detect IL-23 production, which may be attributable to cell damage caused by the siRNA transfection procedure. These results suggest that IκBζ is likely an integral part of the IL-36γ-induced IL-23 upregulation in murine BMDCs.

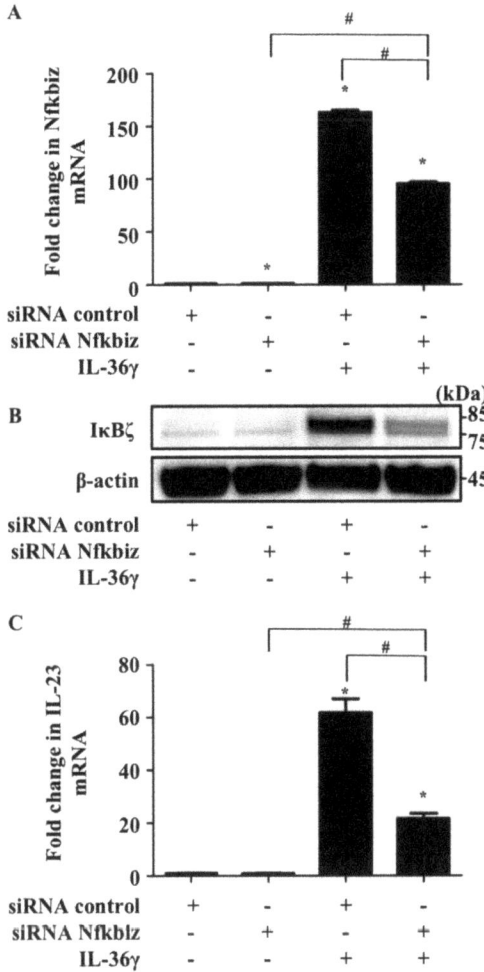

Figure 2. IκBζ is likely an integral part of IL-36γ-induced IL-23 upregulation in BMDCs. Control small interfering RNA (siRNA)- or Nfkbiz siRNA-transfected BMDCs were treated with/without IL-36γ (10 ng/mL) for 1 h and analyzed via quantitative reverse transcription (qRT)-PCR and Western

blotting. +/− indicates whether siRNA or IL-36γ is utilized. (**A**) qRT-PCR. (**B**) Western blotting. (**C**) qRT-PCR. (**A,C**) Data are expressed as the mean ± standard error of the mean (SEM); $n = 3$/group. * Significant difference versus the control siRNA-transfected group with no IL-36γ stimulation ($p < 0.05$). # Significant difference between the Nfkbiz siRNA-transfected and control siRNA-transfected groups that were stimulated with IL-36γ ($p < 0.05$). mRNA levels normalized to Ywhaz mRNA expression are expressed as the fold change versus that in the control group. (**B**) IκBζ expression was evaluated using anti-murine IκBζ antibody. Data are representative of experiments repeated three times with similar results.

3.3. IL-36γ Upregulates Nfkbiz and IL-23 via the Activation of NF-κB Signaling

Next, we examined the mechanism by which IL-36γ upregulates Nfkbiz expression in murine BMDCs. Considering that IL-36 binding to the IL-36 receptor complex leads to the recruitment of MyD88 and activation of NF-κB signaling [16] and that Nfkbiz expression is regulated by phosphorylation of p65, a component of the NF-κB heterodimer [24], we hypothesized that IL-36γ modulated Nfkbiz expression via NF-κB signaling in murine BMDCs. We analyzed p65 phosphorylation in murine BMDCs stimulated with IL-36γ (100 ng/mL) for 10, 20, 30, 40, or 60 min using Western blotting. We confirmed that p65 phosphorylation was induced after 10 min of IL-36γ stimulation (Figure 3A). We further examined whether BAY 11-7082, an inhibitor of p65 phosphorylation, affects the upregulation of Nfkbiz induced by IL-36γ stimulation. We stimulated murine BMDCs with IL-36γ (100 ng/mL) for 1 h in the absence or presence of BAY 11-7082 (10, 50, or 100 μM) and measured Nfkbiz mRNA and IκBζ protein expression by qRT-PCR (Figure 3B) and Western blotting (Figure 3C), respectively. BAY 11-7082 treatment inhibited Nfkbiz upregulation in a concentration-dependent manner (Figure 3B,C). Moreover, we examined whether BAY 11-7082 treatment inhibits the upregulation of IL-23 induced by IL-36γ. We measured IL-23 production in the culture supernatant of BMDCs stimulated with IL-36γ (100 ng/mL) for 24 h in the absence or presence of BAY 11-7082 (10, 50, or 100 μM) using ELISA. BAY 11-7082 treatment also inhibited the upregulation of IL-23 induced by IL-36γ stimulation in a concentration-dependent manner (Figure 3D).

3.4. Metformin Treatment Inhibited the Upregulation of Nfkbiz and IL-23 Induced by IL-36 Stimulation by Impairing NF-κB Signaling

It has been reported that metformin controls NF-κB signaling [25]. Moreover, clinical studies of patients with psoriasis and T2DM have suggested that metformin administration may attenuate the disease activity of psoriasis [19,20]. Therefore, we hypothesized that metformin treatment affects the IL-36γ-induced upregulation of Nfkbiz and IL-23 by modulating NF-κB signaling in murine BMDCs. To test this, we analyzed p65 phosphorylation in BMDCs stimulated with IL-36γ (100 ng/mL) for 10, 20, 30, 40, and 60 min in the absence or presence of metformin (5 mM) using Western blotting. Metformin treatment inhibited p65 phosphorylation induced by IL-36γ (Figure 4A). In addition, we evaluated mRNA and protein expression in murine BMDCs stimulated with IL-36γ (100 ng/mL) for 1 h in the absence or presence of metformin (0.5, 1, or 5 mM). Metformin treatment inhibited the IL-36γ-induced upregulation of Nfkbiz mRNA and IκBζ protein expression in a concentration-dependent manner in BMDCs (Figure 4B,C). Subsequently, metformin treatment was revealed to inhibit the upregulation of IL-23 mRNA expression in BMDCs stimulated with IL-36γ for 1 h in a concentration-dependent manner (Figure 4D). In addition, metformin treatment downregulated IL-23 production in the culture supernatant of BMDCs stimulated with IL-36γ for 24 h in a concentration-dependent manner (Figure 4E).

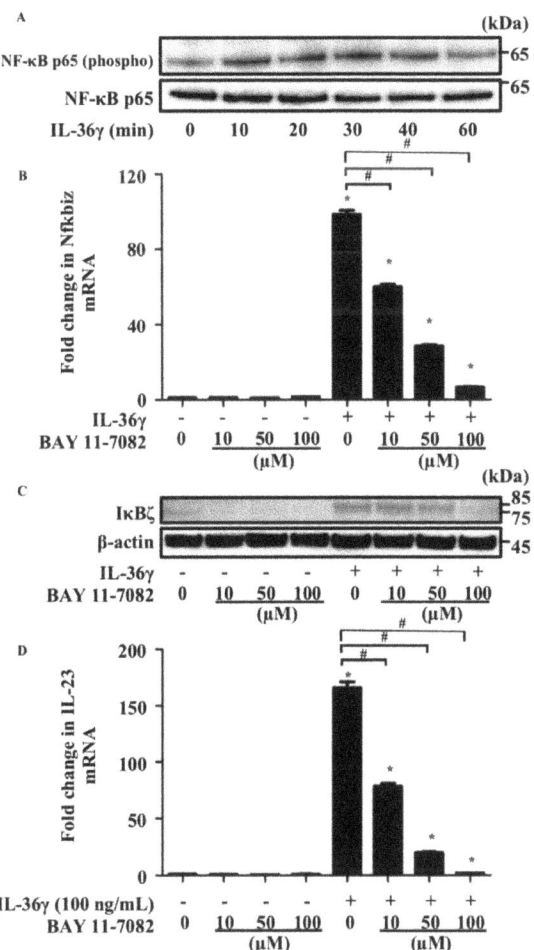

Figure 3. Nfkbiz expression was regulated by p65 phosphorylation in BMDCs. BMDCs were stimulated with IL-36γ (100 ng/mL) for 10, 20, 30, 40, or 60 min (**A**). (**A**) Western blotting. BMDCs were stimulated with/without IL-36γ (100 ng/mL) for 1 h (+/−) in the absence or presence of BAY 11-7082 (10, 50, or 100 μM) (**B**–**D**). (**B**,**D**) Quantitative reverse transcription-PCR. (**C**) Western blotting. (**B**,**D**) Data are expressed as the mean ± standard error of the mean; $n = 3$/group. * Significant difference between the IL-36γ-stimulated and control groups ($p < 0.05$). # Significant difference between the BAY 11-7082-treated and untreated groups that were stimulated with IL-36γ ($p < 0.05$). mRNA levels normalized to Ywhaz mRNA expression were expressed as the fold change versus that in the control group. (**A**,**C**) Data are representative of experiments repeated three times with similar results. +/− indicates whether IL-36γ is utilized.

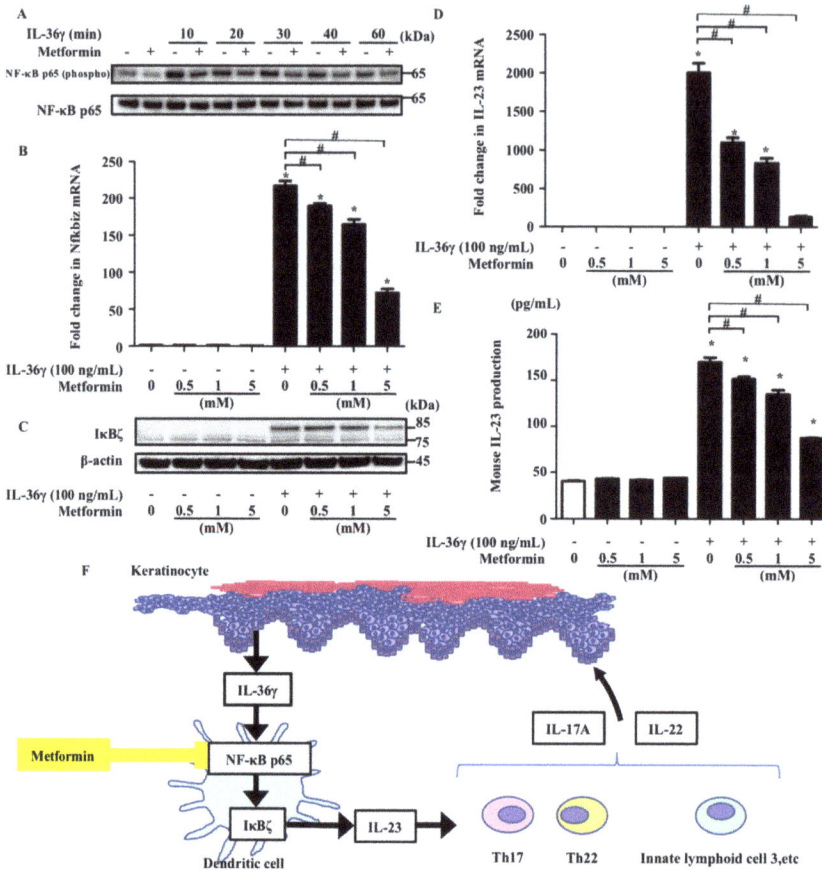

Figure 4. Metformin treatment inhibited IL-36γ-induced upregulation of Nfkbiz and IL-23 by modulating NF-κB signaling in BMDCs. BMDCs stimulated with IL-36γ (100 ng/mL) for 10, 20, 30, 40, or 60 min in the absence or presence of metformin (5 mM) (**A**). (**A**) Western blotting. BMDCs were stimulated with/without IL-36γ (100 ng/mL) for 1 h (+/−) in the absence or presence of metformin (0.5, 1, or 5 mM). (**B,D,E**). (**B,D**) quantitative reverse transcription-PCR. (**E**) ELISA. (**F**) Graphical abstract. Data are expressed as the mean ± standard error of the mean; $n = 3$/group. * Significant difference between the IL-36γ-stimulated and control groups ($p < 0.05$). # Significant differences between the metformin-treated and control groups that were stimulated with IL-36γ ($p < 0.05$). mRNA levels normalized for Ywhaz expression were expressed as fold changes versus that in the control group. (**A,C**) Data are representative of experiments repeated three times with similar results. +/− indicates whether IL-36γ or metformin is utilized.

4. Discussion

IL-36γ is a cytokine associated with the disease activity of psoriasis. Therefore, it is of great interest to identify a strategy that inhibits the responses of downstream inflammatory cytokines. In this study, we obtained evidence that IL-36γ induces Nfkbiz upregulation, which subsequently leads to IL-23 upregulation, in murine BMDCs. Furthermore, we revealed that metformin treatment inhibited IL-23 upregulation via the impairment of Nfkbiz upregulation. To our knowledge, this is the first study providing evidence that metformin can modulate IL-36γ-mediated IL-23 production in DCs, thereby contributing to the prevention of psoriasis. However, the systemic expression of IL-23 following the administration of IL-23 minicircle DNA [26] or transgenic expression of IL-23 derived from keratinocytes [27] can reportedly promote the development of psoriasis. Therefore, the production of IL-23 by cells other than DCs has also been reported to contribute to the pathogenesis of psoriasis, which is a limitation of this study.

We confirmed that IL-36γ (10 or 100 ng/mL) stimulation efficiently induces IL-23 mRNA upregulation in murine BMDCs, which is consistent with previous findings [28,29]. Furthermore, we revealed that IL-36γ stimulation increases IL-23 protein expression using ELISA. Although the concentration of 100 ng/mL is rather high, we considered it reasonable in this experiment system because IL-36γ is activated by neutrophil-derived proteases such as proteinase-3 [30].

IκBζ, a transcriptional regulator of selective NF-κB target genes, has been identified as a crucial mediator of IL-36-driven psoriasis-related gene expression in keratinocytes [21]; however, it is unclear whether IκBζ is involved in the IL-36γ-mediated expression of genes including IL-23 in DCs. Based on the result that depletion of Nfkbiz mRNA expression partially downregulated IL-23 mRNA expression induced by IL-36 stimulation, IκBζ is likely an integral part of IL-36-induced IL-23 upregulation in murine BMDCs. As we utilized siRNA transfection to deplete Nfkbiz mRNA expression, the low depletion efficiency may have resulted in weak repression of IL-23 mRNA expression.

Although several studies suggested that the molecular machinery underlying the regulation of IκBζ could be cell type-specific, it has been reported that the induction of IκBζ by IL-36γ is mediated by MyD88, NF-κB, and STAT3 in human keratinocytes [13,14]. We found that inhibition of NF-κB activity by BAY 11-7082 treatment significantly downregulated IκBζ induction by IL-36γ in murine BMDCs, suggesting that NF-κB activation may be critical in IL-36γ-mediated IκBζ induction in DCs. Furthermore, inhibition of NF-κB activity by metformin treatment had the same effect as BAY 11-7082 treatment. These data support the potential benefits of metformin treatment in patients with type 2 diabetes mellitus (T2DM) and psoriasis. As several studies revealed an association between T2DM and psoriasis [31,32] and suggested a severity-dependent relationship between psoriasis and T2DM [17], the management of T2DM is considered extremely important in the treatment of psoriasis. Metformin treatment has been reported to inhibit several signaling pathways including the mammalian target of rapamycin [33] and mitogen-activated protein kinase signaling [34], in addition to NF-κB signaling. As such, we cannot thus exclude the possibility that other kinases might have been affected by metformin in the experiments. Further studies will be required to clarify this possibility.

We revealed here that metformin exerts anti-inflammatory effects on DCs, at least in part via pathways involving the inhibition of IκBζ production (Figure 4F). Our study presents the novel concept that pharmacological modulation by metformin of IL-36γ-induced IL-23 production via IκBζ inhibition may offer a potential therapeutic approach to psoriasis. It can be hypothesized that oral metformin administration suppresses psoriasis by this mechanism. However, the clinical relevance of IL-23 inhibition by metformin requires further investigation.

Supplementary Materials: The following are available online at https://www.mdpi.com/2077-0383/10/23/5610/s1, Table S1: Murine TaqMan gene expression assay probes.

Author Contributions: T.M.-T. and G.T. designed the experiments. T.M.-T., G.T., M.F. and T.N. wrote the manuscript. G.T., A.H.-H., T.M.-T., A.T.-Y. and M.T. performed the experiments. T.M.-T., G.T. and M.F. analyzed the results. All authors contributed to the interpretation of the research. All authors have read and agreed to the published version of the manuscript.

Funding: This research was funded by grants from the Ministry of Health, Labour and Welfare of Japan (R3-Shokuhin-Shitei-005) and JSPS KAKENHI (grant number 20K08653).

Institutional Review Board Statement: The study was conducted according to the guidelines of the Declaration of Helsinki and approved by the Institutional Review Board of KYUSHU UNIVERSITY (A21-283-0 and 1 June 2021).

Conflicts of Interest: The authors declare no conflict of interest.

References

1. Michalek, I.M.; Loring, B.; John, S.M. A systematic review of worldwide epidemiology of psoriasis. *J. Eur. Acad. Dermatol. Venereol.* **2017**, *31*, 205–212. [CrossRef]
2. Furue, M.; Furue, K.; Tsuji, G.; Nakahara, T. Interleukin-17A and Keratinocytes in Psoriasis. *Int. J. Mol. Sci.* **2020**, *21*, 1275. [CrossRef] [PubMed]
3. Boehncke, W.H.; Schön, M.P. Psoriasis. *Lancet* **2015**, *386*, 983–994. [CrossRef]
4. Yan, B.; Liu, N.; Li, J.; Li, J.; Zhu, W.; Kuang, Y.; Chen, X.; Peng, C. The role of Langerhans cells in epidermal homeostasis and pathogenesis of psoriasis. *J. Cell Mol. Med.* **2020**, *24*, 11646–11655. [CrossRef] [PubMed]
5. Hawkes, J.E.; Yan, B.Y.; Chan, T.C.; Krueger, J.G. Discovery of the IL-23/IL-17 Signaling Pathway and the Treatment of Psoriasis. *J. Immunol.* **2018**, *201*, 1605–1613. [CrossRef]
6. Wohn, C.; Ober-Blöbaum, J.L.; Haak, S.; Pantelyushin, S.; Cheong, C.; Zahner, S.P.; Onderwater, S.; Kant, M.; Weighardt, H.; Holzmann, B.; et al. Langerin(neg) conventional dendritic cells produce IL-23 to drive psoriatic plaque formation in mice. *Proc. Natl. Acad. Sci. USA* **2013**, *110*, 10723–10728. [CrossRef]
7. Riol-Blanco, L.; Ordovas-Montanes, J.; Perro, M.; Naval, E.; Thiriot, A.; Alvarez, D.; Paust, S.; Wood, J.N.; von Andrian, U.H. Nociceptive sensory neurons drive interleukin-23-mediated psoriasiform skin inflammation. *Nature* **2014**, *510*, 157–161. [CrossRef]
8. Lee, E.; Trepicchio, W.L.; Oestreicher, J.L.; Pittman, D.; Wang, F.; Chamian, F.; Dhodapkar, M.; Krueger, J.G. Increased expression of interleukin 23 p19 and p40 in lesional skin of patients with psoriasis vulgaris. *J. Exp. Med.* **2004**, *199*, 125–130. [CrossRef]
9. Di Cesare, A.; Di Meglio, P.; Nestle, F.O. The IL-23/Th17 axis in the immunopathogenesis of psoriasis. *J. Investig. Dermatol.* **2009**, *129*, 1339–1350. [CrossRef]
10. Cai, Y.; Shen, X.; Ding, C.; Qi, C.; Li, K.; Li, X.; Jala, V.R.; Zhang, H.G.; Wang, T.; Zheng, J.; et al. Pivotal role of dermal IL-17-producing gammadelta T cells in skin inflammation. *Immunity* **2011**, *35*, 596–610. [CrossRef]
11. Gordon, K.B.; Duffin, K.C.; Bissonnette, R.; Prinz, J.C.; Wasfi, Y.; Reich, K.; Li, S.; Shen, Y.-K.; Szapary, P.; Randazzo, B.; et al. A Phase 2 Trial of Guselkumab versus Adalimumab for Plaque Psoriasis. *N. Engl. J. Med.* **2015**, *373*, 136–144. [CrossRef] [PubMed]
12. Papp, K.A.; Blauvelt, A.; Bukhalo, M.; Gooderham, M.; Krueger, J.G.; Lacour, J.-P.; Menter, A.; Philipp, S.; Sofen, H.; Tyring, S.; et al. Risankizumab versus Ustekinumab for Moderate-to-Severe Plaque Psoriasis. *N. Engl. J. Med.* **2017**, *376*, 1551–1560. [CrossRef] [PubMed]
13. Reich, K.; Warren, R.B.; Iversen, L.; Puig, L.; Pau-Charles, I.; Igarashi, A.; Ohtsuki, M.; Falqués, M.; Harmut, M.; Rozzo, S.; et al. Long-term efficacy and safety of tildrakizumab for moderate-to-severe psoriasis: Pooled analyses of two randomized phase III clinical trials (reSURFACE 1 and reSURFACE 2) through 148 weeks. *Br. J. Dermatol.* **2020**, *182*, 605–617. [CrossRef] [PubMed]
14. D'Erme, A.M.; Wilsmann-Theis, D.; Wagenpfeil, J.; Hölzel, M.; Ferring-Schmitt, S.; Sternberg, S.; Wittmann, M.; Peters, B.; Bosio, A.; Bieber, T.; et al. IL-36γ (IL-1F9) is a biomarker for psoriasis skin lesions. *J. Investig. Dermatol.* **2015**, *135*, 1025–1032. [CrossRef] [PubMed]
15. Mercurio, L.; Morelli, M.; Scarponi, C.; Eisenmesser, E.Z.; Doti, N.; Pagnanelli, G.; Gubinelli, E.; Mazzanti, C.; Cavani, A.; Ruvo, M.; et al. IL-38 has an anti-inflammatory action in psoriasis and its expression correlates with disease severity and therapeutic response to anti-IL-17A treatment. *Cell Death Dis.* **2018**, *9*, 1104. [CrossRef]
16. Walsh, P.T.; Fallon, P.G. The emergence of the IL-36 cytokine family as novel targets for inflammatory diseases. *Ann. N. Y. Acad. Sci.* **2018**, *1417*, 23–34. [CrossRef]
17. Gelfand, J.M.; Wan, M.T. Psoriasis: A novel risk factor for type 2 diabetes. *Lancet Diabetes Endocrinol.* **2018**, *6*, 919–921. [CrossRef]
18. Brauchli, Y.B.; Jick, S.S.; Curtin, F.; Meier, C.R. Association between use of thiazolidinediones or other oral antidiabetics and psoriasis: A population based case-control study. *J. Am. Acad. Dermatol.* **2008**, *58*, 421–429. [CrossRef]
19. Singh, S.; Bhansali, A. Randomized placebo control study of insulin sensitizers (Metformin and Pioglitazone) in psoriasis patients with metabolic syndrome (Topical Treatment Cohort). *BMC Dermatol.* **2016**, *16*, 12. [CrossRef]
20. Singh, S.; Bhansali, A. Randomized placebo control study of metformin in psoriasis patients with metabolic syndrome (Systemic Treatment Cohort). *Indian J. Endocrinol. Metab.* **2017**, *21*, 581–587. [CrossRef]
21. Müller, A.; Hennig, A.; Lorscheid, S.; Grondona, P.; Schulze-Osthoff, K.; Kramer, D. IκBζ is a key transcriptional regulator of IL-36-driven psoriasis-related gene expression in keratinocytes. *Proc. Natl. Acad. Sci. USA* **2018**, *115*, 10088–10093. [CrossRef]
22. Ovesen, S.K.; Schulze-Osthoff, K.; Iversen, L.; Johansen, C. IkBζ is a Key Regulator of Tumour Necrosis Factor-a and Interleukin-17A-mediated Induction of Interleukin-36g in Human Keratinocytes. *Acta. Derm. Venereol.* **2021**, *101*, adv00386. [CrossRef]
23. Siegert, I.; Schatz, V.; Prechtel, A.T.; Steinkasserer, A.; Bogdan, C.; Jantsch, J. Electroporation of siRNA into mouse bone marrow-derived macrophages and dendritic cells. *Methods Mol. Biol.* **2014**, *1121*, 111–119. [CrossRef] [PubMed]
24. Willems, M.; Dubois, N.; Musumeci, L.; Bours, V.; Robe, P.A. IκBζ: An emerging player in cancer. *Oncotarget* **2016**, *7*, 66310–66322. [CrossRef]
25. Sultuybek, G.K.; Soydas, T.; Yenmis, G. NF-κB as the mediator of metformin's effect on ageing and ageing-related diseases. *Clin. Exp. Pharmacol. Physiol.* **2019**, *46*, 413–422. [CrossRef] [PubMed]
26. Sherlock, J.P.; Joyce-Shaikh, B.; Turner, S.P.; Chao, C.-C.; Sathe, M.; Grein, J.; Gorman, D.M.; Bowman, E.P.; McClanahan, T.K.; Yearley, J.H.; et al. IL-23 induces spondyloarthropathy by acting on ROR-γt$^+$CD3$^+$CD4$^-$CD8$^-$ entheseal resident T cells. *Nat. Med.* **2011**, *18*, 1069–1076. [CrossRef] [PubMed]
27. Chen, L.; Deshpande, M.; Grisotto, M.; Smaldini, P.; Garcia, R.; He, Z.; Gulko, P.S.; Lira, S.A.; Furtado, G.C. Skin expression of IL-23 drives the development of psoriasis and psoriatic arthritis in mice. *Sci. Rep.* **2020**, *10*, 8259. [CrossRef] [PubMed]

28. Vigne, S.; Palmer, G.; Lamacchia, C.; Martin, P.; Talabot-Ayer, D.; Rodriguez, E.; Ronchi, F.; Sallusto, F.; Dinh, H.; Sims, J.E.; et al. IL-36R ligands are potent regulators of dendritic and T cells. *Blood* **2011**, *118*, 5813–5823. [CrossRef] [PubMed]
29. Kovach, M.A.; Singer, B.; Martinez-Colon, G.; Newstead, M.W.; Zeng, X.; Mancuso, P.; Moore, T.A.; Kunkel, S.L.; Peters-Golden, M.; Moore, B.B.; et al. IL-36γ is a crucial proximal component of protective type-1-mediated lung mucosal immunity in Gram-positive and -negative bacterial pneumonia. *Mucosal Immunol.* **2017**, *10*, 1320–1334. [CrossRef]
30. Henry, C.M.; Sullivan, G.P.; Clancy, D.M.; Afonina, I.S.; Kulms, D.; Martin, S.J. Neutrophil-Derived Proteases Escalate Inflammation through Activation of IL-36 Family Cytokines. *Cell Rep.* **2016**, *14*, 708–722. [CrossRef]
31. Yeung, H.; Takeshita, J.; Mehta, N.N.; Kimmel, S.E.; Ogdie, A.; Margolis, D.J.; Shin, D.B.; Attor, R.; Troxel, A.B.; Gelfand, J.M. Psoriasis severity and the prevalence of major medical comorbidity: A population-based study. *JAMA Dermatol.* **2013**, *149*, 1173–1179. [CrossRef] [PubMed]
32. Wan, M.T.; Shin, D.B.; Hubbard, R.A.; Noe, M.H.; Mehta, N.N.; Gelfand, J.M. Psoriasis and the risk of diabetes: A prospective population-based cohort study. *J. Am. Acad. Dermatol.* **2018**, *78*, 315–322. [CrossRef]
33. Nyambuya, T.M.; Dludla, P.V.; Mxinwa, V.; Mokgalaboni, K.; Ngcobo, S.R.; Nkambule, B.B. The impact of metformin and aspirin on T-cell mediated inflammation: A systematic review of in vitro and in vivo findings. *Life Sci.* **2020**, *255*, 117854. [CrossRef] [PubMed]
34. Kim, J.; Kwak, H.J.; Cha, J.Y.; Jeong, Y.S.; Rhee, S.D.; Kim, K.R.; Cheon, H.G. Metformin suppresses lipopolysaccharide (LPS)-induced inflammatory response in murine macrophages via activating transcription factor-3 (ATF-3) induction. *J. Biol. Chem.* **2014**, *289*, 23246–23255. [CrossRef] [PubMed]

Review

Regulatory Roles of Estrogens in Psoriasis

Akimasa Adachi [1,2] and Tetsuya Honda [2,3,*]

1. Department of Dermatology, Tokyo Metropolitan Bokutoh Hospital, Tokyo 130-8575, Japan
2. Department of Dermatology, Kyoto University Graduate School of Medicine, Kyoto 606-8507, Japan
3. Department of Dermatology, Hamamatsu University School of Medicine, Hamamatsu 431-3192, Japan
* Correspondence: hontetsu@hama-med.ac.jp

Abstract: Psoriasis is a common chronic inflammatory skin disease of the interleukin (IL)-23/IL-17 axis. The severity of psoriasis has been reported as higher in men than in women. The immunoregulatory role of female sex hormones has been proposed to be one of the factors responsible for sex differences. Among female sex hormones, estrogens have been suggested to be significantly involved in the development of psoriasis by various epidemiological and in vitro studies. For example, the severity of psoriasis is inversely correlated with serum estrogen levels. In vitro, estrogens suppress the production of psoriasis-related cytokines such as IL-1β and IL-23 from neutrophils and dendritic cells, respectively. Furthermore, a recent study using a mouse psoriasis model indicated the inhibitory role of estrogens in psoriatic dermatitis by suppressing IL-1β production from neutrophils and macrophages. Understanding the role and molecular mechanisms of female sex hormones in psoriasis may lead to better control of the disease.

Keywords: psoriasis; female sex hormone; estrogen; progesterone

1. Introduction

Psoriasis is a common chronic inflammatory disease with well-demarcated red scaly plaques throughout the body [1]. The prevalence of psoriasis is estimated to be approximately 0.5~8.5% of the worldwide population [2]. Although the pathogenesis of psoriasis has not been fully elucidated, it is now widely accepted that the interleukin (IL)-23/IL-17 axis is a central pathway in psoriasis development, especially in plaque-type psoriasis [3]. In psoriatic lesions, IL-23 is primarily produced by inflammatory dendritic cells (DCs) [1]. IL-23, together with IL-1β, induces IL-17A/F and IL-22 production in various IL-17-producing cells, such as Th17/Tc17 and γδT cells [4,5]. IL-17/22 then activates keratinocytes to produce inflammatory molecules/chemokines such as chemokine (C-X-C motif) ligand (CXCL)-1, 2, and 8; chemokine (C-C motif) ligand 2 (CCL-2); and CCL-20, which recruit inflammatory cells including neutrophils, inflammatory macrophages, and T cells to the skin and accelerate psoriatic inflammation [1,6]. T cells, macrophages, and keratinocytes produce tumor necrosis factor-α (TNF-α) and amplify these cytokine networks [6]. Other than these cytokines, IL-36 and IFN-a are mainly involved in the development of pustular psoriasis and paradoxical psoriasis, respectively [7]. In addition to these central pathways, various genetic and environmental factors are involved in the modification of psoriasis development, and female hormones are suggested to be disease-modifying factors [8].

Estrogens are representative female hormones that are produced mainly in the ovaries. Estrogens play an important role in controlling the female sexual cycle, pregnancy, and childbirth. However, estrogens may also be involved in regulating immune cell functions [9]. For example, estrogen suppresses nuclear factor-κ B (NF-κB) and mitogen-activated protein kinase (MAPK) signaling and downregulates inflammatory responses in various cell populations in vitro [9,10]. However, it remains unclear whether these immuneregulatory functions of estrogens play physiologically significant roles in inflammatory diseases, including psoriasis.

In this short review, we summarize the current findings regarding the involvement of estrogen in the pathogenesis of psoriasis.

2. Physiology of Estrogens

2.1. Physiological Levels of Estrogens

Estrogens are a group of steroid hormones present in three major physiological forms: estrone (E1; molecular weight (MW) 270.4 g/mol), 17β-estradiol (E2; MW 272.4 g/mol), and estriol (E3; 288.4 g/mol). Estrogens are mainly produced from cholesterol in the ovaries. Estrogens are also produced in the liver, heart, skin, brain, male testes, adrenal glands, and fat tissues [11]. E2 is the most abundant and potent estrogen at the reproductive age. In males, serum E2 levels are less than 40 pg/mL [12], whereas, in females, serum E2 levels range between 30 and 800 pg/mL during the menstrual cycle and increase up to 20,000 pg/mL during pregnancy [11]. After menopause, the serum E2 levels decrease to <20 pg/mL. In the postmenopausal period, serum E2 levels decrease by 85–90% from the mean premenopausal level [12].

2.2. Estrogen Receptors and Their Signaling

Estrogen signaling is primarily mediated through two estrogen receptors (ERs)—ERα and ERβ—which are expressed in a wide variety of cell types, including neutrophils, monocytes/macrophages, T cells, and DCs [9]. ERα and ERβ genes are encoded by *Esr1* and *Esr2* and these genes are located on 6 and 14 chromosomes, respectively. E2 binds to these receptors to form dimers, which translocate to the nucleus (Figure 1). In the classical genomic pathway, the dimers bind to estrogen response elements (ERE), and activate the target gene expression. In the non-classical pathway, the dimers interact with other transcription factors, such as NF-κB, specificity protein 1 (SP1), activator protein-1 (AP-1), and CCAAT/enhancer binding protein β (C/EBPβ), and prevent their binding to the transcription factor regulatory elements, leading to the inhibition of their target gene expression [13–15]. Of note, these transcriptional factors control the gene expression of many psoriasis-related cytokines and chemokines. For example, NF-κB is involved in the transcription of genes such as IL-23, IL-1β, TNF-α, CCL-2 and CXCL-1; SP1 in IL-1β and TNF-α; and AP-1 and C/EBPβ in IL-23 and IL-36, respectively [16–20].

In addition to these major receptors, G protein-coupled estrogen receptor 1 (GPER1, also known as GPR30), which is located in the endoplasmic reticulum and plasma membrane, binds to E2 with a high affinity [21]. GPER1/GPR30 mediates estrogen signaling through nongenomic responses, including activation of the mitogen-activated protein kinase (MAPK) signaling cascade, cAMP formation, insulin-like growth factor 1 receptor (IGFR), epidermal growth factor receptor (EGFR) and intracellular calcium mobilization [22]. Nuclear ERs mediate signals slowly over hours or days, whereas GPER1 responds much faster, even within seconds [13] (Figure 1).

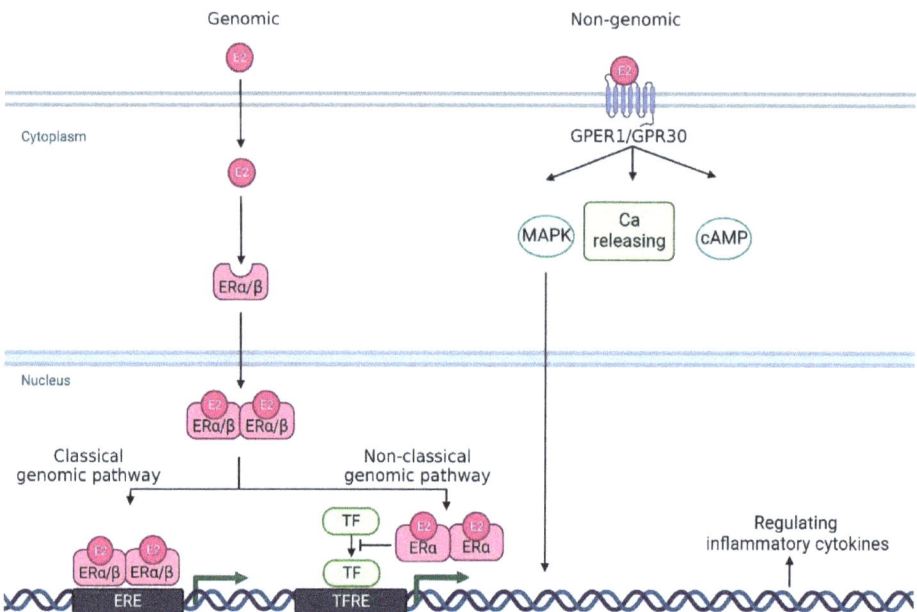

Figure 1. A scheme of estrogen receptors and the intracellular signaling pathway. In genomic pathway, 17β-estradiol (E2) binds to estrogen receptor α and estrogen receptor β in the cytoplasm. It forms dimer and translocates to the nucleus. Then, they bind to estrogen receptor element (ERE) and activate the transcription of downstream genes (classical genomic pathway). Or, they interact with other transcription factor (TF)s, such as NF-κB, specificity protein 1 (SP1), activator protein-1 (AP-1), and CCAAT/enhancer binding protein β (C/EBPβ), and prevent their binding to the transcription factor regulatory element (TFRE) (non-classical genomic pathway), leading to the regulation of their target gene expression. In non-genomic pathway, E2 binds to G protein-coupled estrogen receptor 1 (GPER1) and it regulates mitogen-activated protein kinase (MAPK), calcium (Ca) release, and cyclic adenosine monophosphate (cAMP). Created with Biorender.com.

3. Epidemiological and Case Series Studies about the Possible Involvement of Estrogens in Psoriasis

There are various epidemiological studies investigating the prevalence and severity of psoriasis in men and women. Some studies indicate that the prevalence and severity of psoriasis are higher in men than in women [23–30], especially at the estrogen abundant age [31], while other reports failed to observe significant differences in the prevalence of psoriasis between men and women [32–34] (Table 1). A recent systematic review indicates that the prevenance is similar between men and women, but the severity in women is lower than men [35]. The age of disease onset is also different between men and women. For example, a German study demonstrates that the age of onset has two peaks, one occurring at the age of 16 years in women or 22 years in men, and a second at the age of 60 years in women or 57 years in men [34]. Recent studies indicate that the two peaks for age at onset are around 18–29 and 50–59 years in women, whereas they are around 30–39 and 60–69 or 70–79 years in men [36]. During pregnancy, in which serum levels of female hormones dramatically change, approximately 33–55% of patients with psoriasis show improvement in symptoms, although some patients, especially patients with pustular psoriasis, occasionally show exacerbated symptoms during pregnancy [37]. In contrast, in the postpartum period, approximately 65% of psoriasis patients exhibit worsening of skin lesions associated with decreased levels of female sex hormones [38–43]. Serum levels of E2 and the relative ratio of serum levels of E2 to that of progesterone correlate with psoriasis severity in pregnant patients with psoriasis [38]. Serum E2 levels are inversely correlated with psoriasis severity [44]. Low-dose E2 administration induces improvement in psoriatic arthritis [43], but it is not effective against pustular psoriasis and plaque-type psoriasis [45,46]. On the other hand, it has been reported that tamoxifen, an antiestrogen agent, results in the remission of psoriasis, whose symptoms worsen during a perimenstrual cycle [47]. These studies suggest that estrogens have both proinflammatory and anti-inflammatory roles in psoriasis.

Table 1. A summary of previous reports on the prevalence ratio of psoriasis between men and women.

	Prevalence Ratio of Psoriasis	
	Men	Women
Farber 1974 [32]	46%	54%
Henseler 1985 [34]	50.8%	49.2%
Kawada 2003 [26]	65.80%	34.20%
Takahashi 2009 [25]	66.40%	33.60%
Tsai 2011 [30]	61.60%	38.40%
Furue 2011 [24]	72%	28%
Na 2013 [29]	54.60%	45.40%
Lee 2017 [28]	57.30%	42.70%
Hägg 2017 [23]	59.80%	40.20%
Bayaraa 2018 [31]	67.10%	32.9%
El-komy 2020 [27]	56.30%	43.70%
Armstrong 2021 [33]	48.60%	51.40%

4. In Vitro Studies Regarding the Immuno-Regulatory Action of E2

Keratinocytes and various immune cells orchestrate psoriatic inflammation in psoriatic lesions. In this section, we introduce in vitro studies that investigated the potential anti-inflammatory roles of E2 in each cell population (Table 2).

Table 2. In vitro studies regarding the effects of estrogen on immune cell functions related to psoriatic inflammation.

	Estrogen
Keratinocytes	RANTES↓(physiological to high) [40]
	CCL-2↓(physiological to high) [39]
	CCL-20↓(isoflavone) [42]
	S100A7↓(isoflavone) [42]
	S100A9↓(isoflavone) [42]
Neutrophils	superoxide anion (O_2^-)↓(not mentioned) [48]
	degranulation↓(high) [48]
	apoptosis(physiological to high) [49]
	migration↓(physiological to high) [49]
Monocytes/Macrophages	IL-1β→~↓(high) [50–52]
	TNF-α→~↓(high) [51–53]

Table 2. *Cont.*

	Estrogen
Dendritic cells	IL-23↓(high) [54]
	IL-1β↑(physiological) [55]
	IL-8↑(high) [56]
	CCL-2↑(high) [56]
T cells	IL-17↓(physiological) [57]
	TNF-α↓(high), TNF-α↑(low) [58,59]

RANTES, Regulated on activation, normal T cell expressed and secreted; CCL, CC-chemokine ligand; S100A7, S100 calcium-binding protein A7; S100A9, S100 calcium-binding protein A9; O_2^-, superoxide anion; IL, interleukin; TNF, tumor necrosis factor.

4.1. Keratinocytes

Keratinocytes play a critical role in psoriasis development [50,53,60]. Keratinocytes release multiple factors, such as damage-associated molecular patterns (DAMPs), CCL-20, and CXCL-1, 2, and 8 [1]. In vitro, the production of chemokines, such as RANTES and CCL-2, is inhibited by E2 in normal human keratinocytes [51,52]. Isoflavone genistein, which is the major metabolite of soy that binds to human ERα and ERβ, decreases MAPK, signal transducer and activator of transcription 3 (STAT3), NF-κB, and phosphatidylinositol-3 kinase (PI3K) activation in human keratinocytes, leading to decreased mRNA expression of *CCL20*, *S100A7*, and *S100A9* induced by IL-17A and TNF-α [48,49,54]. These results suggest that E2 downregulates keratinocyte activation in psoriatic lesions.

4.2. Neutrophils, Monocytes, and Macrophages

Infiltration of neutrophils into the epidermis is one of the characteristic histological findings in psoriasis. Although the actual roles of neutrophils/monocytes/macrophages in psoriasis development are still not fully understood, there are some case studies suggesting disease-promoting roles of neutrophils/monocytes/macrophages in psoriasis. For example, psoriatic lesions have been reported to significantly improve during drug-induced agranulocytosis [55]. Granulocyte and monocyte apheresis therapy ameliorates the symptoms of psoriasis [56]. In mouse studies, depletion of neutrophils has been shown to attenuate psoriasis symptoms [55–59]. These studies suggest that neutrophils, monocytes, and macrophages facilitate the development of psoriasis.

Some studies have investigated the effects of E2 on cytokine production from neutrophils/monocytes/macrophages, but the results are not necessarily consistent among reports. For example, physiological to supraphysiological levels of E2 downregulated TNF-α and IL-1β production from human monocytes and macrophages, whereas no inhibitory effects of physiological to supraphysiological levels of E2 were observed in other studies [9,61–64]. E2 may exert bidirectional effects on TNF-α and IL-1β production by monocytes and macrophages, depending on its concentration.

In addition to the effects on cytokine production, the inhibitory roles of E2 on neutrophil functions, such as superoxide anion (O_2^-) generation, degranulation, and apoptosis, have been reported [65,66].

4.3. DCs

DCs play a critical role in the development of psoriasis by producing IL-23 and TNF-α [6]. In vitro, supraphysiological levels of E2 impair IL-23 production from murine bone marrow-derived DCs [67], suggesting that E2 plays a regulatory role in psoriasis development, especially during pregnancy. In contrast, the physiological levels of E2 facilitate IL-1β production in murine vaginal CD11c+DCs [68] and CXCL-8 and CCL-2 production in human monocyte-derived DCs [69], suggesting that the influence of E2 on DC functions differs depending on the concentration and type of DCs.

4.4. T cells

T cells (Th17/Tc17) produce pro-inflammatory cytokines such as IL-17A and TNF-α in psoriatic lesions and significantly contribute to psoriatic inflammation [6]. To date, few studies have investigated the role of E2 in Th17/Tc17 cell functions, but some in vitro studies have suggested inhibitory roles of E2 on Th17 cell differentiation and activation [70].

In vitro, physiological levels of E2 inhibited Th17 differentiation through downregulation of retinoid orphan receptor gamma t (Rorγt) expression in murine splenic T cells [70–72]. The effect of E2 on IL-17 production in Th17/Tc17 cells has not been investigated, but it has been reported that supraphysiological levels of E2 inhibit TNF-α production in human T cells, suggesting that E2 at high concentrations, such as during pregnancy, may downregulate TNF-α production from Th17 cells in psoriatic lesions. However, it has also been reported that E2, at physiological concentrations, enhances TNF-α production [73,74]. The molecular mechanisms that determine the concentration-dependent effects of E2 on T-cell function remain unclear.

Other than Th17 differentiation, involvement of estrogen on Th1/Th2 differentiation has been reported [75]. For example, physiological levels of E2 inhibited Th1 differentiation through downregulation of T-bet, and shifted toward Th2 differentiation in murine T cells in the lymph nodes and spleen [72,76]. Since Th1-type immune responses play facilitating roles in psoriasis while Th2-type immune responses counterbalance Th17-type immune response [77], estrogens may also play inhibitory roles in psoriasis by down-regulating Th1 and up-regulating Th2 differentiation.

5. In Vivo Studies Regarding the Role of E2 on Psoriatic Inflammation

As mentioned above, the possible inhibitory or facilitating roles of E2 in psoriatic inflammation have been suggested by various epidemiological and in vitro studies [78]. However, it remains unclear whether and how E2 plays a role in psoriatic inflammation in vivo. Currently, two in vivo studies have investigated the role of E2 in psoriatic inflammation [79]. Iwano et al. examined the role of E2 in psoriatic inflammation using an imiquimod-induced psoriasis model. Male BALB/c mice were used in the psoriasis model and E2 was administered exogenously. The mice treated with E2 showed exacerbated dermatitis. Administration of an ERα agonist also exacerbated dermatitis. Furthermore, the production of IL-23 by DCs was enhanced by E2 and an ERα agonist in vitro. Based on these data, it was suggested that E2 plays a pro-inflammatory role in psoriasis by inducing IL-23 through ERα [79].

In contrast, we observed anti-psoriatic roles of E2 in the same mouse model [80]. To investigate the role of E2 in psoriatic inflammation in vivo, we applied ovariectomized female C57BL/6 mice, in which the endogenous production of female hormones, including E2, is almost impaired, to an imiquimod-induced psoriasis model. Ovariectomized mice exhibited exacerbated psoriatic inflammation, whereas exogenous administration of E2 reversed the exacerbation, suggesting that E2 plays an anti-psoriatic role physiologically. The anti-psoriatic effects of E2 were mediated through ERα and ERβ in neutrophils and macrophages. Mechanistically, E2 downregulated IL-1β production in neutrophils and macrophages, leading to decreased IL-17A production in γδT cells. The inhibitory effect of E2 on IL-1β production has also been observed in human polymorphonuclear and mononuclear cells. This result may explain the fluctuating IL-1β levels during the female reproductive cycle in humans, in which IL-1β levels are higher during the luteal phase (low serum E2 level) and lower during the follicular phase (high E2 level) [71,81–83]. Together, these results suggest that E2 plays a suppressive role in psoriatic inflammation in mice through the regulation of neutrophil and macrophage functions such as IL-1β production. It remains unclear why different effects of E2 were observed in the two studies. E2 may play both pro- and anti-psoriatic roles in a context-dependent manner (Figure 2), as suggested in previous in vitro studies.

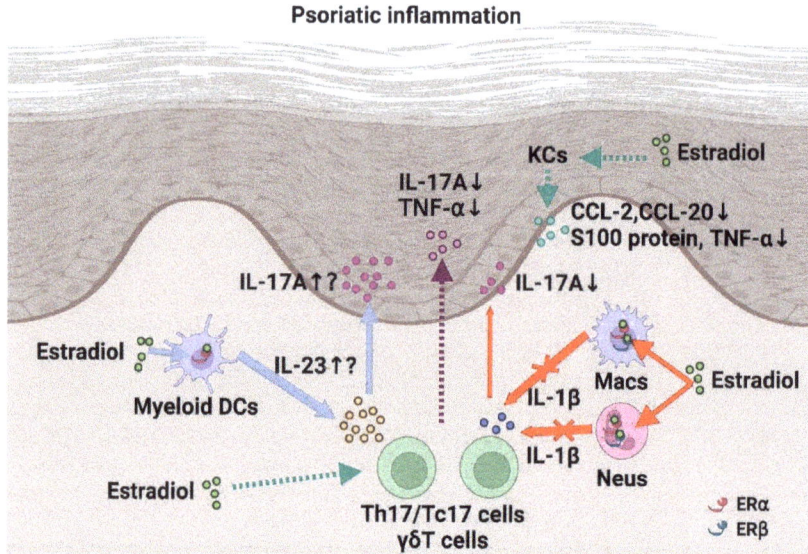

Figure 2. A scheme of possible functions and the mechanisms of estrogen in psoriatic inflammation. E2 play anti-psoriatic functions by downregulating IL-1β production from neutrophils (Neus) and monocytes/macrophages (Macs) through ERα and ERβ. However, in a certain condition, E2 may play facilitating role on psoriatic inflammation by inducing IL-23 production from dendritic cells (DCs) through ERα. Solid lines show the findings from in vivo studies and dotted lines show the findings from in vitro or other disease model studies. Created with Biorender.com.

6. Concluding Remarks

The immunoregulatory mechanisms of E2 in psoriasis, which have mostly been investigated in in vitro studies, have gradually been elucidated in vivo using a mouse psoriasis model. Recognition by patients and clinicians of the potential impact of sex hormones including E2 would lead to a better management of psoriasis symptoms, especially in women. Furthermore, data in the mouse psoriasis model suggest that an appropriate activation of estrogen receptor-signaling is a potential novel therapeutic strategy in psoriasis. However, there are some important issues to be solved before estrogens can be used as a treatment for psoriasis. First, since systemic estrogen therapy has various undesired side effects such as an increased risk of thrombosis and endometrial cancer, and that psoriasis patients tend to develop cardiovascular diseases, topical estrogen therapy, rather than systemic therapy, may be practical. Second, since there are many differences in the pathogenesis between mouse and human psoriasis models, we need to be cautious when applying the findings of mouse studies to human psoriasis. For example, neutrophils and macrophages are the major sources of IL-1β in a murine psoriasis model, while keratinocytes may be the primary source of IL-1β in human psoriasis [5]. Thus, the anti-psoriatic effects of E2 through the inhibition of IL-1β production by neutrophils and macrophages may be limited in human psoriasis. The molecular mechanisms that switch the functions of E2 from pro-inflammatory to anti-inflammatory in psoriasis remain unclear and should be further investigated. Investigation of the involvement of other female hormones such as progesterone in psoriasis is also of interest. In fact, during pregnancy, psoriasis symptoms improve in some patients, whereas they worsen in others, suggesting the existence of female hormones that facilitate psoriasis. In addition, it has been reported that the administration of progesterone flares pustular psoriasis [37,84], suggesting that progesterone may play a facilitating role in psoriasis. Thus, there still remains many unsolved issues on the roles of sex hormones in psoriasis and for the translation of the findings to clinical practice.

Nevertheless, elucidation of these issues may lead to the development of novel treatment strategies for psoriasis from the perspective of sex hormones.

Author Contributions: Conceptualization, A.A. and T.H.; resources, A.A. and T.H.; writing—original draft preparation, A.A. and T.H.; writing—review and editing, T.H.; visualization, A.A.; supervision, T.H.; funding acquisition, A.A. and T.H. All authors have read and agreed to the published version of the manuscript.

Funding: This research received no external funding.

Institutional Review Board Statement: Not applicable.

Informed Consent Statement: Not applicable.

Conflicts of Interest: The authors have declared that no conflict of interest exists.

References

1. Nestle, F.O.; Kaplan, D.H.; Barker, J. Psoriasis. *N. Engl. J. Med.* **2009**, *361*, 496–509. [CrossRef] [PubMed]
2. Parisi, R.; Symmons, D.P.M.; Griffiths, C.E.M.; Ashcroft, D.M. Global epidemiology of psoriasis: A systematic review of incidence and prevalence. *J. Investig. Dermatol.* **2013**, *133*, 377–385. [CrossRef] [PubMed]
3. McGeachy, M.J.; Cua, D.J.; Gaffen, S.L. The IL-17 Family of Cytokines in Health and Disease. *Immunity* **2019**, *50*, 892–906. [CrossRef]
4. Cai, Y.; Shen, X.; Ding, C.; Qi, C.; Li, K.; Li, X.; Jala, V.R.; Zhang, H.-g.; Wang, T.; Zheng, J.; et al. Pivotal Role of Dermal IL-17-Producing γδ T Cells in Skin Inflammation. *Immunity* **2011**, *35*, 596–610. [CrossRef] [PubMed]
5. Cai, Y.; Xue, F.; Quan, C.; Qu, M.; Liu, N.; Zhang, Y.; Fleming, C.; Hu, X.; Zhang, H.; Weichselbaum, R.; et al. A Critical Role of the IL-1β–IL-1R Signaling Pathway in Skin Inflammation and Psoriasis Pathogenesis. *J. Investig. Dermatol.* **2019**, *139*, 146–156. [CrossRef] [PubMed]
6. Greb, J.E.; Goldminz, A.M.; Elder, J.T.; Lebwohl, M.G.; Gladman, D.D.; Wu, J.J.; Mehta, N.N.; Finlay, A.Y.; Gottlieb, A.B. Psoriasis. *Nat. Rev. Dis. Prim.* **2016**, *2*, 1–17. [CrossRef] [PubMed]
7. Griffiths, C.E.M.; Armstrong, A.W.; Gudjonsson, J.E.; Barker, J.N.W.N. Psoriasis. *Lancet* **2021**, *397*, 1301–1315. [CrossRef]
8. Kanda, N.; Watanabe, S. Regulatory roles of sex hormones in cutaneous biology and immunology. *J. Dermatol. Sci.* **2005**, *38*, 1–7. [CrossRef]
9. Klein, S.L.; Flanagan, K.L. Sex differences in immune responses. *Nat. Rev. Immunol.* **2016**, *16*, 626–638. [CrossRef]
10. Hall, O.J.; Klein, S.L. Progesterone-based compounds affect immune responses and susceptibility to infections at diverse mucosal sites. *Mucosal Immunol.* **2017**, *10*, 1097–1107. [CrossRef]
11. Straub, R.H. The complex role of estrogens in inflammation. *Endocr. Rev.* **2007**, *28*, 521–574. [CrossRef]
12. Stanczyk, F.Z.; Clarke, N.J. Measurement of estradiol-challenges ahead. *J. Clin. Endocrinol. Metab.* **2014**, *99*, 56–58. [CrossRef] [PubMed]
13. Kovats, S. Estrogen receptors regulate innate immune cells and signaling pathways. *Cell. Immunol.* **2015**, *294*, 63–69. [CrossRef] [PubMed]
14. Ghisletti, S.; Meda, C.; Maggi, A.; Vegeto, E. 17β-Estradiol Inhibits Inflammatory Gene Expression by Controlling NF-κB Intracellular Localization. *Mol. Cell. Biol.* **2005**, *25*, 2957–2968. [CrossRef] [PubMed]
15. Björnström, L.; Sjöberg, M. Mechanisms of estrogen receptor signaling: Convergence of genomic and nongenomic actions on target genes. *Mol. Endocrinol.* **2005**, *19*, 833–842. [CrossRef] [PubMed]
16. Chadjichristos, C.; Ghayor, C.; Kypriotou, M.; Martin, G.; Renard, E.; Ala-Kokko, L.; Suske, G.; De Crombrugghe, B.; Pujol, J.P.; Galéra, P. Sp1 and Sp3 transcription factors mediate interleukin-1β down-regulation of human type II collagen gene expression in articular chondrocytes. *J. Biol. Chem.* **2003**, *278*, 39762–39772. [CrossRef] [PubMed]
17. Novoszel, P.; Holcmann, M.; Stulnig, G.; De Sa Fernandes, C.; Zyulina, V.; Borek, I.; Linder, M.; Bogusch, A.; Drobits, B.; Bauer, T.; et al. Psoriatic skin inflammation is promoted by c-Jun/AP-1-dependent CCL2 and IL-23 expression in dendritic cells. *EMBO Mol. Med.* **2021**, *13*, 1–18. [CrossRef]
18. Wang, S.; Wang, W.; Wesley, R.A.; Danner, R.L. A Sp1 binding site of the tumor necrosis factor α promoter functions as a nitric oxide response element. *J. Biol. Chem.* **1999**, *274*, 33190–33193. [CrossRef]
19. Nerlich, A.; Ruangkiattikul, N.; Laarmann, K.; Janze, N.; Dittrich-Breiholz, O.; Kracht, M.; Goethe, R. C/EBPβ is a transcriptional key regulator of IL-36α in murine macrophages. *Biochim. Biophys. Acta—Gene Regul. Mech.* **2015**, *1849*, 966–978. [CrossRef]
20. Liu, T.; Zhang, L.; Joo, D.; Sun, S.C. NF-κB signaling in inflammation. *Signal Transduct. Target. Ther.* **2017**, *2*, 1–9. [CrossRef]
21. Notas, G.; Kampa, M.; Castanas, E. G Protein-Coupled Estrogen Receptor in Immune Cells and Its Role in Immune-Related Diseases. *Front. Endocrinol.* **2020**, *11*, 579420. [CrossRef] [PubMed]
22. Revankar, C.M.; Cimino, D.F.; Sklar, L.A.; Arterburn, J.B.; Prossnitz, E.R. A transmembrane intracellular estrogen receptor mediates rapid cell signaling. *Science* **2005**, *307*, 1625–1630. [CrossRef] [PubMed]

23. Hägg, D.; Sundström, A.; Eriksson, M.; Schmitt-Egenolf, M. Severity of Psoriasis Differs Between Men and Women: A Study of the Clinical Outcome Measure Psoriasis Area and Severity Index (PASI) in 5438 Swedish Register Patients. *Am. J. Clin. Dermatol.* **2017**, *18*, 583–590. [CrossRef] [PubMed]
24. Furue, M.; Yamazaki, S.; Jimbow, K.; Tsuchida, T.; Amagai, M.; Tanaka, T.; Matsunaga, K.; Muto, M.; Morita, E.; Akiyama, M.; et al. Prevalence of dermatological disorders in Japan: A nationwide, cross-sectional, seasonal, multicenter, hospital-based study. *J. Dermatol.* **2011**, *38*, 310–320. [CrossRef] [PubMed]
25. Takahashi, H.; Takahashi, I.; Tsuji, H.; Ibe, M.; Kinouchi, M.; Hashimoto, Y.; Ishida-Yamamoto, A.; Matsuo, S.; Ohkuma, N.; Ohkawara, A.; et al. Analysis of psoriatic patients registered in Asahikawa Medical College Hospital from 1983 to 2007. *J. Dermatol.* **2009**, *36*, 632–637. [CrossRef]
26. Kawada, A.; Tezuka, T.; Nakamizo, Y.; Kimura, H.; Nakagawa, H.; Ohkido, M.; Ozawa, A.; Ohkawara, A.; Kobayashi, H.; Harada, S.; et al. A survey of psoriasis patients in Japan from 1982 to 2001. *J. Dermatol. Sci.* **2003**, *31*, 59–64. [CrossRef]
27. El-Komy, M.H.M.; Mashaly, H.; Sayed, K.S.; Hafez, V.; El-Mesidy, M.S.; Said, E.R.; Amer, M.A.; AlOrbani, A.M.; Saadi, D.G.; El-Kalioby, M.; et al. Clinical and epidemiologic features of psoriasis patients in an Egyptian medical center. *JAAD Int.* **2020**, *1*, 81–90. [CrossRef]
28. Lee, J.Y.; Kang, S.; Park, J.S.; Jo, S.J. Prevalence of psoriasis in Korea: A population-based epidemiological study using the Korean national health insurance database. *Ann. Dermatol.* **2017**, *29*, 761–767. [CrossRef]
29. Na, S.J.; Jo, S.J.; Youn, J. Il Clinical study on psoriasis patients for past 30 years (1982-2012) in Seoul National University Hospital Psoriasis Clinic. *J. Dermatol.* **2013**, *40*, 731–735. [CrossRef]
30. Tsai, T.F.; Wang, T.S.; Hung, S.T.; Tsai, P.I.C.; Schenkel, B.; Zhang, M.; Tang, C.H. Epidemiology and comorbidities of psoriasis patients in a national database in Taiwan. *J. Dermatol. Sci.* **2011**, *63*, 40–46. [CrossRef]
31. Bayaraa, B.; Imafuku, S. Relationship between environmental factors, age of onset and familial history in Japanese patients with psoriasis. *J. Dermatol.* **2018**, *45*, 715–718. [CrossRef] [PubMed]
32. Farber, E.M.; Nall, M.L. The natural history of psoriasis in 5600 patients. *Dermatologica* **1974**, *148*, 1–18. [CrossRef] [PubMed]
33. Armstrong, A.W.; Mehta, M.D.; Schupp, C.W.; Gondo, G.C.; Bell, S.J.; Griffiths, C.E.M. Psoriasis Prevalence in Adults in the United States. *JAMA Dermatol.* **2021**, *157*, 940–946. [CrossRef] [PubMed]
34. Henseler, T.; Christophers, E. Psoriasis of early and late onset: Characterization of two types of psoriasis vulgaris. *J. Am. Acad. Dermatol.* **1985**, *13*, 450–456. [CrossRef]
35. Guillet, C.; Seeli, C.; Nina, M.; Maul, L.V.; Maul, J.-T. The impact of gender and sex in psoriasis: What to be aware of when treating women with psoriasis. *Int. J. Women's Dermatol.* **2022**, *8*, e010. [CrossRef] [PubMed]
36. Parisi, R.; Iskandar, I.Y.K.; Kontopantelis, E.; Augustin, M.; Griffiths, C.E.M.; Ashcroft, D.M. National, regional, and worldwide epidemiology of psoriasis: Systematic analysis and modelling study. *BMJ* **2020**, *369*, 369. [CrossRef] [PubMed]
37. Murphy, F.R.; Stolman, L.P. Generalized Pustular Psoriasis. *Arch. Dermatol.* **1979**, *115*, 1215–1216. [CrossRef]
38. Murase, J.E.; Chan, K.K.; Garite, T.J.; Cooper, D.M.; Weinstein, G.D. Hormonal effect on psoriasis in pregnancy and post partum. *Arch. Dermatol.* **2005**, *141*, 601–606. [CrossRef]
39. Raychaudhuri, S.P.; Navare, T.; Gross, J.; Raychaudhuri, S.K. Clinical course of psoriasis during pregnancy. *Int. J. Dermatol.* **2003**, *42*, 518–520. [CrossRef] [PubMed]
40. Mowad, C.M.; Margolis, D.J.; Halpern, A.C.; Suri, B.; Synnestvedt, M.; Guzzo, C.A. Hormonal Influences on Women with Psoriasis. *Cutis* **1998**, *61*, 257–260.
41. Park, B.S.; Youn, J. Il Factors influencing psoriasis: An analysis based upon the extent of involvement and clinical type. *J. Dermatol.* **1998**, *25*, 97–102. [CrossRef] [PubMed]
42. Boyd, A.S.; Morris, L.F.; Phillips, C.M.; Menter, M.A. Psoriasis and pregnancy: Hormone and immune system interaction. *Int. J. Dermatol.* **1996**, *35*, 169–172. [CrossRef] [PubMed]
43. McHugh, N.J.; Laurent, M.R. The effect of pregnancy on the onset of psoriatic arthritis. *Br. J. Rheumatol.* **1989**, *28*, 50–52. [CrossRef] [PubMed]
44. Cemil, B.C.; Cengiz, F.P.; Atas, H.; Ozturk, G.; Canpolat, F. Sex hormones in male psoriasis patients and their correlation with the Psoriasis Area and Severity Index. *J. Dermatol.* **2015**, *42*, 500–503. [CrossRef]
45. Braverman, I.M.; Cohen, I.; O'keefe, E. Metabolic and Ultrastructural Studies in a Patient With Pustular Psoriasis (von Zumbusch). *Arch. Dermatol.* **1972**, *105*, 189–196. [CrossRef]
46. Spangler, A.S.; Antoniades, H.N.; Sotman, S.L.; Inderbitizin, T.M. Enhancement of the anti-inflammatory action of hydrocortisone by estrogen. *J. Clin. Endocrinol. Metab.* **1969**, *29*, 650–655. [CrossRef]
47. Boyd, A.S.; King, J. Tamoxifen-induced remission of psoriasis. *J. Am. Acad. Dermatol.* **1999**, *41*, 887–889. [CrossRef]
48. Smolinska, E.; Moskot, M.; Jakóbkiewicz-Banecka, J.; Wegrzyn, G.; Banecki, B.; Szczerkowska-Dobosz, A.; Purzycka-Bohdan, D.; Gabig-Ciminska, M. Molecular action of isoflavone genistein in the human epithelial cell line HaCaT. *PLoS ONE* **2018**, *13*, e0192157. [CrossRef]
49. Bocheńska, K.; Moskot, M.; Smolińska-Fijołek, E.; Jakóbkiewicz-Banecka, J.; Szczerkowska-Dobosz, A.; Słomiński, B.; Gabig-Cimińska, M. Impact of isoflavone genistein on psoriasis in in vivo and in vitro investigations. *Sci. Rep.* **2021**, *11*, 1–16. [CrossRef]
50. Dainichi, T.; Kitoh, A.; Otsuka, A.; Nakajima, S.; Nomura, T.; Kaplan, D.H.; Kabashima, K. The epithelial immune microenvironment (EIME) in atopic dermatitis and psoriasis. *Nat. Immunol.* **2018**, *19*, 1286–1298. [CrossRef]

51. Kanda, N.; Watanabe, S. 17β-Estradiol Inhibits MCP-1 Production in Human Keratinocytes. *J. Investig. Dermatol.* **2003**, *120*, 1058–1066. [CrossRef] [PubMed]
52. Kanda, N.; Watanabe, S. 17β-estradiol inhibits the production of RANTES in human keratinocytes. *J. Investig. Dermatol.* **2003**, *120*, 420–427. [CrossRef] [PubMed]
53. Li, H.; Yao, Q.; Mariscal, A.G.; Wu, X.; Hülse, J.; Pedersen, E.; Helin, K.; Waisman, A.; Vinkel, C.; Thomsen, S.F.; et al. Epigenetic control of IL-23 expression in keratinocytes is important for chronic skin inflammation. *Nat. Commun.* **2018**, *9*, 1–8. [CrossRef] [PubMed]
54. Wang, A.; Wei, J.; Lu, C.; Chen, H.; Zhong, X.; Lu, Y.; Li, L.; Huang, H.; Dai, Z.; Han, L. Genistein suppresses psoriasis-related inflammation through a STAT3–NF-κB-dependent mechanism in keratinocytes. *Int. Immunopharmacol.* **2019**, *69*, 270–278. [CrossRef]
55. Toichi, E.; Tachibana, T.; Furukawa, F. Rapid improvement of psoriasis vulgaris during drug-induced agranulocytosis. *J. Am. Acad. Dermatol.* **2000**, *43*, 391–395. [CrossRef]
56. Ikeda, S.; Takahashi, H.; Suga, Y.; Eto, H.; Etoh, T.; Okuma, K.; Takahashi, K.; Kanbara, T.; Seishima, M.; Morita, A.; et al. Therapeutic depletion of myeloid lineage leukocytes in patients with generalized pustular psoriasis indicates a major role for neutrophils in the immunopathogenesis of psoriasis. *J. Am. Acad. Dermatol.* **2013**, *68*, 609–617. [CrossRef]
57. Sumida, H.; Yanagida, K.; Kita, Y.; Abe, J.; Matsushima, K.; Nakamura, M.; Ishii, S.; Sato, S.; Shimizu, T. Interplay between CXCR2 and BLT1 Facilitates Neutrophil Infiltration and Resultant Keratinocyte Activation in a Murine Model of Imiquimod-Induced Psoriasis. *J. Immunol.* **2014**, *192*, 4361–4369. [CrossRef]
58. Han, G.; Havnaer, A.; Lee, H.H.; Carmichael, D.J.; Martinez, L.R. Biological depletion of neutrophils attenuates pro-inflammatory markers and the development of the psoriatic phenotype in a murine model of psoriasis. *Clin. Immunol.* **2020**, *210*, 108294. [CrossRef]
59. Morimura, S.; Oka, T.; Sugaya, M.; Sato, S. CX3CR1 deficiency attenuates imiquimod-induced psoriasis-like skin inflammation with decreased M1 macrophages. *J. Dermatol. Sci.* **2016**, *82*, 175–188. [CrossRef]
60. Matsumoto, R.; Sugimoto, Y.; Kabashima, K.; Matsumoto, R.; Dainichi, T.; Tsuchiya, S.; Nomura, T.; Kitoh, A. Epithelial TRAF6 drives IL-17–mediated psoriatic inflammation. *JCI Insight* **2018**, *3*, 121175. [CrossRef]
61. Ito, A.; Bebo, B.F.; Matejuk, A.; Zamora, A.; Silverman, M.; Fyfe-Johnson, A.; Offner, H. Estrogen Treatment Down-Regulates TNF-α Production and Reduces the Severity of Experimental Autoimmune Encephalomyelitis in Cytokine Knockout Mice. *J. Immunol.* **2001**, *167*, 542–552. [CrossRef] [PubMed]
62. Carruba, G.; D'Agostino, P.; Miele, M.; Calabrò, M.; Barbera, C.; Di Bella, G.; Milano, S.; Ferlazzo, V.; Caruso, R.; La Rosa, M.; et al. Estrogen regulates cytokine production and apoptosis in PMA-differentiated, macrophage-like U937 cells. *J. Cell. Biochem.* **2003**, *90*, 187–196. [CrossRef] [PubMed]
63. Bouman, A.; Schipper, M.; Heineman, M.J.; Faas, M. 17β-Estradiol and progesterone do not influence the production of cytokines from lipopolysaccharide-stimulated monocytes in humans. *Fertil. Steril.* **2004**, *82*, 1212–1219. [CrossRef] [PubMed]
64. Rogers, A.; Eastell, R. The effect of 17β-estradiol on production of cytokines in cultures of peripheral blood. *Bone* **2001**, *29*, 30–34. [CrossRef]
65. Buyon, J.P.; Korchak, H.M.; Rutherford, L.E.; Ganguly, M.; Weissmann, G. Female hormones reduce neutrophil responsiveness in vitro. *Arthritis Rheum.* **1984**, *27*, 623–630. [CrossRef] [PubMed]
66. Molloy, E.J.; O'Neill, A.J.; Grantham, J.J.; Sheridan-Pereira, M.; Fitzpatrick, J.M.; Webb, D.W.; Watson, R.W.G. Sex-specific alterations in neutrophil apoptosis: The role of estradiol and progesterone. *Blood* **2003**, *102*, 2653–2659. [CrossRef]
67. Relloso, M.; Aragoneses-Fenoll, L.; Lasarte, S.; Bourgeois, C.; Romera, G.; Kuchler, K.; Corbí, A.L.; Muñoz-Fernández, M.A.; Nombela, C.; Rodríguez-Fernández, J.L.; et al. Estradiol impairs the Th17 immune response against Candida albicans. *J. Leukoc. Biol.* **2012**, *91*, 159–165. [CrossRef]
68. Anipindi, V.C.; Bagri, P.; Roth, K.; Dizzell, S.E.; Nguyen, P.V.; Shaler, C.R.; Chu, D.K.; Jiménez-Saiz, R.; Liang, H.; Swift, S.; et al. Estradiol Enhances CD4+ T-Cell Anti-Viral Immunity by Priming Vaginal DCs to Induce Th17 Responses via an IL-1-Dependent Pathway. *PLoS Pathog.* **2016**, *12*, 1–27. [CrossRef]
69. Bengtsson, Å.K.; Ryan, E.J.; Giordano, D.; Magaletti, D.M.; Clark, E.A. 17β-estradiol (E2) modulates cytokine and chemokine expression in human monocyte-derived dendritic cells. *Blood* **2004**, *104*, 1404–1410. [CrossRef]
70. Chen, R.-Y.; Fan, Y.-M.; Zhang, Q.; Liu, S.; Li, Q.; Ke, G.-L.; Li, C.; You, Z. Estradiol Inhibits Th17 Cell Differentiation through Inhibition of RORγT Transcription by Recruiting the ERα/REA Complex to Estrogen Response Elements of the RORγT Promoter. *J. Immunol.* **2015**, *194*, 4019–4028. [CrossRef]
71. Bouman, A.; Jan Heineman, M.; Faas, M.M. Sex hormones and the immune response in humans. *Hum. Reprod. Update* **2005**, *11*, 411–423. [CrossRef] [PubMed]
72. Lélu, K.; Laffont, S.; Delpy, L.; Paulet, P.-E.; Périnat, T.; Tschanz, S.A.; Pelletier, L.; Engelhardt, B.; Guéry, J.-C. Estrogen Receptor α Signaling in T Lymphocytes Is Required for Estradiol-Mediated Inhibition of Th1 and Th17 Cell Differentiation and Protection against Experimental Autoimmune Encephalomyelitis. *J. Immunol.* **2011**, *187*, 2386–2393. [CrossRef] [PubMed]
73. Ralston, S.H.; Russell, R.G.G.; Gowen, M. Estrogen inhibits release of tumor necrosis factor from peripheral blood mononuclear cells in postmenopausal women. *J. Bone Miner. Res.* **1990**, *5*, 983–988. [CrossRef] [PubMed]
74. Gilmore, W.; Weiner, L.P.; Correale, J. Effect of estradiol on cytokine secretion by proteolipid protein-specific T cell clones isolated from multiple sclerosis patients and normal control subjects. *J. Immunol.* **1997**, *158*, 446–451. [PubMed]

75. Khan, D.; Ansar Ahmed, S. The immune system is a natural target for estrogen action: Opposing effects of estrogen in two prototypical autoimmune diseases. *Front. Immunol.* **2016**, *6*, 1–8. [CrossRef]
76. Haghmorad, D.; Salehipour, Z.; Nosratabadi, R.; Rastin, M.; Kokhaei, P.; Mahmoudi, M.B.; Amini, A.A.; Mahmoudi, M. Medium-dose estrogen ameliorates experimental autoimmune encephalomyelitis in ovariectomized mice. *J. Immunotoxicol.* **2016**, *13*, 885–896. [CrossRef]
77. Yamanaka, K.; Yamamoto, O.; Honda, T. Pathophysiology of psoriasis: A review. *J. Dermatol.* **2021**, *48*, 722–731. [CrossRef]
78. Danesh, M.; Murase, J.E. The immunologic effects of estrogen on psoriasis: A comprehensive review. *Int. J. Women's Dermatol.* **2015**, *1*, 104–107. [CrossRef]
79. Iwano, R.; Iwashita, N.; Takagi, Y.; Fukuyama, T. Estrogen receptor α activation aggravates imiquimod-induced psoriasis-like dermatitis in mice by enhancing dendritic cell interleukin-23 secretion. *J. Appl. Toxicol.* **2020**, *40*, 1353–1361. [CrossRef]
80. Adachi, A.; Honda, T.; Egawa, G.; Kanameishi, S.; Takimoto, R.; Miyake, T.; Hossain, M.R.; Komine, M.; Ohtsuki, M.; Gunzer, M.; et al. Estradiol suppresses psoriatic inflammation in mice by regulating neutrophil and macrophage functions. *J. Allergy Clin. Immunol.* **2022**. [CrossRef]
81. Bouman, A.; Moes, H.; Heineman, M.J.; De Leij, L.F.M.H.; Faas, M.M. The immune response during the luteal phase of the ovarian cycle: Increasing sensitivity of human monocytes to endotoxin. *Fertil. Steril.* **2001**, *76*, 555–559. [CrossRef]
82. Cannon, J.G.; Dinarello, C.A. Increased plasma interleukin-1 activity in women after ovulation. *Science* **1984**, *227*, 1247–1249. [CrossRef] [PubMed]
83. Brännström, M.; Fridén, B.E.; Jasper, M.; Norman, R.J. Variations in peripheral blood levels of immunoreactive tumor necrosis factor α (TNFα) throughout the menstrual cycle and secretion of TNFα from the human corpus luteum. *Eur. J. Obstet. Gynecol. Reprod. Biol.* **1999**, *83*, 213–217. [CrossRef]
84. Shelley, W.B. Generalized Pustular Psoriasis Induced by Potassium Iodide. *Jama* **1967**, *201*, 1009. [CrossRef]

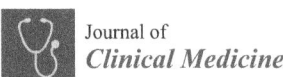

Review

Adherence and Persistence to Biological Drugs for Psoriasis: Systematic Review with Meta-Analysis

Eugenia Piragine [1,2], Davide Petri [3], Alma Martelli [1], Agata Janowska [4], Valentina Dini [4], Marco Romanelli [4], Vincenzo Calderone [1] and Ersilia Lucenteforte [3,*]

1. Department of Pharmacy, University of Pisa, 56126 Pisa, Italy; eugenia.piragine@farm.unipi.it (E.P.); alma.martelli@unipi.it (A.M.); vincenzo.calderone@unipi.it (V.C.)
2. School of Specialization in Hospital Pharmacy, University of Pisa, 56126 Pisa, Italy
3. Department of Clinical and Experimental Medicine, University of Pisa, 56126 Pisa, Italy; davide.petri@unipi.it
4. Department of Dermatology, University of Pisa, 56126 Pisa, Italy; agata.janowska@unipi.it (A.J.); valentina.dini@unipi.it (V.D.); marco.romanelli@unipi.it (M.R.)
* Correspondence: ersilia.lucenteforte@unipi.it; Tel.: +39-050-2218785

Abstract: Despite the large number of biologics currently available for moderate-to-severe psoriasis, poor adherence and persistence to therapy represent the main issues for both the clinical and economic management of psoriasis. However, the data about adherence and persistence to biologics in psoriasis patients are conflicting. Our aim was to produce summary estimates of adherence and persistence to biologics in adult patients with psoriasis. We performed a systematic review and meta-analysis of observational studies, searching two databases (PubMed and Embase). Sixty-two records met the inclusion criteria, and a meta-analysis was conducted on fifty-five studies. Overall, the proportion of adherent and persistent patients to biological therapy was 0.61 (95% confidence interval: 0.48–0.73) and 0.63 (0.57–0.68), respectively. The highest proportions were found for ustekinumab, while the lowest ones were found for etanercept. The proportions of adherence and persistence to biological drugs in psoriasis patients are sub-optimal. Notably, both proportions largely differ between drugs, suggesting that a more rational use of biologics might ensure better management of psoriasis.

Keywords: psoriasis; biological drugs; anti-TNF-α; anti-IL-17; anti-IL-12/23; adherence; persistence

1. Introduction

Psoriasis affects about 30 million adults worldwide [1]. Genetic factors, as well as lifestyle (smoking, alcohol consumption, and diet), certain drugs, environmental factors, and various metabolic conditions, can promote the development and progression of psoriasis [2,3]. Although the etiopathogenesis of psoriasis is multifactorial, its clinical manifestation mainly results from both uncontrolled keratinocyte proliferation and the overproduction of inflammatory mediators, such as tumor necrosis factor-α (TNF-α), interleukin (IL)-17, IL-12, and IL-23. In particular, the activation of these pro-inflammatory molecules triggers a vicious circle that progressively exacerbates psoriasis [2].

Due to its peculiar clinical manifestation, psoriasis has a negative psychological impact on patients, deeply affecting their quality of life [4]. Moreover, patients with psoriasis usually have several comorbidities that further aggravate their clinical condition [1]. Therefore, adequate pharmacological treatment might ameliorate both disease severity and, indirectly, the psychosocial sphere of the individual.

The therapeutic armamentarium currently available for the management of psoriasis is mainly represented by anti-inflammatory drugs and immunomodulators. In particular, topical (i.e., corticosteroids, vitamin D3 derivatives, and keratolytic products) and systemic drugs, such as methotrexate and retinoids, are commonly used in the mild-to-moderate forms of psoriasis, while targeted biological drugs are recommended for patients with severe forms who fail to respond to first-line therapy. TNF-α inhibitors were the first

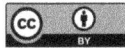

Citation: Piragine, E.; Petri, D.; Martelli, A.; Janowska, A.; Dini, V.; Romanelli, M.; Calderone, V.; Lucenteforte, E. Adherence and Persistence to Biological Drugs for Psoriasis: Systematic Review with Meta-Analysis. *J. Clin. Med.* **2022**, *11*, 1506. https://doi.org/10.3390/jcm11061506

Academic Editors: Mayumi Komine and Stamatis Gregoriou

Received: 4 February 2022
Accepted: 7 March 2022
Published: 9 March 2022

Publisher's Note: MDPI stays neutral with regard to jurisdictional claims in published maps and institutional affiliations.

Copyright: © 2022 by the authors. Licensee MDPI, Basel, Switzerland. This article is an open access article distributed under the terms and conditions of the Creative Commons Attribution (CC BY) license (https://creativecommons.org/licenses/by/4.0/).

biologics to obtain marketing authorization and reimbursement for psoriasis, and they include etanercept (ETN), infliximab (INF), and adalimumab (ADA) [5]. Other biologics are IL17A inhibitors (ixekizumab, IXE; secukinumab, SECU) [6] and ustekinumab (UST), which is an anti-IL12/23 human monoclonal antibody [7].

Despite the large number of therapeutic options for the clinical management of psoriasis, two key contributors to both treatment failure and scarce relapse control are poor adherence and persistence to therapy. Adherence reflects "the extent to which a patient acts in accordance with the prescribed interval, and dose of a dosing regimen", while persistence, also known as drug survival, is "the duration of time from initiation to discontinuation of therapy" [8]. In addition, suboptimal adherence and persistence deeply impact the economic management of psoriasis in healthcare systems [9], especially for the more expensive drugs (i.e., biologics). Therefore, improving medication-taking behaviors may help patients to better control therapy, as well as limiting the economic health expenditure. Currently, the data about adherence and persistence to biological therapy in psoriasis patients are scarce and conflicting, and previous systematic reviews, although quite recent [8,10], do not provide an exhaustive and quantitative synthesis of the literature. Moreover, real-world data about adherence and persistence to individual biologics are discordant, thus hindering the rational use of these drugs in clinical practice.

Hence, the aim of this systematic review and meta-analysis is to provide overall, updated adherence and persistence proportions to biologics, as well as reporting a stratification of results based on the individual biological drugs.

2. Materials and Methods

The protocol for this systematic review and meta-analysis was registered in the PROSPERO database (CRD42021245065).

2.1. Eligibility Criteria

We included prospective, retrospective, and cross-sectional observational studies evaluating adherence and persistence (or drug survival) to biologic drugs among participants aged 18 years or older with psoriasis. We considered studies irrespective of patient gender, comorbidities, or concomitant drugs. Biological drugs belonging to the following 3 classes were considered: TNF-α inhibitors (ETN, ADA, INF); IL17A inhibitors (IXE, SECU); and IL12/23 inhibitors (UST). The outcomes were adherence and persistence to biologics, as reported in the included studies.

2.2. Information Sources and Search Strategy

We searched Medline and EMBASE for studies published from inception to 18 January 2021. The search strategy (Supplementary Material S1) reports psoriasis as the first term; drug or therapy adherence, persistence, compliance, and switching as the second term; and the considered biologic drugs as the third term (etanercept, ustekinumab, adalimumab, infliximab, ixekizumab, and secukinumab). The three terms were combined using the Boolean operator "AND".

2.3. Selection Process

Titles and abstracts of papers identified by the search strategy were screened by two authors independently, E.P. and D.P. Each paper was categorized as not relevant or potentially included according to the eligibility criteria. Any disagreement was discussed with another author, E.L.

The full text of the potentially includible articles was retrieved or, if not available, directly requested from the authors of the study. Two authors (E.P. and D.P.) checked the full texts for the eligibility criteria and excluded studies not fitting them.

The selection process was managed using bibliographic management software Mendeley Desktop (v1.19.6, Mendeley Ltd., London, UK).

2.4. Data Extraction Process

We extracted the following information: study design, outcome (adherence or persistence), and objective; number and general characteristics of participants included in the studies, such as age, gender, comorbidities, and concomitant drugs (drugs used for the treatment of psoriasis, as well as other drugs); definition of adherence/persistence as reported in the study; number of adherent/persistent patients; and reasons for discontinuation/switching. Furthermore, the data relating to any stratifications were retrieved. The data extraction was carried out by two authors independently, E.P. and D.P., and any discrepancies were resolved through consultation with a third reviewer, E.L.

For the data collection, spreadsheet software Microsoft Excel was used (version 2102 build 13801.20864).

2.5. Study Risk of Bias Assessment

The methodological quality of included studies was assessed according to risk of bias in prevalence studies developed by Hoy et al. [11]. The tool considers ten domains concerning characteristics of prevalence studies, each rated in terms of risk of bias and applicability to research question. Risk of bias was judged from 0 (high risk) to 10 (low risk). The risk of bias was evaluated by two authors independently, E.P. and D.P., and any discrepancies were resolved through consultation with a third reviewer, E.L.

2.6. Effect Measures

We evaluated the study-specific prevalence of adherence or persistence (drug survival) to biologics by calculating the proportion of adherent or persistent subjects on the total number of participants for each study. Where the study provided adherence/persistence as a percentage or where the non-adherence/non-persistence was provided, appropriate calculations were performed.

2.7. Synthesis Methods

As adherence and persistence refer to two different concepts that cannot be matched and pooled, we separately analyzed these parameters, as previously reported by others [12]. In detail, three outcomes were evaluated in our meta-analysis: (1) adherence; (2) good adherence, generally reported as the medication possession ratio (MPR) or proportion of days covered (PDC) $\geq 80\%$; and (3) persistence.

Study-specific means of adherence were pooled using random effect models and the generic inverse variance method. Study-specific adherence/persistence proportions were pooled using random effect models with Freeman–Tukey transformation.

The heterogeneity for both methods was quantified through the Higgins heterogeneity index (I^2) and was tested through the chi-square test for mean adherence and Cochran's Q test for adherence/persistence proportion.

Subgroup analyses were conducted according to study design (retrospective observational, prospective observational, or cross-sectional), type of biologics, the type of biologic users (biological-naïve subjects, i.e., subjects who have never used a biological drug, and biological-experienced subjects, i.e., subjects who have already had experience with this type of treatment), and study quality (high quality, score ≥ 8, vs. low quality, score < 8). Differences between groups was considered statistically significant if the heterogeneity test was significant.

p-value < 0.10 was considered statistically significant.

The "metagen" and "metaprop" routines within the META package in R (version 4.12) was used for analyses [13].

3. Results

3.1. Systematic Review

A flowchart of the search is presented in Figure 1. We identified 1285 records from the PUBMED search and 2698 from EMBASE. In total, 62 studies, including 169,371 participants, met the inclusion criteria and were included in the qualitative synthesis. Three studies [14–16] did not show data on persistence or the number of persistent patients, while one did not show data on adherence [17]; two studies were conducted on patients not only affected by psoriasis [18,19] and did not report adherence data for psoriasis patients; one study [20] did not report the number of patients treated with each biological drug but only adherence as percentage. Fifty-five studies [21–75] on 161,748 participants were included in the quantitative synthesis (meta-analyses).

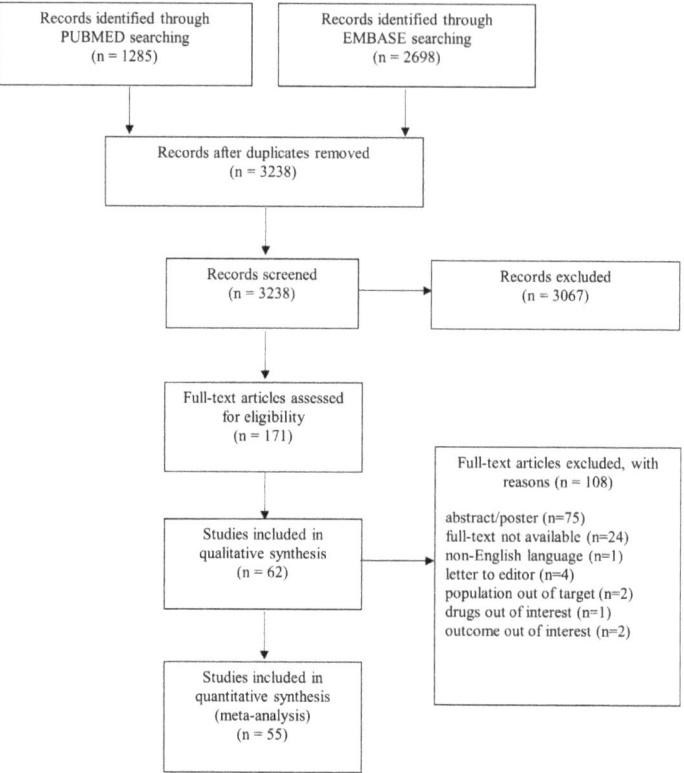

Figure 1. Flowchart of search.

In 13 studies [24,25,28,32,34,35,38,39,55,64,66,70,75], the sample was composed of patients with other chronic inflammatory autoimmune conditions, including osteoarticular diseases (such as ankylosing spondylitis and rheumatoid arthritis), bowel diseases (such as ulcerative colitis and Crohn's disease), and psoriatic arthritis. The extraction of data, in this case, focused on the cohorts of patients suffering from psoriasis regardless of other conditions.

Among the included studies (Table 1), 5 studies presented data on adherence [22,27, 33,44,53], 16 studies on good adherence [21,25–27,32,33,35,40,44,46,49,53,63,68,71,73], 46 studies on persistence data [21,23–25,27–31,33,34,36–39,41–45,47–62,64–70,72,74,75], and 8 studies reported data on both adherence and persistence [21,25,27,33,44,49,53,68]. Regarding study design (Table S1), 51 were retrospective cohort studies [15,18,19,21–49,51–57,59–62,64,66–68,70,72,74,75], 5 were prospective cohort studies [14,50,58,65,69], and 6 were cross-sectional studies [16,17,20,63,71,73]. The mean age of the participants was 47 years, of which about 45% were female. Thirty-two studies reported no use of concomitant drugs [14, 16–19,21,23–26,28–31,34,37,39,42,51,52,55,58,61,62,64,67,68,70,71,73,75]. Twenty-four studies presented data on biological-naïve patients [26–32,37–39,41,43,46,48,50,51,53,55,60,61,

66,68,74,75], while four studies [37,39,50,75] reported data on biological-experienced patients. Twenty-eight studies reported data on ADA adherence/persistence [26,27,29, 31–33,35,36,39,40,48–53,55,61,63–70,74,75], fifteen on INF [27,29,36,39,47,49,50,52,53,55,57, 64,67,70,75], twenty-five on ETN [22,26,27,29–32,36,39,40,48–53,55,56,63,66–68,70,74,75], four on IXE [28,33,44,54], ten on SECU [24,28,32,34,44,59,61,68–70], and twenty-one on UST [23,26,27,31,32,39,40,48,50,51,53,60,61,63,64,67–70,72,75]. Finally, forty-five studies were included in biological drug subgroup analysis [21,23,24,26–36,39,40,42–44,46–56,59–61,63–70,72–75] and twenty-eight in experienced/naïve subgroup analysis [26–32,35,37–39,41,43,46,48,50,51,53,55,60,61,66,68,74,75].

Table 1. Details of calculation methods in considered outcomes.

	No. of Studies (No. of Patients)
Adherence	
MPR/PDC mean	
during a period of 12 months	2 (4832) [27,53]
during a period of >12 months	3 (6297) [22,33,44]
Good adherence	
MPR/PDC ≥ 80%	
during a period of 12 months	6 (29,256) [25–27,49,53,68]
during a period of >12 months	5 (11,516) [32,33,35,40,44]
Other definitions during different or not-specified periods [a]	5 (4480) [21,46,63,71,73]
Persistence	
No discontinuation or gap [a] or switch	
during a period of <12 months	2 (1179) [23,72]
during a period of 12 months	24 (114,864) [24,27,28,31,37–39,43,45,48,49,51,53–55,60–62,64–66,68,74,75]
during a period of >12 months	11 (24,246) [29,33,34,41,42,44,50,56,58,59,67,69]
during a not-specified period	1 (84) [52]
Still on treatment	
after a period of <12 months	1 (378) [25]
after a period of 12 months or more	4 (2336) [30,36,47,57]
Other definitions during different or not-specified periods	2 (13,714) [21,70]

[a] different permissible gaps (from 7 to 150 days).

Table 1 shows details on adherence, good adherence, and persistence. The measures were highly heterogeneous: 5 studies gave the mean of adherence using MPR or PDC measures defined during different periods; 16 studies gave the proportion of adherent patients by mainly using (11 out of 16) the cut-off of 80% of MPR or PDC measures defined during different periods; 46 gave the proportion of persistent patients by mainly using (38 out of 64) discontinuation or switch or no gap (from 7 to 150 days) concepts defined during different periods.

3.2. Risk of Bias in Studies

Seventeen studies [18,25–27,32,39,45,46,48,49,53,59,61,62,67–69] obtained a total score of 10 in quality assessment based on the scale of Hoy et al. [11], while three studies [34,42,73] scored less or equal than 6 points. Details on single domains can be found in Table S2.

3.3. Results of Synthesis

3.3.1. Adherence

The meta-analysis conducted on five studies including 11,129 patients showed a mean adherence of 65% (95% confidence interval, CI: 61–70%, Figure S1) with considerable heterogeneity (I^2 = 99%). Among 16 studies including 45,252 patients, the proportion of good adherence was 61% (48–73, Figure 2), with considerable heterogeneity (I^2 = 100.0%). Only 2 out of 16 studies reported the reasons for non-adherence, which were loss of efficacy and adverse events. Qualitative descriptions of the reasons are shown in Table S3.

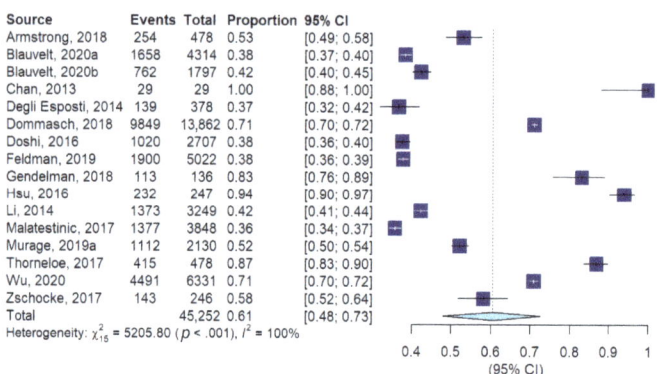

Figure 2. Forest plot of proportions, and their 95% confidence intervals, of adherent patients.

Regarding the stratification according to the type of biologic drug, the highest adherence proportion (Table 2, Figures 3 and 4) was observed for UST (72%, 48–91), followed by INF (63%, 44–80), ADA (62%, 47–76), SECU (52%, 35–68), ETN (50%, 36–65), and, finally, IXE (46%, 43–48). The difference between groups was statistically significant (p-value = 0.04). ADA, ETN, and UST represent the three biological drugs most considered in the included studies, as the use of each of them was evaluated in a considerable number of studies compared to the others: 10 studies for the first drug [26,27,32,33,35,40,49,53,63,68], 8 for the second [26,27,32,40,49,53,63,68], and 7 for the third [26,27,32,40,53,63,68].

Table 2. Pooled proportions of adherent patients stratified according to study design, type of biological drug, and type of patient.

	No. of Studies	No. of Patients	Adherence, % [CI 95%]	I^2	Q	p-Value for Heterogeneity within Strata	p-Value for Heterogeneity between Strata
Overall	16	45,252	61 [48; 73]	99.7%	5205.80	0	
Study design							
Cross-sectional	3	753	85 [55; 100]	98%	89.03	<0.0001	0.06
Retrospective cohort	13	44,499	54 [43; 66]	100%	4905.70	<0.0001	
Biological drug							
ADA	10	19,340	62 [47; 76]	100.0%	2263.54	0	
ETN	8	11,376	50 [36; 65]	100.0%	1444.93	<0.0001	
INF	3	650	63 [44; 80]	94.0%	33.15	<0.0001	
UST	7	6179	72 [48; 91]	99.0%	1087.17	<0.0001	0.04
IXE	2	1291	46 [43; 48]	0.0%	0.28	0.5976	
SECU	3	2036	52 [35; 68]	98.0%	128.11	<0.0001	
Not specified	5	4380	61 [33; 85]	97.0%	129.88	<0.0001	
Type of patient							
Biological naïve	6	33,301	52 [39; 65]	99.8%	3107.32	0	0.29
Not specified	12	12,912	63 [47; 78]	99.1%	1198.03	<0.0001	

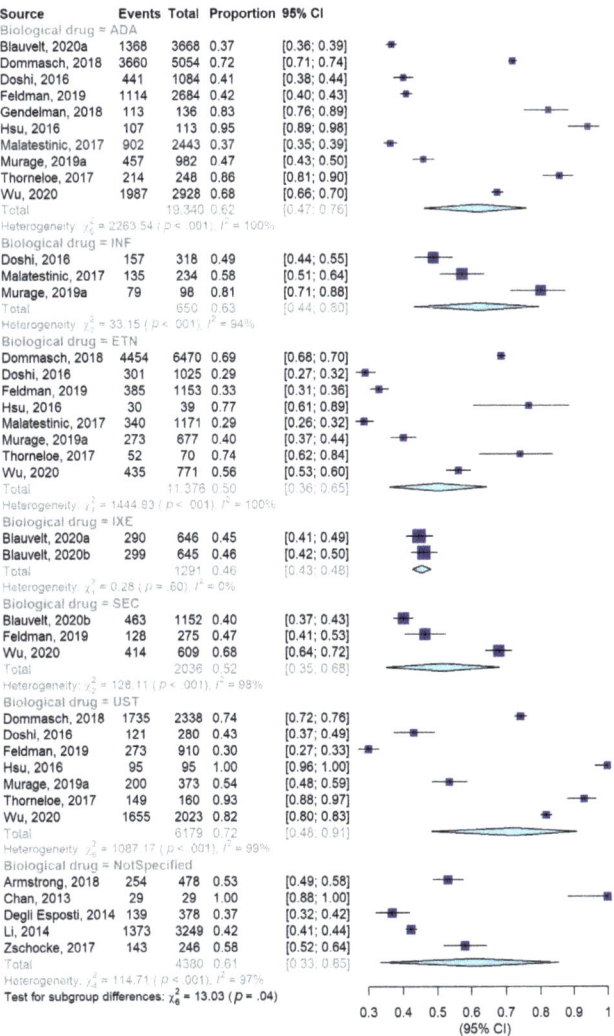

Figure 3. Forest plot of proportions, and their 95% confidence intervals, of adherent patients stratified according to biological drugs.

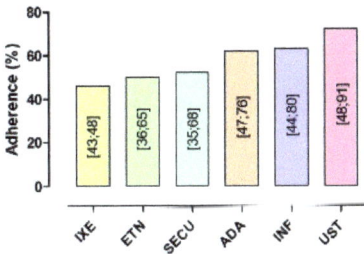

Figure 4. Percentage of adherent patients according to biological drugs. Confidence intervals (95%) are reported within the vertical bars.

There were differences stratifying by study design, with the cross-sectional design (85%; 55–100) showing a higher adherence compared to the retrospective cohort design (54%; 43–66) (*p*-value from subgroup test = 0.06) (Table 2 and Figure S2); however, only 3 studies had a cross-sectional design in contrast with 13 retrospective cohort studies. There were no differences stratifying by biological-naïve patients and not-specified patients (*p*-value = 0.24) (Table 2 and Figure S3) or stratifying by risk of bias (*p*-value = 0.40) (Figure S4).

3.3.2. Persistence

The meta-analysis conducted on 46 studies including 156,801 patients showed a persistence proportion of 63% (57–68, Figure 5), with considerable heterogeneity (I^2 = 100%). Less than half of the studies (19 out of 46) reported the reasons for drug discontinuation or switching. The most common reasons were loss of efficacy and adverse events (nine studies) followed by ineffectiveness (three studies). Qualitative descriptions of the reasons are shown in Table S3.

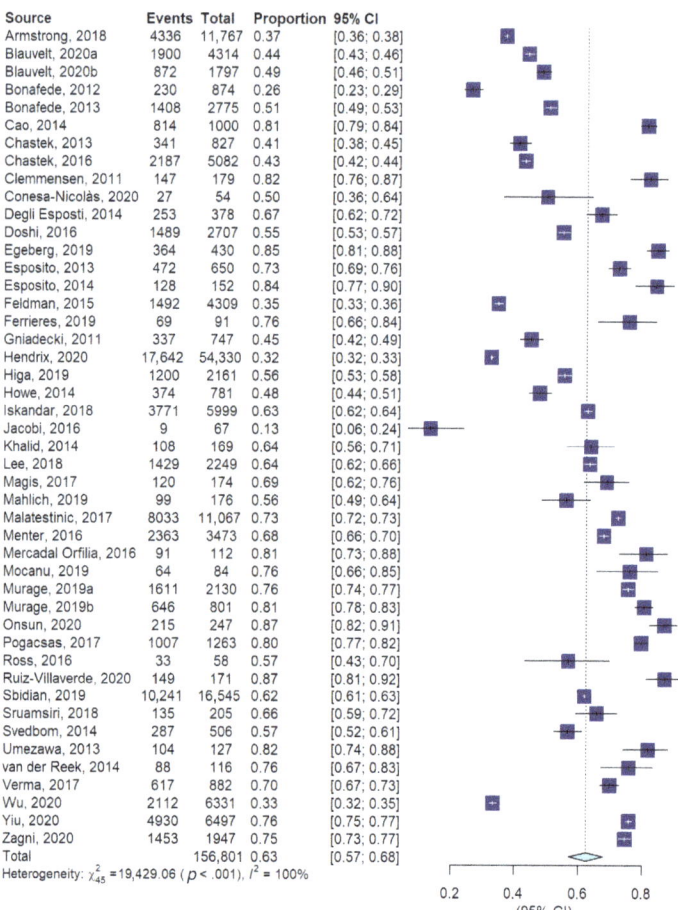

Figure 5. Forest plot of proportions, and their 95% confidence intervals, of persistent patients.

Regarding the stratification according to the type of biological drug, the highest persistence (Table 3, Figures 6 and 7) was found for UST (77%, 70–84), followed by SECU (72%, 58–84), IXE (70%, 52–85), INF (64%, 60–68), ADA (57%, 50–63), and ETN (53%, 42–65).

The heterogeneity between groups was statistically significant (p-value < 0.01). ADA, ETN, and UST represent the three biological drugs most considered in the included studies, as the use of each of them was evaluated in a considerable number of studies compared to the others: 22 studies for the first drug [29,31,36,39,48,50–52,55,61,64–67,69,70,74,75], 19 for the second [29–31,36,39,48,50–52,55,56,66,67,70,74,75], and 17 for the third [23,31,39,48,50, 51,60,61,64,67,69,70,72,75].

Table 3. Pooled proportions of persistent patients stratified according to study design, type of biological drug, and type of patient.

	No. of Studies	No. of Patients	Persistence, %, [CI 95%]	I^2	Q	p-Value for Heterogeneity within Strata	p-Value for Heterogeneity between Strata
Overall	46	156,801	63 [57; 68]	100.0%	19,429.06	0	
Study design							
Retrospective cohort	42	146,657	62 [56; 68]	100.0%	16,496.95	0	0.07
Prospective cohort	4	10,144	71 [63; 77]	96.1%	76.69	<0.001	
Biological drug							
ADA	22	21,176	57 [50; 63]	99.0%	2428.85	0	
ETN	19	12,914	53 [42; 65]	99.0%	2770.05	0	
INF	14	1465	64 [60; 68]	56.0%	29.85	0.0049	
UST	17	11,869	77 [70; 84]	98.0%	1045.48	<0.001	<0.001
IXE	4	2155	70 [52; 85]	98.0%	176.12	<0.001	
SECU	9	3053	72 [58; 84]	99.0%	585.42	<0.001	
Not specified	12	90,014	55 [44; 66]	100.0%	9286.07	0	
Type of patient							
Biological naïve	21	66,821	56 [49; 64]	100.0%	5408.54	0	
Biological experienced	4	43,097	50 [35; 65]	100.0%	1638.78	<0.001	0.05
Not specified	25	46,583	67 [60; 74]	100.0%	5961.35	0	

Different persistence proportions (p-value from heterogeneity test = 0.05) were observed among 21 studies on biological-naïve patients (56%, 49–64), 4 studies on biological-experienced patients (50%, 35–65), and 25 studies where it was not specified (67%, 60–74) (Table 3 and Figure S5). There were also statistical differences in study design stratification (p-value from subgroup test = 0.07) (Table 3 and Figure S6). However, only 4 studies had a cross-sectional design in contrast with 42 retrospective cohort studies. There were no statistical differences in the risk of bias stratification (p-value = 0.78) (Figure S7).

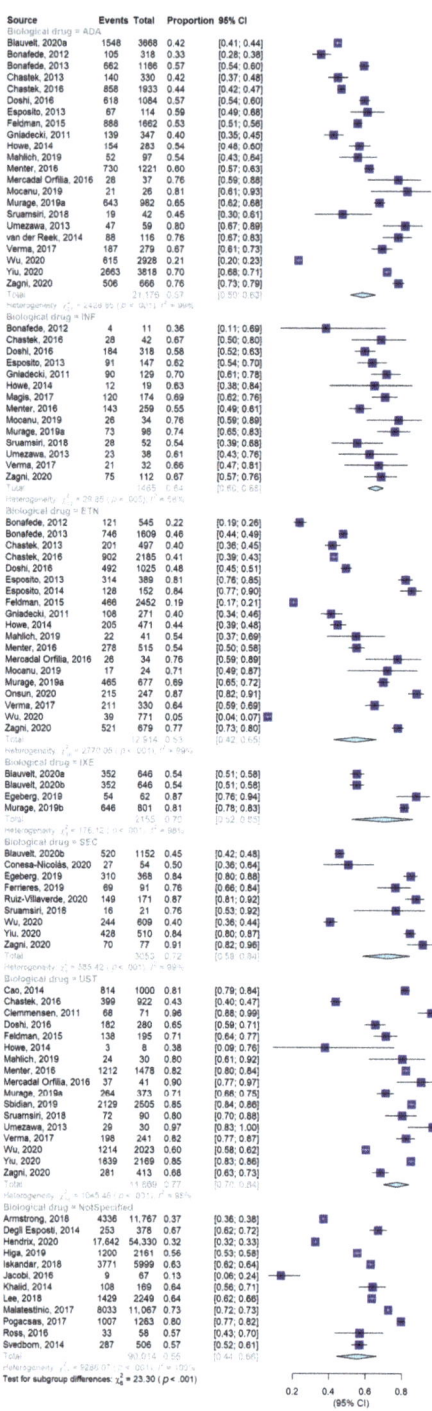

Figure 6. Forest plot of proportions, and their 95% confidence intervals, of persistent patients stratified according to biological drugs.

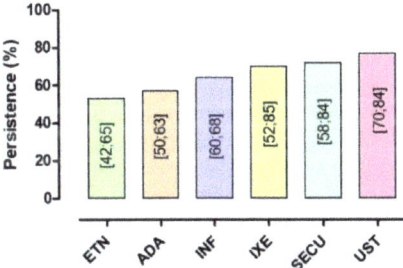

Figure 7. Percentage of persistent patients according to biological drugs. Confidence intervals (95%) are reported within vertical bars.

4. Discussion

We systematically reviewed data from 55 studies including 161,748 psoriatic patients and showed that 61% of patients were adherent to biologic therapy and 63% were persistent. Our findings are consistent with those reported in previous studies. In a systematic review on inflammatory bowel disease [76], 23–62% of patients were found adherent to biologics. Another systematic review on rheumatoid arthritis [77] reported a median adherence value of 63% for both ETN and ADA. Finally, two recent meta-analyses on psoriasis showed that 66% of patients were persistent at 1 year [78] and 53.2% at two years [79].

In the studies included in our systematic review, the main reported reasons for drug discontinuation, switching, or non-adherence were loss of efficacy and adverse events. However, many other aspects could affect the patient's behavior toward biological therapy. The female gender, recent disease onset, smoking, the presence of comorbidities, and a lack of efficacy of the previous treatments have been reported as predictors of non-persistence/non-adherence [42,71,80–82]. On the contrary, the presence of psoriatic arthritis has been generally associated with sustained drug survival of biological agents [69,81].

The variability in the included studies is reflected in the heterogeneity of our analysis. We found that biological-naïve patients were more persistent than biological-experienced patients. However, only four studies evaluated persistence in biological-experienced patients. Moreover, we observed a high percentage of adherent and persistent patients among cross-sectional and prospective cohort studies, respectively, compared to retrospective cohort ones. This is expected, even if only three studies evaluating adherence had a cross-sectional design and four studies evaluating persistence had a prospective cohort design. We did not investigate whether the inclusion of different definitions of the concepts of adherence and persistence influenced our results because few studies used the same definition. This represents a limitation of our study, as well as other meta-analyses aimed at pooling adherence and persistence. The proposal of a unified set of definitions might be useful to make the results of future studies more consistent and comparable [83].

At present, the data about adherence and persistence to individual biological drugs are quite scarce. This evaluation is essential to guide clinicians toward a more rational therapeutic choice, which is fundamental for both medical and economic purposes. In our study, the highest adherence was found for the human antibody UST (72%), followed by INF (63%), ADA (62%), SECU (52%), ETN (50%), and IXE (46%). Similar proportions were found for persistence as, in descending order, they were UST with 77%, SECU with 72%, IXE with 70%, INF with 64%, ADA with 57%, and ETN with 53%.

The variability in both adherence and persistence to specific biologics could derive, to a minimal extent, from the differences in the efficacy of treatments, which can reasonably affect patients' satisfaction and, consequently, adherence/persistence to therapy. Future studies are required to elucidate on comparative efficacy because few data derived from direct "head-to-head" comparisons, and short-term efficacy outcomes were mainly evaluated [84–87]. A role for body mass index (BMI) in the patient's attitude toward biological treatment has been recently proposed [88,89]. Indeed, the efficacy of TNF-α inhibitors and

UST is reduced in obese/overweight patients with psoriasis [90–92], with consequences for both adherence and persistence [93,94].

The difference between adherence and persistence to biological therapies can be certainly explained by discussing the origin, therapeutic class, administration route and timing, and toxicity profile of the biologics. Firstly, the immunogenic potential of chimeric antibodies (i.e., INF) might cause acute anaphylactic reactions following infusion, as well as hypersensitivity reactions (such as influenza-like syndrome, local skin reactions, and pyrexia) [95]. These phenomena can be counteracted with concomitant immunosuppressive therapy, with serious consequences on patient compliance and medication adherence/persistence [96]. On the contrary, pharmacological treatment with fully human antibodies (ADA, SECU, and UST) is less associated with anti-drug antibody production, although residual immunogenicity has been reported even for the most innovative biological drugs [97].

All biological drugs share the common risk of mild-to-moderate adverse events, including headache, cutaneous and upper respiratory tract infections, and injection site reactions, which can dramatically reduce quality of life [98]. Generally, these reactions do not require additional therapy, but they can be prevented by combining biological drugs with immunomodulators [99], with predictable detrimental effects on the patient's compliance. Notably, TNF-α inhibitors are generally associated with a higher risk of severe infections, and they can induce hypersensitivity reactions [100] and dermatological disorders [101]. Hence, the peculiar toxicity profile of TNF-α inhibitors might explain, at least in part, the sub-optimal medication adherence to ETN, ADA, and INF in psoriatic patients.

Among the TNF-α inhibitors, ETN is self-administered using pre-filled syringes or pens up to twice a week. Both self-administration and short intervals between administrations might reduce compliance [102]. ADA is administered subcutaneously every 2 weeks. Therefore, the interval between administrations is longer than that reported for ETN, partially justifying the better adherence and persistence proportions to ADA rather than ETN. Finally, INF is intravenously administered at weeks 0, 2, and 6 after initiation and then at an 8- to 12-week interval [103]. The outpatient administration of INF ensures periodic support is provided to psoriasis patients, as well as contributing to a more assiduous monitoring of therapy by clinicians. Importantly, patients with scheduled appointments do not forget to take drugs, and they do not make mistakes, which instead can occur in self-administered therapy.

Concerning IL17A inhibitors, SECU is self-administered once a week for 4 weeks and then every 4 weeks [104], while IXE is self-administered every 2 weeks for the first 12 weeks and then once a month [105].

The highest adherence and persistence proportions were found for the IL12/23 inhibitor UST (72% for adherence and 77% for persistence). UST is characterized by high efficacy in the treatment of moderate-to-severe forms of psoriasis [106] and a favorable safety profile [107]. Moreover, it is administered every 12 weeks, exclusively under the guidance of an experienced physician. Both the longest administration interval and the supervision of a healthcare provider might favorably impact adherence and persistence [108]. The subcutaneous administration of UST using pre-filled syringes or pens might also explain the wide difference in the adherence and persistence proportions from another biological drug administered in hospitals or clinics, namely, INF (63% vs. 64%, respectively). Indeed, the latter therapy requires a slow 2 h infusion followed by an additional monitoring period of 2 h; it is a demotivating protocol that might partially contribute to scarce medication adherence and persistence.

In accordance with our findings, a comparative meta-analysis showed that UST has the longest persistence at 5 years after initiation compared with TNF-α inhibitors (ETN, ADA, and INF) [79]. In a meta-analysis of real-world evidence, UST appeared as the biological drug less frequently discontinued due to loss of efficacy [78], thus confirming its clinical relevance in the pharmacological treatment of psoriasis. On the contrary, ETN showed the worst persistence and the highest number of therapy interruptions for low efficacy, supporting the results of our meta-analysis.

Even if UST is one of the most expensive biological drugs, it is endowed with one of the most favorable cost-efficacy profiles among the biological drugs for psoriasis [109]. Indeed, both sustained adherence and persistence and a sporadic dose regimen reduce the direct costs of treatment in the long term [110], but great attention should be paid to obese patients requiring high dosage [111]. In addition, UST is associated with minor indirect costs for the healthcare system, as it reduces hospital visits for non-responders; treatment failure; and resultant drug switching, which is associated with a 7–17% increase in annual costs [112]. There are, however, some crucial aspects that must be considered before initiating biological therapy with UST. Of course, UST must be avoided in patients with hypersensitivity to this biological drug or any of the excipients [110]. Moreover, health insurance coverage does not apply in all cases in real clinical practice. This latter aspect is reported to be responsible for short-term intermittent treatment with UST [113], as uninsured patients cannot afford the economic burden of continuous treatment with this biologic drug. Hence, the expansion of insurance coverage might ameliorate both patients' satisfaction and adherence/persistence toward biological therapy. Finally, patient preferences should also be considered before starting therapy with UST, as involving patients in treatment decisions can influence both adherence to treatment and the outcomes of therapy [114].

5. Conclusions

The adherence and persistence to biological therapy in psoriasis patients are suboptimal; however, the initial therapeutic choice might be crucial to ensure better medication adherence/persistence. Psoriasis patients are more adherent and persistent to therapies with a favorable safety profile and that are characterized by less frequent administrations (i.e., UST). However, several aspects regarding comorbidities, insurance coverage, patient preferences, and costs must be considered before initiating therapy with UST. We suggest that constant real-life therapeutic discussions between health providers (dermatologists, general practitioners, pharmacists, and nurses) and their patients, as well as specific support programs, might promote the optimal levels of adherence and persistence to biological drugs for both clinical and economic purposes.

Our study has several strengths, including the high number of studies identified and the large sample size, which gives consistency to the results. Our study also has some limitations, such as having considered work from all over the world; therefore, it cannot be excluded that adherence and persistence to treatment may have a link with reimbursement policies that vary from country to country. In addition, the follow-up period was variable from study to study, although most papers were aligned in considering 12 months as the follow-up period. We are also aware that we had to exclude some studies because of the lack of usable data, even though they met all inclusion and exclusion criteria. The age and sex of the participants could influence adherence/persistence; however, in the studies included in our meta-analysis, patients were very similar in terms of age and sex. Finally, although we included all drugs approved before May 2021 (data of our literature search) to manage moderate-to-severe psoriasis, we did not include studies investigating new groups of drugs, for example, selective inhibitors of IL-23 in a recently published study [115], and this represents a limitation of our systematic review.

Supplementary Materials: The following supporting information can be downloaded at: https://www.mdpi.com/article/10.3390/jcm11061506/s1, Supplementary Material S1: Search strategy; Table S1: Summary of findings of included studies; Table S2. Risk of bias for prevalence studies; Figure S1: Forest plot of mean adherence; Table S3: Qualitative description of the main reasons for biological drug discontinuation or switching; Figure S2: Forest plot of proportions of adherent patients with psoriasis to biological drugs stratified by study design; Figure S3: Forest plot of proportions of adherent patients with psoriasis to biological drugs stratified by type of patient; Figure S4: Forest plot of proportions of adherent patients with psoriasis to biological drugs stratified by risk of bias; Figure S5: Forest plot of proportions of prevalent patients with psoriasis to biological drugs stratified by type of patient; Figure S6: Forest plot of proportions of prevalent patients with psoriasis to biological drugs stratified by study design; Figure S7: Forest plot of proportions of prevalent patients with psoriasis to biological drugs stratified by risk of bias.

Author Contributions: Conceptualization, A.M., V.C. and E.L.; methodology, D.P. and E.L.; formal analysis, D.P. and E.L.; data curation, E.P. and D.P.; writing—original draft preparation, E.P. and D.P.; writing—review and editing, E.P., D.P., A.M., A.J., V.D., M.R., V.C. and E.L.; supervision, V.C. and E.L. All authors have read and agreed to the published version of the manuscript.

Funding: This research was funded by the University research project PRA 2020–2022 #PRA_2020_57.

Institutional Review Board Statement: Not applicable.

Informed Consent Statement: Not applicable.

Data Availability Statement: The data that support the findings of this study are available from the corresponding author upon reasonable request.

Acknowledgments: This work is dedicated to the memory of the Corrado Blandizzi, who spent his life dedicated to experimental teaching and research.

Conflicts of Interest: E.L. was involved as an investigator of an observational study funded by the pharmaceutical company Galapagos in compliance with the ENCEPP Code of Conduct. E.L. has carried out consultancy for Angelini. E.P., D.P., A.M. and V.C. have no relevant or non-financial interest to disclose.

References

1. Parisi, R.; Iskandar, I.Y.K.; Kontopantelis, E.; Augustin, M.; Griffiths, C.E.M.; Ashcroft, D.M. National, regional, and worldwide epidemiology of psoriasis: Systematic analysis and modelling study. *BMJ* **2020**, *369*, m1590. [CrossRef] [PubMed]
2. Kamiya, K.; Kishimoto, M.; Sugai, J.; Komine, M.; Ohtsuki, M. Risk factors for the development of psoriasis. *Int. J. Mol. Sci.* **2019**, *20*, 4347. [CrossRef] [PubMed]
3. Ito, T.; Takahashi, H.; Kawada, A.; Iizuka, H.; Nakagawa, H. Epidemiological survey from 2009 to 2012 of psoriatic patients in Japanese Society for Psoriasis Research. *J. Dermatol.* **2018**, *45*, 251–333. [CrossRef] [PubMed]
4. Bhosle, M.J.; Kulkarni, A.; Feldman, S.R.; Balkrishnan, R. Quality of life in patients with psoriasis. *Health Qual. Life Outcomes* **2006**, *4*, 35. [CrossRef]
5. Silva, L.C.R.; Ortigosa, L.C.M.; Benard, G. Anti-TNF-α agents in the treatment of immune-mediated inflammatory diseases: Mechanisms of action and pitfalls. *Immunotherapy* **2010**, *2*, 817–833. [CrossRef]
6. Giunta, A.; Ventura, A.; Chimenti, M.S.; Bianchi, L.; Esposito, M. Spotlight on ixekizumab for the treatment of moderate-to-severe plaque psoriasis: Design, development, and use in therapy. *Drug Des. Devel. Ther.* **2017**, *2017*, 1643–1651. [CrossRef]
7. Ergen, E.N.; Yusuf, N. Inhibition of interleukin-12 and/or interleukin-23 for the treatment of psoriasis: What is the evidence for an effect on malignancy? *Exp. Dermatol.* **2018**, *27*, 737–747. [CrossRef]
8. Belinchón, I.; Rivera, R.; Blanch, C.; Comellas, M.; Lizán, L. Adherence, satisfaction and preferences for treatment in patients with psoriasis in the European union: A systematic review of the literature. *Patient Prefer. Adherence* **2016**, *10*, 2357–2367. [CrossRef]
9. De Vera, M.A.; Mailman, J.; Galo, J.S. Economics of Non-Adherence to Biologic Therapies in Rheumatoid Arthritis. *Curr. Rheumatol. Rep.* **2014**, *16*, 460. [CrossRef]
10. Aleshaki, J.S.; Cardwell, L.A.; Muse, M.E.; Feldman, S.R. Adherence and resource use among psoriasis patients treated with biologics. *Expert Rev. Pharm. Outcomes Res.* **2018**, *18*, 609–617. [CrossRef]
11. Hoy, D.; Brooks, P.; Woolf, A.; Blyth, F.; March, L.; Bain, C.; Baker, P.; Smith, E.; Buchbinder, R. Assessing risk of bias in prevalence studies: Modification of an existing tool and evidence of interrater agreement. *J. Clin. Epidemiol.* **2012**, *65*, 934–939. [CrossRef] [PubMed]
12. Ozaki, A.F.; Choi, A.S.; Le, Q.T.; Ko, D.T.; Han, J.K.; Park, S.S.; Jackevicius, C.A. Real-World Adherence and Persistence to Direct Oral Anticoagulants in Patients with Atrial Fibrillation: A Systematic Review and Meta-Analysis. *Circ. Cardiovasc. Qual. Outcomes* **2020**, *13*, e005969. [CrossRef] [PubMed]
13. Balduzzi, S.; Rücker, G.; Schwarzer, G. How to perform a meta-analysis with R: A practical tutorial. *Evid. Based Ment. Health* **2019**, *22*, 153–160. [CrossRef] [PubMed]
14. Dávila-Seijo, P.; Dauden, E.; Carretero, G.; Ferrandiz, C.; Vanaclocha, F.; Gómez-García, F.-J.; Herrera-Ceballos, E.; De la Cueva-Dobao, P.; Belinchón, I.; Sánchez-Carazo, J.-L.; et al. Survival of classic and biological systemic drugs in psoriasis: Results of the BIOBADADERM registry and critical analysis. *J. Eur. Acad. Dermatol. Venereol.* **2016**, *30*, 1942–1950. [CrossRef]
15. Gniadecki, R.; Bang, B.; Bryld, L.E.; Iversen, L.; Lasthein, S.; Skov, L. Comparison of long-term drug survival and safety of biologic agents in patients with psoriasis vulgaris. *Br. J. Dermatol.* **2015**, *172*, 244–252. [CrossRef]

16. Yeung, H.; Wan, J.; Van Voorhees, A.S.; Callis Duffin, K.; Krueger, G.G.; Kalb, R.E.; Weisman, J.D.; Sperber, B.R.; Brod, B.A.; Schleicher, S.M.; et al. Patient-reported reasons for the discontinuation of commonly used treatments for moderate to severe psoriasis. *J. Am. Acad. Dermatol.* **2013**, *68*, 64–72. [CrossRef]
17. Wang, Q.; Luo, Y.; Lv, C.; Zheng, X.; Zhu, W.; Chen, X.; Shen, M.; Kuang, Y. Nonadherence to Treatment and Patient-Reported Outcomes of Psoriasis During the COVID-19 Epidemic: A Web-Based Survey. *Patient Prefer. Adherence* **2020**, *14*, 1403–1409. [CrossRef]
18. Bergman, M.; Patel, P.; Chen, N.; Jing, Y.; Saffore, C.D. Evaluation of Adherence and Persistence Differences Between Adalimumab Citrate-Free and Citrate Formulations for Patients with Immune-Mediated Diseases in the United States. *Rheumatol. Ther.* **2020**, *8*, 109–118. [CrossRef]
19. Marshall, J.K.; Bessette, L.; Shear, N.H.; Lebovic, G.; Glass, J.; Millson, B.; Gaetano, T.; Gazel, S.; Latour, M.G.; Laliberté, M.-C.; et al. Canada's Study of Adherence Outcomes in Patients Receiving Adalimumab: 3-year Results from the COMPANION Study. *Clin. Ther.* **2018**, *40*, 1024–1032. [CrossRef]
20. Ichiyama, S.; Ito, M.; Funasaka, Y.; Abe, M.; Nishida, E.; Muramatsu, S.; Nishihara, H.; Kato, H.; Morita, A.; Imafuku, S.; et al. Assessment of medication adherence and treatment satisfaction in Japanese patients with psoriasis of various severities. *J. Dermatol.* **2018**, *45*, 727–731. [CrossRef]
21. Armstrong, A.W.; Foster, S.A.; Comer, B.S.; Lin, C.-Y.; Malatestinic, W.; Burge, R.; Goldblum, O. Real-world health outcomes in adults with moderate-to-severe psoriasis in the United States: A population study using electronic health records to examine patient-perceived treatment effectiveness, medication use, and healthcare resource utilization. *BMC Dermatol.* **2018**, *18*, 4. [CrossRef] [PubMed]
22. Bhosle, M.J.; Feldman, S.R.; Camacho, F.T.; Timothy Whitmire, J.; Nahata, M.C.; Balkrishnan, R. Medication adherence and health care costs associated with biologics in Medicaid-enrolled patients with psoriasis. *J. Dermatolog. Treat.* **2006**, *17*, 294–301. [CrossRef] [PubMed]
23. Clemmensen, A.; Spon, M.; Skov, L.; Zachariae, C.; Gniadecki, R. Responses to ustekinumab in the anti-TNF agent-naïve vs. anti-TNF agent-exposed patients with psoriasis vulgaris. *J. Eur. Acad. Dermatol. Venereol.* **2011**, *25*, 1037–1040. [CrossRef] [PubMed]
24. Conesa-Nicolás, E.; García-Lagunar, M.H.; Núñez-Bracamonte, S.; García-Simón, M.S.; Mira-Sirvent, M.C. Persistence of secukinumab in patients with psoriasis, psoriatic arthritis, and ankylosing spondylitis. *Farm. Hosp.* **2020**, *45*, 16–21. [CrossRef] [PubMed]
25. Degli Esposti, L.; Sangiorgi, D.; Perrone, V.; Radice, S.; Clementi, E.; Perone, F.; Buda, S. Adherence and resource use among patients treated with biologic drugs: Findings from BEETLE study. *Clinicoecon. Outcomes Res.* **2014**, *6*, 401–407. [CrossRef] [PubMed]
26. Dommasch, E.D.; Lee, M.P.; Joyce, C.J.; Garry, E.M.; Gagne, J.J. Drug utilization patterns and adherence in patients on systemic medications for the treatment of psoriasis: A retrospective, comparative cohort study. *J. Am. Acad. Dermatol.* **2018**, *79*, 1061–1068.e1. [CrossRef]
27. Doshi, J.A.; Takeshita, J.; Pinto, L.; Li, P.; Yu, X.; Rao, P.; Viswanathan, H.N.; Gelfand, J.M. Biologic therapy adherence, discontinuation, switching, and restarting among patients with psoriasis in the US Medicare population. *J. Am. Acad. Dermatol.* **2016**, *74*, 1057–1065.e4. [CrossRef]
28. Egeberg, A.; Bryld, L.E.; Skov, L. Drug survival of secukinumab and ixekizumab for moderate-to-severe plaque psoriasis. *J. Am. Acad. Dermatol.* **2019**, *81*, 173–178. [CrossRef]
29. Esposito, M.; Gisondi, P.; Cassano, N.; Ferrucci, G.; Del Giglio, M.; Loconsole, F.; Giunta, A.; Vena, G.A.; Chimenti, S.; Girolomoni, G. Survival rate of antitumour necrosis factor-α treatments for psoriasis in routine dermatological practice: A multicentre observational study. *Br. J. Dermatol.* **2013**, *169*, 666–672. [CrossRef]
30. Esposito, M.; Gisondi, P.; Cassano, N.; Babino, G.; Cannizzaro, M.V.; Ferrucci, G.; Chimenti, S.; Giunta, A. Treatment adherence to different etanercept regimens, continuous vs. intermittent, in patients affected by plaque-type psoriasis. *Drug Dev. Res.* **2014**, *75* (Suppl. 1), S31–S34. [CrossRef]
31. Feldman, S.R.; Zhao, Y.; Navaratnam, P.; Friedman, H.S.; Lu, J.; Tran, M.H. Patterns of medication utilization and costs associated with the use of etanercept, adalimumab, and ustekinumab in the management of moderate-to-severe psoriasis. *J. Manag. Care Spec. Pharm.* **2015**, *21*, 201–209. [CrossRef] [PubMed]
32. Feldman, S.R.; Zhang, J.; Martinez, D.J.; Lopez-Gonzalez, L.; Marchlewicz, E.H.; Shrady, G.; Mendelsohn, A.M.; Zhao, Y. Real-world treatment patterns and healthcare costs of biologics and apremilast among patients with moderate-to-severe plaque psoriasis by metabolic condition status. *J. Dermatolog. Treat.* **2021**, *32*, 203–211. [CrossRef] [PubMed]
33. Blauvelt, A.; Shi, N.; Burge, R.; Malatestinic, W.N.; Lin, C.-Y.; Lew, C.R.; Zimmerman, N.M.; Goldblum, O.M.; Zhu, B.; Murage, M.J. Comparison of real-world treatment patterns among patients with psoriasis prescribed ixekizumab or secukinumab. *J. Am. Acad. Dermatol.* **2020**, *82*, 927–935. [CrossRef] [PubMed]
34. Ferrières, L.; Konstantinou, M.P.; Bulai Livideanu, C.; Hegazy, S.; Tauber, M.; Amelot, F.; Paul, C. Long-term continuation with secukinumab in psoriasis: Association with patient profile and initial psoriasis clearance. *Clin. Exp. Dermatol.* **2019**, *44*, e230–e234. [CrossRef]
35. Gendelman, O.; Weitzman, D.; Rosenberg, V.; Shalev, V.; Chodick, G.; Amital, H. Characterization of adherence and persistence profile in a real-life population of patients treated with adalimumab. *Br. J. Clin. Pharmacol.* **2018**, *84*, 786–795. [CrossRef]

36. Gniadecki, R.; Kragballe, K.; Dam, T.N.; Skov, L. Comparison of drug survival rates for adalimumab, etanercept and infliximab in patients with psoriasis vulgaris. *Br. J. Dermatol.* **2011**, *164*, 1091–1096. [CrossRef]
37. Hendrix, N.; Marcum, Z.A.; Veenstra, D.L. Medication persistence of targeted immunomodulators for plaque psoriasis: A retrospective analysis using a U.S. claims database. *Pharmacoepidemiol. Drug Saf.* **2020**, *29*, 675–683. [CrossRef]
38. Higa, S.; Devine, B.; Patel, V.; Baradaran, S.; Wang, D.; Bansal, A. Psoriasis treatment patterns: A retrospective claims study. *Curr. Med. Res. Opin.* **2019**, *35*, 1727–1733. [CrossRef]
39. Howe, A.; Ten Eyck, L.; Dufour, R.; Shah, N.; Harrison, D.J. Treatment patterns and annual drug costs of biologic therapies across indications from the Humana commercial database. *J. Manag. Care Spec. Pharm.* **2014**, *20*, 1236–1244. [CrossRef]
40. Hsu, D.Y.; Gniadecki, R. Patient Adherence to Biologic Agents in Psoriasis. *Dermatology* **2016**, *232*, 326–333. [CrossRef]
41. Iskandar, I.Y.K.; Warren, R.B.; Lunt, M.; Mason, K.J.; Evans, I.; McElhone, K.; Smith, C.H.; Reynolds, N.J.; Ashcroft, D.M.; Griffiths, C.E.M. Differential Drug Survival of Second-Line Biologic Therapies in Patients with Psoriasis: Observational Cohort Study from the British Association of Dermatologists Biologic Interventions Register (BADBIR). *J. Investig. Dermatol.* **2018**, *138*, 775–784. [CrossRef] [PubMed]
42. Jacobi, A.; Rustenbach, S.J.; Augustin, M. Comorbidity as a predictor for drug survival of biologic therapy in patients with psoriasis. *Int. J. Dermatol.* **2016**, *55*, 296–302. [CrossRef] [PubMed]
43. Khalid, J.M.; Fox, K.M.; Globe, G.; Maguire, A.; Chau, D. Treatment patterns and therapy effectiveness in psoriasis patients initiating biologic therapy in England. *J. Dermatolog. Treat.* **2014**, *25*, 67–72. [CrossRef] [PubMed]
44. Blauvelt, A.; Shi, N.; Burge, R.; Malatestinic, W.N.; Lin, C.-Y.; Lew, C.R.; Zimmerman, N.M.; Goldblum, O.M.; Zhu, B.; Murage, M.J. Comparison of Real-World Treatment Patterns Among Psoriasis Patients Treated with Ixekizumab or Adalimumab. *Patient Prefer. Adherence* **2020**, *14*, 517–527. [CrossRef] [PubMed]
45. Lee, S.; Xie, L.; Wang, Y.; Vaidya, N.; Baser, O. Evaluating the Effect of Treatment Persistence on the Economic Burden of Moderate to Severe Psoriasis and/or Psoriatic Arthritis Patients in the U.S. Department of Defense Population. *J. Manag. Care Spec. Pharm.* **2018**, *24*, 654–663. [CrossRef] [PubMed]
46. Li, Y.; Zhou, H.; Cai, B.; Kahler, K.H.; Tian, H.; Gabriel, S.; Arcona, S. Group-based trajectory modeling to assess adherence to biologics among patients with psoriasis. *Clinicoecon. Outcomes Res.* **2014**, *6*, 197–208. [CrossRef]
47. Magis, Q.; Jullien, D.; Gaudy-Marqueste, C.; Baumstark, K.; Viguier, M.; Bachelez, H.; Guibal, F.; Delaporte, E.; Karimova, E.; Montaudié, H.; et al. Predictors of long-term drug survival for infliximab in psoriasis. *J. Eur. Acad. Dermatol. Venereol.* **2017**, *31*, 96–101. [CrossRef]
48. Mahlich, J.; Alba, A.; El Hadad, L.; Leisten, M.-K.; Peitsch, W.K. Drug Survival of Biological Therapies for Psoriasis Treatment in Germany and Associated Costs: A Retrospective Claims Database Analysis. *Adv. Ther.* **2019**, *36*, 1684–1699. [CrossRef]
49. Malatestinic, W.; Nordstrom, B.; Wu, J.J.; Goldblum, O.; Solotkin, K.; Lin, C.-Y.; Kistler, K.; Fraeman, K.; Johnston, J.; Hawley, L.L.; et al. Characteristics and Medication Use of Psoriasis Patients Who May or May Not Qualify for Randomized Controlled Trials. *J. Manag. Care Spec. Pharm.* **2017**, *23*, 370–381. [CrossRef]
50. Menter, A.; Papp, K.A.; Gooderham, M.; Pariser, D.M.; Augustin, M.; Kerdel, F.A.; Fakharzadeh, S.; Goyal, K.; Calabro, S.; Langholff, W.; et al. Drug survival of biologic therapy in a large, disease-based registry of patients with psoriasis: Results from the Psoriasis Longitudinal Assessment and Registry (PSOLAR). *J. Eur. Acad. Dermatol. Venereol.* **2016**, *30*, 1148–1158. [CrossRef]
51. Mercadal Orfila, G.; Ventayol Bosch, P.; Maestre Fullana, M.A.; Serrano López De Las Hazas, J.; Fernández Cortés, F.; Palomero Massanet, A.; García Álvarez, Á. Persistence and cost of biologic agents for psoriasis: Retrospective study in the Balearic Islands. *Eur. J. Clin. Pharm.* **2016**, *18*, 163–170.
52. Mocanu, M.; Toader, M.-P.; Rezus, E.; Taranu, T. Aspects concerning patient adherence to anti-TNFα therapy in psoriasis: A decade of clinical experience. *Exp. Ther. Med.* **2019**, *18*, 4987–4992. [CrossRef] [PubMed]
53. Murage, M.J.; Anderson, A.; Casso, D.; Oliveria, S.A.; Ojeh, C.K.; Muram, T.M.; Merola, J.F.; Zbrozek, A.; Araujo, A.B. Treatment patterns, adherence, and persistence among psoriasis patients treated with biologics in a real-world setting, overall and by disease severity. *J. Dermatolog. Treat.* **2019**, *30*, 141–149. [CrossRef] [PubMed]
54. Murage, M.J.; Gilligan, A.M.; Tran, O.; Goldblum, O.; Burge, R.; Lin, C.-Y.; Qureshi, A. Ixekizumab treatment patterns and healthcare utilization and costs for patients with psoriasis. *J. Dermatolog. Treat.* **2021**, *32*, 56–63. [CrossRef] [PubMed]
55. Bonafede, M.; Fox, K.M.; Watson, C.; Princic, N.; Gandra, S.R. Treatment patterns in the first year after initiating tumor necrosis factor blockers in real-world settings. *Adv. Ther.* **2012**, *29*, 664–674. [CrossRef] [PubMed]
56. Onsun, N.; Güneş, B.; Yabacı, A. Retention and survival rate of etanercept in psoriasis over 15 years and patient outcomes during the COVID-19 pandemic: The real-world experience of a single center. *Dermatol. Ther.* **2021**, *34*, e14623. [CrossRef]
57. Pogácsás, L.; Borsi, A.; Takács, P.; Remenyik, É.; Kemény, L.; Kárpáti, S.; Holló, P.; Wikonkál, N.; Gyulai, R.; Károlyi, Z.; et al. Long-term drug survival and predictor analysis of the whole psoriatic patient population on biological therapy in Hungary. *J. Dermatolog. Treat.* **2017**, *28*, 635–641. [CrossRef]
58. Ross, C.; Marshman, G.; Grillo, M.; Stanford, T. Biological therapies for psoriasis: Adherence and outcome analysis from a clinical perspective. *Australas. J. Dermatol.* **2016**, *57*, 137–140. [CrossRef]
59. Ruiz-Villaverde, R.; Rodriguez-Fernandez-Freire, L.; Galán-Gutierrez, M.; Armario-HIta, J.C.; Martinez-Pilar, L. Drug survival, discontinuation rates, and safety profile of secukinumab in real-world patients: A 152-week, multicenter, retrospective study. *Int. J. Dermatol.* **2020**, *59*, 633–639. [CrossRef]

60. Sbidian, E.; Mezzarobba, M.; Weill, A.; Coste, J.; Rudant, J. Persistence of treatment with biologics for patients with psoriasis: A real-world analysis of 16545 biologic-naïve patients from the French National Health Insurance database (SNIIRAM). Br. J. Dermatol. **2019**, *180*, 86–93. [CrossRef]
61. Sruamsiri, R.; Iwasaki, K.; Tang, W.; Mahlich, J. Persistence rates and medical costs of biological therapies for psoriasis treatment in Japan: A real-world data study using a claims database. *BMC Dermatol.* **2018**, *18*, 5. [CrossRef] [PubMed]
62. Svedbom, A.; Dalén, J.; Mamolo, C.; Cappelleri, J.C.; Petersson, I.F.; Ståhle, M. Treatment patterns with topicals, traditional systemics and biologics in psoriasis—A Swedish database analysis. *J. Eur. Acad. Dermatol. Venereol.* **2015**, *29*, 215–223. [CrossRef] [PubMed]
63. Thorneloe, R.J.; Griffiths, C.E.M.; Emsley, R.; Ashcroft, D.M.; Cordingley, L. Intentional and Unintentional Medication Non-Adherence in Psoriasis: The Role of Patients' Medication Beliefs and Habit Strength. *J. Investig. Dermatol.* **2018**, *138*, 785–794. [CrossRef] [PubMed]
64. Umezawa, Y.; Nobeyama, Y.; Hayashi, M.; Fukuchi, O.; Ito, T.; Saeki, H.; Nakagawa, H. Drug survival rates in patients with psoriasis after treatment with biologics. *J. Dermatol.* **2013**, *40*, 1008–1013. [CrossRef]
65. van den Reek, J.M.P.A.; Tummers, M.; Zweegers, J.; Seyger, M.M.B.; van Lümig, P.P.M.; Driessen, R.J.B.; van de Kerkhof, P.C.M.; Kievit, W.; de Jong, E.M.G.J. Predictors of adalimumab drug survival in psoriasis differ by reason for discontinuation: Long-term results from the Bio-CAPTURE registry. *J. Eur. Acad. Dermatol. Venereol.* **2015**, *29*, 560–565. [CrossRef]
66. Bonafede, M.; Johnson, B.H.; Fox, K.M.; Watson, C.; Gandra, S.R. Treatment patterns with etanercept and adalimumab for psoriatic diseases in a real-world setting. *J. Dermatolog. Treat.* **2013**, *24*, 369–373. [CrossRef]
67. Verma, L.; Mayba, J.N.; Gooderham, M.J.; Verma, A.; Papp, K.A. Persistency of Biologic Therapies for Plaque Psoriasis in 2 Large Community Practices. *J. Cutan. Med. Surg.* **2018**, *22*, 38–43. [CrossRef]
68. Wu, B.; Muser, E.; Teeple, A.; Pericone, C.D.; Feldman, S.R. Treatment adherence and persistence of five commonly prescribed medications for moderate to severe psoriasis in a U.S. commercially insured population. *J. Dermatolog. Treat.* **2021**, *32*, 595–602. [CrossRef]
69. Yiu, Z.Z.N.; Mason, K.J.; Hampton, P.J.; Reynolds, N.J.; Smith, C.H.; Lunt, M.; Griffiths, C.E.M.; Warren, R.B. Drug survival of adalimumab, ustekinumab and secukinumab in patients with psoriasis: A prospective cohort study from the British Association of Dermatologists Biologics and Immunomodulators Register (BADBIR). *Br. J. Dermatol.* **2020**, *183*, 294–302. [CrossRef]
70. Zagni, E.; Colombo, D.; Fiocchi, M.; Perrone, V.; Sangiorgi, D.; Andretta, M.; De Sarro, G.; Nava, E.; Degli Esposti, L. Pharmaco-utilization of biologic drugs in patients affected by psoriasis, psoriatic arthritis and ankylosing spondylitis in an Italian real-world setting. *Expert Rev. Pharm. Outcomes Res.* **2020**, *20*, 491–497. [CrossRef]
71. Zschocke, I.; Ortland, C.; Reich, K. Evaluation of adherence predictors for the treatment of moderate to severe psoriasis with biologics: The importance of physician-patient interaction and communication. *J. Eur. Acad. Dermatol. Venereol.* **2017**, *31*, 1014–1020. [CrossRef] [PubMed]
72. Cao, Z.; Carter, C.; Wilson, K.L.; Schenkel, B. Ustekinumab dosing, persistence, and discontinuation patterns in patients with moderate-to-severe psoriasis. *J. Dermatolog. Treat.* **2015**, *26*, 113–120. [CrossRef] [PubMed]
73. Chan, S.A.; Hussain, F.; Lawson, L.G.; Ormerod, A.D. Factors affecting adherence to treatment of psoriasis: Comparing biologic therapy to other modalities. *J. Dermatolog. Treat.* **2013**, *24*, 64–69. [CrossRef] [PubMed]
74. Chastek, B.; Fox, K.M.; Watson, C.; Kricorian, G.; Gandra, S.R. Psoriasis treatment patterns with etanercept and adalimumab in a United States health plan population. *J. Dermatolog. Treat.* **2013**, *24*, 25–33. [CrossRef]
75. Chastek, B.; White, J.; Van Voorhis, D.; Tang, D.; Stolshek, B.S. A Retrospective Cohort Study Comparing Utilization and Costs of Biologic Therapies and JAK Inhibitor Therapy Across Four Common Inflammatory Indications in Adult US Managed Care Patients. *Adv. Ther.* **2016**, *33*, 626–642. [CrossRef]
76. Khan, S.; Rupniewska, E.; Neighbors, M.; Singer, D.; Chiarappa, J.; Obando, C. Real-world evidence on adherence, persistence, switching and dose escalation with biologics in adult inflammatory bowel disease in the United States: A systematic review. *J. Clin. Pharm. Ther.* **2019**, *44*, 495–507. [CrossRef]
77. Murage, M.J.; Tongbram, V.; Feldman, S.R.; Malatestinic, W.N.; Larmore, C.J.; Muram, T.M.; Burge, R.T.; Bay, C.; Johnson, N.; Clifford, S.; et al. Medication adherence and persistence in patients with rheumatoid arthritis, psoriasis, and psoriatic arthritis: A systematic literature review. *Patient Prefer. Adherence* **2018**, *12*, 1483–1503. [CrossRef]
78. Lin, P.-T.; Wang, S.-H.; Chi, C.-C. Drug survival of biologics in treating psoriasis: A meta-analysis of real-world evidence. *Sci. Rep.* **2018**, *8*, 16068. [CrossRef]
79. Mourad, A.I.; Gniadecki, R. Biologic Drug Survival in Psoriasis: A Systematic Review & Comparative Meta-Analysis. *Front. Med.* **2020**, *7*, 625755.
80. Geale, K.; Lindberg, I.; Paulsson, E.C.; Wennerström, E.C.M.; Tjärnlund, A.; Noel, W.; Enkusson, D.; Theander, E. Persistence of biologic treatments in psoriatic arthritis: A population-based study in Sweden. *Rheumatol. Adv. Pract.* **2020**, *4*, rkaa070. [CrossRef]
81. Warren, R.B.; Smith, C.H.; Yiu, Z.Z.N.; Ashcroft, D.M.; Barker, J.N.W.N.; Burden, A.D.; Lunt, M.; McElhone, K.; Ormerod, A.D.; Owen, C.M.; et al. Differential Drug Survival of Biologic Therapies for the Treatment of Psoriasis: A Prospective Observational Cohort Study from the British Association of Dermatologists Biologic Interventions Register (BADBIR). *J. Investig. Dermatol.* **2015**, *135*, 2632–2640. [CrossRef] [PubMed]
82. Kaur, P.; Pannu, H.S.; Malhi, A.K. Comprehensive Study of Continuous Orthogonal Moments—A Systematic Review. *ACM Comput. Surv.* **2019**, *52*, 1–30. [CrossRef]

83. Raebel, M.A.; Schmittdiel, J.; Karter, A.J.; Konieczny, J.L.; Steiner, J.F. Standardizing terminology and definitions of medication adherence and persistence in research employing electronic databases. *Med. Care* **2013**, *51*, S11–S21. [CrossRef] [PubMed]
84. Mahil, S.K.; Ezejimofor, M.C.; Exton, L.S.; Manounah, L.; Burden, A.D.; Coates, L.C.; de Brito, M.; McGuire, A.; Murphy, R.; Owen, C.M.; et al. Comparing the efficacy and tolerability of biologic therapies in psoriasis: An updated network meta-analysis. *Br. J. Dermatol.* **2020**, *183*, 638–649. [CrossRef] [PubMed]
85. Sawyer, L.M.; Malottki, K.; Sabry-Grant, C.; Yasmeen, N.; Wright, E.; Sohrt, A.; Borg, E.; Warren, R.B. Assessing the relative efficacy of interleukin-17 and interleukin-23 targeted treatments for moderate-to-severe plaque psoriasis: A systematic review and network meta-analysis of PASI response. *PLoS ONE* **2019**, *14*, e0220868. [CrossRef]
86. Sbidian, E.; Chaimani, A.; Afach, S.; Doney, L.; Dressler, C.; Hua, C.; Mazaud, C.; Phan, C.; Hughes, C.; Riddle, D.; et al. Systemic pharmacological treatments for chronic plaque psoriasis: A network meta-analysis. *Cochrane Database Syst. Rev.* **2020**, *1*, CD011535. [CrossRef]
87. Reich, K.; Burden, A.D.; Eaton, J.N.; Hawkins, N.S. Efficacy of biologics in the treatment of moderate to severe psoriasis: A network meta-analysis of randomized controlled trials. *Br. J. Dermatol.* **2012**, *166*, 179–188. [CrossRef]
88. Kisielnicka, A.; Szczerkowska-Dobosz, A.; Nowicki, R. The influence of body weight of patients with chronic plaque psoriasis on biological treatment response. *Adv. Dermatol. Allergol. Dermatol. Alergol.* **2020**, *37*, 168–173. [CrossRef]
89. Anghel, F.; Nitusca, D.; Cristodor, P. Body Mass Index Influence for the Personalization of the Monoclonal Antibodies Therapy for Psoriasis. *Life* **2021**, *11*, 1316. [CrossRef]
90. Giunta, A.; Babino, G.; Ruzzetti, M.; Manetta, S.; Chimenti, S.; Esposito, M. Influence of body mass index and weight on etanercept efficacy in patients with psoriasis: A retrospective study. *J. Int. Med. Res.* **2016**, *44*, 72–75. [CrossRef]
91. Singh, S.; Facciorusso, A.; Singh, A.G.; Casteele, N.V.; Zarrinpar, A.; Prokop, L.J.; Grunvald, E.L.; Curtis, J.R.; Sandborn, W.J. Obesity and response to anti-tumor necrosis factor-α agents in patients with select immune-mediated inflammatory diseases: A systematic review and meta-analysis. *PLoS ONE* **2018**, *13*, e0195123. [CrossRef] [PubMed]
92. Yanaba, K.; Umezawa, Y.; Ito, T.; Hayashi, M.; Kikuchi, S.; Fukuchi, O.; Saeki, H.; Nakagawa, H. Impact of obesity on the efficacy of ustekinumab in Japanese patients with psoriasis: A retrospective cohort study of 111 patients. *Arch. Dermatol. Res.* **2014**, *306*, 921–925. [CrossRef]
93. Di Lernia, V.; Tasin, L.; Pellicano, R.; Zumiani, G.; Albertini, G. Impact of body mass index on retention rates of anti-TNF-alfa drugs in daily practice for psoriasis. *J. Dermatolog. Treat.* **2012**, *23*, 404–409. [CrossRef] [PubMed]
94. Zweegers, J.; van den Reek, J.M.P.A.; van de Kerkhof, P.C.M.; Otero, M.E.; Kuijpers, A.L.A.; Koetsier, M.I.A.; Arnold, W.P.; Berends, M.A.M.; Weppner-Parren, L.; Ossenkoppele, P.M.; et al. Body mass index predicts discontinuation due to ineffectiveness and female sex predicts discontinuation due to side-effects in patients with psoriasis treated with adalimumab, etanercept or ustekinumab in daily practice: A prospective, comparative, long-. *Br. J. Dermatol.* **2016**, *175*, 340–347. [CrossRef] [PubMed]
95. Hansel, T.T.; Kropshofer, H.; Singer, T.; Mitchell, J.A.; George, A.J.T. The safety and side effects of monoclonal antibodies. *Nat. Rev. Drug Discov.* **2010**, *9*, 325–338. [CrossRef] [PubMed]
96. Afif, W.; Loftus, E.V.J.; Faubion, W.A.; Kane, S.V.; Bruining, D.H.; Hanson, K.A.; Sandborn, W.J. Clinical utility of measuring infliximab and human anti-chimeric antibody concentrations in patients with inflammatory bowel disease. *Am. J. Gastroenterol.* **2010**, *105*, 1133–1139. [CrossRef]
97. Harding, F.A.; Stickler, M.M.; Razo, J.; DuBridge, R.B. The immunogenicity of humanized and fully human antibodies: Residual immunogenicity resides in the CDR regions. *MAbs* **2010**, *2*, 256–265. [CrossRef] [PubMed]
98. Loft, N.D.; Vaengebjerg, S.; Halling, A.-S.; Skov, L.; Egeberg, A. Adverse events with IL-17 and IL-23 inhibitors for psoriasis and psoriatic arthritis: A systematic review and meta-analysis of phase III studies. *J. Eur. Acad. Dermatol. Venereol.* **2020**, *34*, 1151–1160. [CrossRef]
99. Matsui, T.; Umetsu, R.; Kato, Y.; Hane, Y.; Sasaoka, S.; Motooka, Y.; Hatahira, H.; Abe, J.; Fukuda, A.; Naganuma, M.; et al. Age-related trends in injection site reaction incidence induced by the tumor necrosis factor-α (TNF-α) inhibitors etanercept and adalimumab: The Food and Drug Administration adverse event reporting system, 2004–2015. *Int. J. Med. Sci.* **2017**, *14*, 102–109. [CrossRef]
100. Campi, P.; Benucci, M.; Manfredi, M.; Demoly, P. Hypersensitivity reactions to biological agents with special emphasis on tumor necrosis factor-alpha antagonists. *Curr. Opin. Allergy Clin. Immunol.* **2007**, *7*, 393–403. [CrossRef]
101. Sfikakis, P.P.; Iliopoulos, A.; Elezoglou, A.; Kittas, C.; Stratigos, A. Psoriasis induced by anti-tumor necrosis factor therapy: A paradoxical adverse reaction. *Arthritis Rheum.* **2005**, *52*, 2513–2518. [CrossRef] [PubMed]
102. Kerensky, T.A.; Gottlieb, A.B.; Yaniv, S.; Au, S. Etanercept: Efficacy and safety for approved indications. *Expert Opin. Drug Saf.* **2012**, *11*, 121–139. [CrossRef] [PubMed]
103. Leman, J.; Burden, A. Treatment of severe psoriasis with infliximab. *Ther. Clin. Risk Manag.* **2008**, *4*, 1165–1176. [CrossRef] [PubMed]
104. Yang, E.J.; Beck, K.M.; Liao, W. Secukinumab in the treatment of psoriasis: Patient selection and perspectives. *Psoriasis Auckl.* **2018**, *8*, 75–82. [CrossRef] [PubMed]
105. Craig, S.; Warren, R.B. Ixekizumab for the treatment of psoriasis: Up-to-date. *Expert Opin. Biol. Ther.* **2020**, *20*, 549–557. [CrossRef]
106. Leonardi, C.L.; Kimball, A.B.; Papp, K.A.; Yeilding, N.; Guzzo, C.; Wang, Y.; Li, S.; Dooley, L.T.; Gordon, K.B. Efficacy and safety of ustekinumab, a human interleukin-12/23 monoclonal antibody, in patients with psoriasis: 76-week results from a randomised, double-blind, placebo-controlled trial (PHOENIX 1). *Lancet* **2008**, *371*, 1665–1674. [CrossRef]

107. Ghosh, S.; Gensler, L.S.; Yang, Z.; Gasink, C.; Chakravarty, S.D.; Farahi, K.; Ramachandran, P.; Ott, E.; Strober, B.E. Ustekinumab Safety in Psoriasis, Psoriatic Arthritis, and Crohn's Disease: An Integrated Analysis of Phase II/III Clinical Development Programs. *Drug Saf.* **2019**, *42*, 751–768. [CrossRef]
108. Sandoval, L.F.; Huang, K.E.; Feldman, S.R. Adherence to ustekinumab in psoriasis patients. *J. Drugs Dermatol.* **2013**, *12*, 1090–1092.
109. Chi, C.-C.; Wang, S.-H. Efficacy and cost-efficacy of biologic therapies for moderate to severe psoriasis: A meta-analysis and cost-efficacy analysis using the intention-to-treat principle. *Biomed Res. Int.* **2014**, *2014*, 862851. [CrossRef]
110. Rouse, N.C.; Farhangian, M.E.; Wehausen, B.; Feldman, S.R. The cost-effectiveness of ustekinumab for moderate-to-severe psoriasis. *Expert Rev. Pharm. Outcomes Res.* **2015**, *15*, 877–884. [CrossRef]
111. D'Souza, L.S.; Payette, M.J. Estimated cost efficacy of systemic treatments that are approved by the US Food and Drug Administration for the treatment of moderate to severe psoriasis. *J. Am. Acad. Dermatol.* **2015**, *72*, 589–598. [CrossRef] [PubMed]
112. Feldman, S.R.; Evans, C.; Russell, M.W. Systemic treatment for moderate to severe psoriasis: Estimates of failure rates and direct medical costs in a north-eastern US managed care plan. *J. Dermatolog. Treat.* **2005**, *16*, 37–42. [CrossRef] [PubMed]
113. Choi, C.W.; Choi, J.Y.; Kim, B.R.; Youn, S.W. Economic Burden Can Be the Major Determining Factor Resulting in Short-Term Intermittent and Repetitive Ustekinumab Treatment for Moderate-to-Severe Psoriasis. *Ann. Dermatol.* **2018**, *30*, 179–185. [CrossRef] [PubMed]
114. Xu, Y.; Sudharshan, L.; Hsu, M.-A.; Koenig, A.S.; Cappelleri, J.C.; Liu, W.F.; Smith, T.W.; Pasquale, M.K. Patient preferences associated with therapies for psoriatic arthritis: A conjoint analysis. *Am. Health Drug Benefits* **2018**, *11*, 408–416. [PubMed]
115. Torres, T.; Puig, L.; Vender, R.; Lynde, C.; Piaserico, S.; Carrascosa, J.M.; Gisondi, P.; Daudén, E.; Conrad, C.; Mendes-Bastos, P.; et al. Drug Survival of IL-12/23, IL-17 and IL-23 Inhibitors for Psoriasis Treatment: A Retrospective Multi-Country, Multicentric Cohort Study. *Am. J. Clin. Dermatol.* **2021**, *22*, 567–579. [CrossRef]

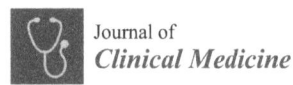

Review

Role of Janus Kinase Inhibitors in Therapy of Psoriasis

Sylwia Słuczanowska-Głąbowska, Anna Ziegler-Krawczyk, Kamila Szumilas and Andrzej Pawlik *

Department of Physiology, Pomeranian Medical University in Szczecin, 70-111 Szczecin, Poland; sylwia@pum.edu.pl (S.S.-G.); ania.ziegler@op.pl (A.Z.-K.); kamila.szumilas@pum.edu.pl (K.S.)
* Correspondence: pawand@poczta.onet.pl

Abstract: Janus kinases inhibitors are molecules that target Janus kinases—signal transducers and activators of transcription (JAK/STAT). They inhibit this intracellular signal pathway, blocking the gene transcription of crucial proinflammatory cytokines that play a central role in the pathogenesis of many inflammatory and autoimmune diseases, including psoriasis. This process reduces psoriatic inflammation. The JAK inhibitors are divided into two generations. The first generation of JAK inhibitors blocks two or more different Janus kinases. The second generation is more specified and blocks only one type of Janus kinase and has less side effects than the first generation. Tofacitinib, ruxolitinib and baricitinib belong to first generation JAK inhibitors and decernotinib and filgotinib belong to second group. This narrative review summarizes the role of Janus kinase inhibitors in the therapy of psoriasis. Oral JAK inhibitors show promise for efficacy and safety in the treatment of psoriasis. Studies to date do not indicate that JAK inhibitors are superior to recent biologic drugs in terms of efficacy. However, JAK inhibitors, due to their lack of increased incidence of side effects compared to other biologic drugs, can be included in the psoriasis treatment algorithm because they are orally taken. Nevertheless, further studies are needed to evaluate long-term treatment effects with these drugs.

Keywords: psoriasis; Janus kinases; therapy

1. Introduction

Psoriasis vulgaris is a common inflammatory, chronic skin disease that affects 2% to 3% of the world population. It is a disease with periods of exacerbation and remission. Psoriasis vulgaris has a genetic basis and multigenetic inheritance. Many factors play a role in the development of psoriasis, among which are distinguished: environmental and immunological factors. However, the influence of genetic conditions and multigene background is underlined.

There are two types of psoriasis. Type I is associated with autosomal dominant inheritance, occurring in up to 40 years of age and is associated with HLA-Cw6 tissue compatibility antigens, as well as B13 and B57. Type II appears for the first time between 50 and 70 years of age and is associated with HLA antigens Cw6, Cw2 and B27. Thus far, no specific gene responsible for psoriasis has been found, and HLA-Cw6 alleles are also found in the normal population [1–3].

The most common variant of this disease, affecting 85–90% of patients, is plaque psoriasis. In addition, there is palmoplantar psoriasis, erythrodermic psoriasis, and inverse psoriasis as well as generalized pustular psoriasis, which is alternatively termed von Zumbush type. In addition to isolated skin lesions, 25% of patients with psoriasis and joint lesions are diagnosed with psoriatic arthritis [1].

The skin lesions of psoriasis are erythematous scaly plaques, which are preferentially disposed at extensor sites and in areas of mechanic stress such as the knees and elbows. They are characterized by hyperplasia and parakeratosis with accumulation of inflammatory cells in the dermis. In addition, scalp, nails and inverse regions can also be affected [4].

The inflammatory response in psoriasis is mainly driven by T cells, especially T helper cells (Th17), and is mediated by different cytokines, especially TNF-α, IL-17, IL-23 but also other cytokines such as IFN-γ, IL-2, IL-6, IL-8, IL-17, IL-18 and IL-22. The IL-23 is crucial in the pathogenesis of psoriasis and causes Th17 cells to produce IL-17 and IL-22. They induce changes in the skin characteristic for psoriasis. Psoriasis severity is generally characterized by the Psoriasis Area and Severity Index (PASI), which is usually presented as a percentage response rate [2,4,5].

There is a wide range of treatment possibilities for psoriasis. The treatments include mainly topical medicines such as ointments with urea, salicylic acid and cygnoline, glucocorticosteroids and vitamin D derivatives and phototherapy. In moderate to severe cases of psoriasis, oral drugs such as acitretin and immunosuppressive drugs such as methotrexate and cyclosporine were given. In recent years, new groups of medicine were used in the treatment of psoriasis, which are biologics. The biologic drugs targeting TNF, IL-12/IL-23, and IL-17 have been approved for the treatment of psoriasis in the last few years, but not all patients respond to treatment with biologics. The biologics are efficient, well tolerated, and safe for treatment of psoriasis but are expensive [4,6–8]. The Janus kinase (JAK) inhibitors are a new class of drugs that can be used in systemic treatment of psoriasis, and they are less expensive.

1.1. Janus Kinases

Janus kinase (JAK) is the non-receptor tyrosine kinase that transduces signals from multitudes of cytokines and growth factors and plays a major role in the pathogenesis of many inflammatory and autoimmune diseases, including psoriasis [4,9]. The JAKs are intracellular enzymes that bind to the cytoplasmic domains of cytokine receptors [10,11]. In recent years, there have been many trials about modulating the key intracellular components of cytokine signaling through Janus kinases (JAK) [2,4,12].

Cytokines are a group of proteins consisting of different structures. They act on different signal transductions, as a result of joining receptors, and they are grouped depending on the receptor to which they join. The binding of cytokines to their receptors initiates an inflammatory signal that can be mediated by JAK. The large group of cytokines such as IL-2, IL-4, IL-6, IL-7, IL-9, IL-12, IL-15, IL-21, IL-22 and IL23 as well as interferons such as INF-gamma bind to type I and II cytokine receptors [13,14].

When cytokines bind to receptors, the intracellular JAKs are recruited and joined in pairs to the intracellular part of the cytokine receptors, and then, they are activated. The dimerization of JAKs formats heterodimers, autophosphorylate, and attracts STAT (signal transducer and activator of transcription) protein. Afterward, the activated STAT proteins dimerize and translocate to the cell nucleus, where they regulate gene transcription of different cytokines, including proinflammatory cytokines that play role in pathogenesis of psoriasis [6,14–17] (Figure 1).

JAK was discovered in the end of the last century [18]. In mammals, there are four JAK proteins: JAK1, JAK2, JAK3, and TYK2 (tyrosine kinase 2) [11] and seven STATs [4,11]. JAK1, JAK2, and TYK2 are involved in cell growth processes in different cell types, they partake in their development and differentiation, while JAK3 is critical to hematopoiesis [14,15,19,20]. JAKs are crucial for intracellular signaling of lymphocytes. Their dysfunction is involved with impairment of immune cells [15,21]. The JAK/STAT signaling pathway is typically found in many inflammatory skin diseases including psoriasis [10,13]. It was shown that JAK1 expression correlates with duration of psoriasis and Psoriasis Area and Severity Index (PASI) score [7].

Different JAKs are associated with specific cytokine receptors and influence different aspects of immune cell development and function. JAK1 is associated with INF, IL-6 and Il-10 receptors and with receptors containing the common gamma chain during JAK2 with hematopoetic receptors as well as the IL-12 and IL-23 receptors. JAK3 is associated with major cytokines for lymphocyte function IL-2, IL-4, IL-7, IL-9, IL-15 and IL-21 receptors. The TYK2 is conjuncted with JAK2 and associated with INF, IL-12 and IL-23 receptors [17,21,22].

Mutations of JAK cause dysfunction of cells and diseases such as essential thrombocytopenia, myelofibrosis, polycythemia vera, severe combined immunodeficiency, autoimmune diseases and others [14,16,20,23].

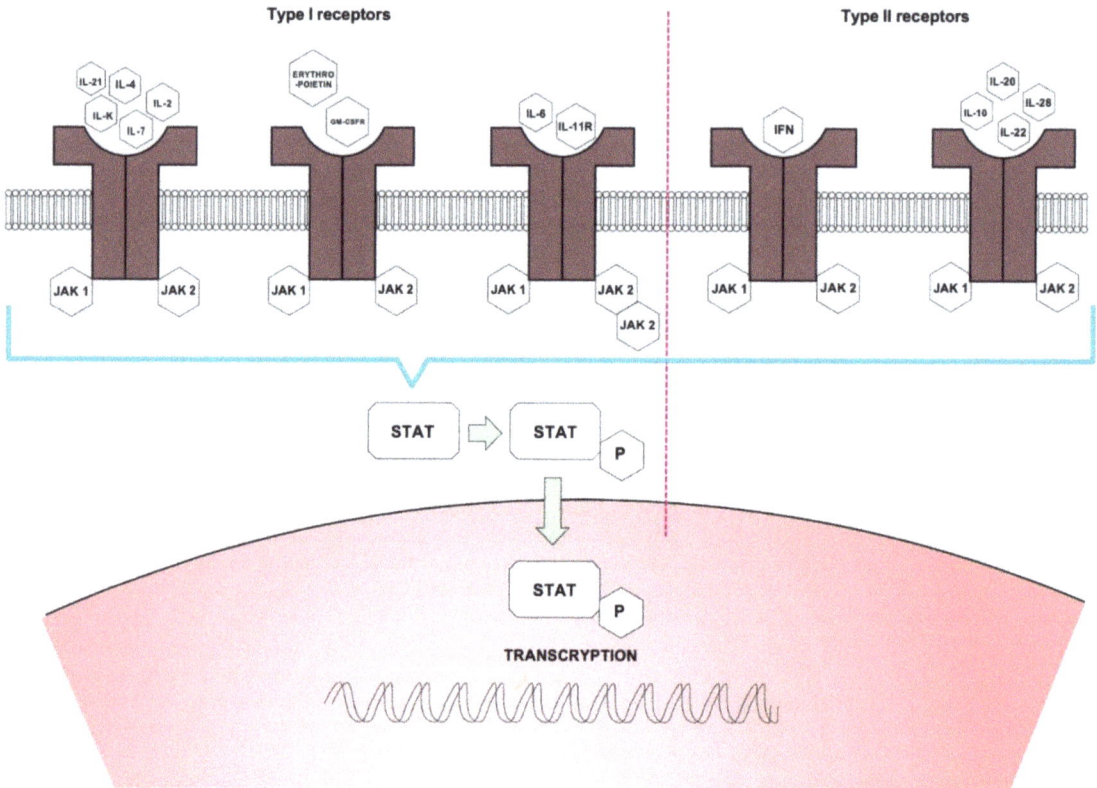

Figure 1. Mechanisms of action of Janus kinases. JAK—Janus kinase, STAT—signal transducer and activator of transcription; P—phosphoric acid, GM-CSF—Granulocyte-macrophage colony-stimulating factor, IFN—Interferon.

1.2. Janus Kinase Inhibitors

JAK inhibitors improve the treatment of many inflammatory diseases, including psoriasis [18]. JAK inhibitors are the molecules targeting the Janus kinase—a signal transducer and activator of transcription (JAK/STAT). They block this intracellular signal pathway by blocking the gene transcription of crucial proinflammatory cytokines, which play a central role in the pathogenesis of many inflammatory and autoimmune diseases including psoriasis [9,10] (Figure 2). This process reduces psoriatic inflammation [14,16,23]. JAK inhibitors target JAKs inside the cell [14,24]. The JAK inhibitors are divided into two generations. The first generation of JAK inhibitors target two or more different JAKs. The second generation is more specified and target only one type of JAK and has less side effects than the first generation [14,25]. Tofacitinib, ruxolitinib and baricitinib belong to first generation of JAK inhibitors and the decernotinib and filgotinib to the second group [13,14,25].

1.3. JAK Inhibitors in Psoriasis Treatment

Knowledge about biologics used for psoriasis (such as ustekinumab, secukinumab, ixekizumab, risankizumab) targeting the IL23/IL17 axis, shows that there is also therapeutical potential of JAK inhibitors associated with receptors for these cytokines. The blocking by JAK inhibitors of cytokines pathway may suppress the expression of many cytokines important for pathogenesis of psoriasis [4,14,25,26]. For example, IL-23, the crucial interleukin in the pathogenesis of psoriasis, transduces the signal by JAK2 and TYK2 [14,27] and can be a target for the treatment of psoriasis [4].

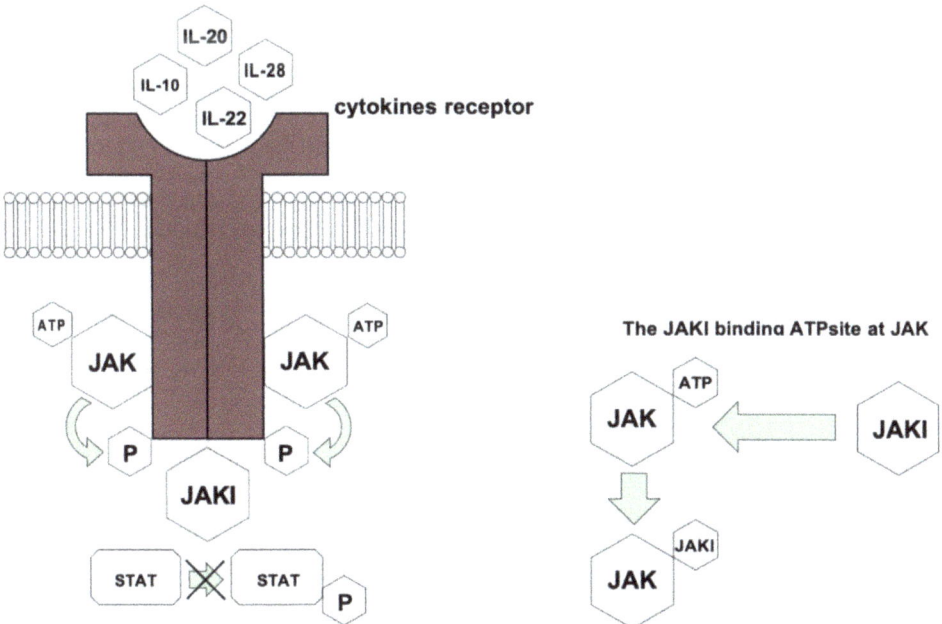

Figure 2. Mechanisms of action of Janus kinase inhibitors. JAK—Janus kinase, JAKI—Janus kinase inhibitor, STAT—signal transducer and activator of transcription; P—phosphoric acid, ATP—Adenosine triphosphate.

The JAK inhibitors are currently under clinical investigation for oral and topical treatment in psoriasis [4,10,13,28]. Currently, the three JAK inhibitors, tofacitinib, baricitinib, and ruxolitinib, have been approved for clinical use in psoriasis in the United States of America and Europe [4,29].

1.4. Tofacitinib—General Information and Clinical Trials

Tofacitinib is the most studied JAK inhibitor in cutaneous diseases. It is now being explored in skin diseases and do not respond to or sustain intolerable adverse effects as an immunosuppressive and biologic treatment [10,11]. Compared to immunosuppressives and biologics treatment, tofacitinib is easy to administer and can be used orally or topically [11]. Besides being used in psoriasis [4,29], tofacitinib is being used as an off-label indication in alopecia areata, vitiligo and atopic dermatitis [11,15,30]. It is also used in treatment in skin diseases such as moderate to severe active rheumatoid arthritis [15,31–34], psoriatic arthritis [15,32,35], and ulcerative colitis [15,36].

Tofacitinib, a first-generation JAK inhibitor, blocks tyrosine kinases of the Janus family such as JAK1 and JAK3, with affinity for JAK2 and TYK 2 [10,15,37]. Tofacitinib is rapidly eliminated. The peak level of tofacitinib occurs within 30 min, and the half-life is 3 h. It is metabolized mainly by the liver, primarily mediated by CYP3A4 with minor contribution from CYP2C19, and metabolized at a low percentage in kidneys. It is excreted renally [11,31,38–40]. In pregnancy, is not well established and can be used only if benefits outweigh the potential risks. There is a reported small amount of cases of pregnant women who received tofacitinib [11,41]. Tofacitinib is secreted in breast milk and breastfeeding is avoided during treatment [11]. In the pediatric population, studies are not robust. This drug cannot be used in those less than 18 years of age [11].

Tofacitinib is the most studied JAK inhibitor used to heal chronic plaque psoriasis orally [14,19,23]. It was shown that treatment with tofacitinib (10 mg twice daily) decreases epidermal thickness, reduces of the number of T cells infiltrating the skin, and suppresses the IL-23/Th17 pathway [11].

The action of this drug is decreased during concurrent administration of the potent CYP3A4 inducers (e.g., Rifampicin) and is increased during concurrent administration of potent inhibitors of CYP3A4 (e.g., ketoconazole and flukonazole). The immunosuppressive drugs, e.g., azathioprine, tacrolimus, and cyclosporine, are avoided during treatment with tofacitinib because of increased risk of immunosuppression. In addition, disease-modifying anti-rheumatic drugs and biologics are not well studied and are not recommended for co-administration because of an increased risk of immunosuppression [11]. The therapy with tofacitinib should not be started in the following conditions: active infection, hematological abnormalities, severe hepatic impartment, and hypersensitivity to the active substance or to any excipients [11].

The effectiveness of oral administration of tofacitinib was confirmed in the treatment of moderate to severe plaque psoriasis phase III trials [42,43]. The effectiveness and safety of tofacitinib (in dose 5 and 10 mg twice daily) was described in two phase III trials in patients with active psoriasis arthritis. In these trials, tofacinitib was in combination with methotrexate, sulfasalazine and leflunomide [33,34,44].

Tofacitinib was also be used as a topical treatment. The topical application of 2% tofacitinib ointment decreased possible systemic adverse effects. It was tested in a phase II trial. It was observed to have a better effect than placebo [24,45].

1.4.1. PIVOTAL 1 and PIVOTAL 2—Phase III Studies of Tofacitinib Treatment

The most important studies of tofacitinib were Pivotal 1 and 2. The duration of these trials was 52 weeks. These were phase III double-blinded studies, which compared tofacitinib 5 mg twice daily and 10 mg twice daily with placebo. The Pivotal 1 study was conducted in 74 centers and the Pivotal 2 study in 94 centers, both in the USA, Canada, Colombia, Germany, Hungary, Japan (Pivotal 1 only), Mexico, Poland, Puerto Rico (Pivotal 2 only), Serbia, Taiwan and Ukraine. Inclusion criteria was age over 18 years, diagnosis of plaque-type psoriasis for over 12 months before the first dose of tofacitinib, Psoriasis Area and Severity Index (PASI) score over 12, psoriatic lesion involvement greater than 10% body surface area (BSA) and Physician's Global Assessment (PGA) score of 3 (moderate) or 4 (severe). PGA is a five-point scale that shows global consideration of erythema, induration, and scaling of psoriatic lesions. Patients had to be candidates for systemic therapy or phototherapy independently of use of prior systemic agents. Exclusion criteria: nonplaque psoriasis systemic, infections, evidence of active, latent or improperly treated Mycobacterium tuberculosis infection, present drug-induced psoriasis, malignancy or history of malignancies, and receiving of efalizumab previously [46]. Patients were recruited by the investigators and were randomized 2:2:1 to administer tofacitinib: 5 mg—745 patients, 10 mg—741 patients or placebo—373 patients, twice daily.

End points consisted of the proportion of patients achieving PASI 90 at week 16, the percentage change from baseline in BSA at week 16, change from baseline Dermatology Life Quality Index (DLQI) total score at week 16, the proportion of patients achieving PGA response at week 4, change from baseline DLQI total score at week 4, the proportion of patients achieving PASI 75 at week 4, and percentage change from baseline Nail Psoriasis Severity Index (NAPSI) at week 16 in patients with nail psoriasis at baseline. Another secondary efficacy end point included time to PASI 75 or PGA response to week 16. Patients who received placebo were randomized at week 16 to be given tofacitinib 5 or 10 mg twice daily—it continued until week 52. Patients who did not achieve PASI 75 or PGA score of "clear" or "almost clear" at week 28 were drawn back [42,43].

In this study, it was observed during Pivotal 1 and Pivotal 2, with similar protocols, that the efficacy of oral tofacitinib, with the 10 mg twice daily, was more efficacious than the 5 mg daily. The psoriasis patients who received tofacitinib in 5 or 10 mg twice daily achieved PASI75 at week 16 in higher percentages (OPT Pivotal 1, 5 mg: 39.9%; 10 mg: 59.2% and OPT Pivotal 2, 5 mg: 46.0%; 10 mg: 59.6%), compared with those receiving placebo (OPT PIVOTAL 1: 6.2%; OPT PIVOTAL 2: 11.4%). The proportions of patients achieving PGA responses at week 16 with tofacitinib 5 and 10 mg twice daily were in OPT Pivotal 1: 41.9% and 59.2% versus placebo 9.0%, and in OPT PIVOTAL 2: 46.0% and 59.1% versus placebo 10.9%. These results were maintained until month 24. Discontinuation of treatment by tofacitinib was associated with a risk of return of lesions, but restart of the treatment rapidly decreased psoriatic inflammation. Retreatment recovery efficacy existed in ~60% of the patients. The reason for this is unknown [4,7,10,42,43,47–52]. In conclusion, tofacitinib 5 and 10 mg twice daily showed clinically relevant efficacy versus placebo over a 16-week period [42,43].

1.4.2. OPT Compare—Phase III Studies of Tofacitinib Treatment

Another phase III trial was OPT Compare. It was conducted to compare tofacitinib 5 mg twice daily or 10 mg twice daily with etanercept 50 mg twice weekly and placebo. It was a randomized multicenter study that proved that the efficacy of tofacitinib 10 mg twice daily is non-inferior at week 12 to the efficacy of etanercept 50 mg twice weekly in psoriasis. The primary end point was evaluated at week 12. Only adult patients with chronic stable plaque psoriasis (for $\geq$12 months) participated in this trial. The patients were recruited from 122 investigational dermatology centuries from different countries. They were candidates for phototherapy or systemic treatment. The inclusion criteria were a Psoriasis Area and Severity Index (PASI) score $\geq$12, a Physician's Global Assessment (PGA) of moderate or severe, and no response to at least one conventional systemic therapy or a contraindication or intolerance to this therapy [7,13].

Between November 2010 and September 2012, 1106 patients were grouped in a proportion of 3:3:3:1. In the first group, the patients received 5mg of tofacitinib twice per day, in the second—10 mg twice daily, in the third—50 mg of etanercept twice a week and in the last group—placebo. In this trial, PASI75 was achieved at week 12 by 39.5% patients of the first group, 63.6% of the second group, 58.8% of the third group and 5.6% of the group with placebo. The PGA was better in 47.1% of patients in the first group, in 68.2% in the second, in 66.3% in the third group and in 15.0% in the placebo group. All active groups achieved a Dermatology Life Quality Index score of 0 or 1 in significantly higher percentages compared with placebo ($p < 0.0001$, for all comparisons). The 10 mg tofacitinib-treated group achieved an Itch Severity Item score of 0 or 1 in a greater percentage of patients compared with etanercept, from week 2 up until week 12 ($p < 0.05$ for all comparisons) [14,20,44,53]. Improvement in nail psoriasis, as assessed by the Nail Psoriasis Severity Index score, was also observed during treatment with tofacinitib (5 or 10 mg daily) at week 16 and was generally maintained until week 52 [3,42,47,53,54]. Number of adverse events was similar in all four groups [53].

1.4.3. Adverse Events of Tofacitinib

The adverse events of tofacitinib included skin infections, skin malignancy and cancers of prostate, lungs, breast and pancreas, lymphomas and lymphoproliferative disorders, infections of respiratory system and urinary tract, activation of latent tuberculosis and reactivation of hepatitis B infection, opportunistic infection, pulmonary cryptococcosis, histoplasmosis, gastrointestinal perforations and obstruction. The laboratory adverse events included decreased hemoglobin levels, RBC, neutrophil and lymphocyte count, and elevation of SGPT, SGOT, CPK, HDL, LDL, TG and cholesterol levels. There was urticaria, angioedema, rash, headache, polyneuropathy and hypertension observed in certain examples [11].

During phase III studies (tofacitinib 5 and 10 mg), 10–15% patients with active psoriasis arthritis were observed to have increased lipid levels. These changes were dose-dependent. The highest fluctuations were related to HDL, LDL and total cholesterol [50,55–57]. Hypertriglyceridemia and metabolic syndrome were higher in patients with psoriasis arthritis than in patients with rheumatoid arthritis treated by tofacitinib [50,58,59]. Studies showed that tofacitinib does not increase cardiovascular disease risk. Similar results were observed in studies with secuckinumab and ustekinumab [41,50,54,60–63]. During clinical trials estimating the safety of tofacitinib taken 5 or 10 mg twice daily compared with a TNF inhibitor in patients with rheumatoid arthritis, increased risks of pulmonary embolism and mortality in patients who received tofacitinib 10 mg twice daily were noticed [14,64,65]. These symptoms were also observed during another independent study that compared tofacitinib with TNF inhibitors [14,66].

During trials PIVOTAL 1 and PIVOTAL 2 in the period to week 16, both doses of tofacitinib were well tolerated. In approximately 900 patients per study, the rates of adverse events were low and similar in all groups of patients. Nausea, headache and diarrhea rates were mildly elevated compared with placebo. There were no opportunistic infections and gastrointestinal perforations. The risk of infection during taking tofacitinib was similar to that of treatments with another biologics [23,24,42,43,67]. It was observed that tofacitinib increased the risk of herpes zoster virus infection comparatively to placebo [14,68]. Three patients among 363 treated by 5 mg and five patients among 360 patients treated by 10 mg reported herpes zoster in OPT PIVOTAL 1. In OPT PIVOTAL 2, there were three patients among 382 patients treated by 5 mg and one among 381 patients treated by 10 mg. All these infections were mild or moderate. Three patients discontinued the study due to herpes zoster events. There was one case of genital herpes in OPT PIVOTAL 1 (10 mg twice daily) and none in OPT PIVOTAL 2. During trials, there were no cases of tuberculosis or other opportunistic infection, no evidence of multidermatomal (more than two dermatomes) or systemic herpes zoster and also no Cytomegalovirus and Epstein–Barr infections [14,42,69].

The most frequent infections were nasopharyngitis, which occurred in OPT PIVOTAL 1, occurring in 5.5% of patients treated with 5 mg tofacitinib, 8.6% patients treated with 10 mg tofacitinib, and 11.3% with placebo. In OPT PIVOTAL 2, it occurred in 8.4% patients treated with 5 mg tofacitinib, 7.9% patients treated with 10 mg tofacitinib, and 5.6% with placebo. Quantity of diarrhea (2.2–4.5%) and headache (4.2–6.9%) were higher with tofacitinib than placebo (0–1.7% and 2.8–3.1%, respectively). Incidence of nausea during taking of tofacitinib was similar to placebo (0.5–2.8%) [43].

During the first 16 weeks of research, there were four patients with tumors (excluding nonmelanoma skin cancer) in OPT PIVOTAL 1 (malignant melanoma, malignant melanoma, esophageal carcinoma, prostate cancer) and none in OPT PIVOTAL 2. There was one case of basal cell carcinoma and one case of squamous cell carcinoma (10 mg twice daily) in OPT PIVOTAL 2 [42,43].

In a study with tofacitinib levels of HDL cholesterol, LDL cholesterol and triglycerides were higher during 4 week observations. In the next period (from 4th to 16th week), the levels were stable. It was not connected with increases in cardiovascular risk. Major adverse cardiovascular cases were reported in two patients receiving tofacitinib 5 mg twice daily, one receiving 10 mg twice daily and none with placebo; all cases were unrelated to the treatment by tofacitinib [14,43,69].

Higher levels of median cholesterol and creatinine phosphokinase (CPK) and lower levels of median hemoglobin were confirmed with tofacitinib during OPT PIVOTAL 1 and OPT PIVOTAL 2. Seven patients had a CPK level of >10 times the upper limit of normal. Among these patients, there were observed moderate myalgia, mild neck pain, and mild arthralgia. No rhabdomyolysis was reported. Mild decreases of blood lymphocyte and hemoglobin were reported in patients with psoriasis healed by tofacitinib; however, these changes decreased and were usually reversible. No severe anemia was confirmed [14,65,70].

1.5. Baricitinib—General Information and Clinical Trials

Baricitinib selectively inhibits JAK1/JAK2 tyrosine kinases [71]. Baricitinib has also been tested in clinical double-blind, placebo-controlled, dose-ranging phase 2b studies [4,45].

Before described studies, patients were qualified to be candidates for phototherapy or systemic therapy. Inclusion criteria were: age $\geq$18 years old, chronic plaque psoriasis for $\geq$6 months, $\geq$12% of body surface involved with psoriatic lesions, PASI scores of $\geq$12 and static Physician's Global Assessment (sPGA) scores of $\geq$3 on a 6-point scale at study entry. Exclusion criteria were history of serious infections or illnesses, active infections, serious comorbid cardiac or hepatic conditions, immunocompromised states, previous treatment with an oral JAK inhibitor, treatment with a biologic agent or monoclonal antibody within 8 weeks before study, treatment with systemic psoriasis therapy or phototherapy within 4 weeks before study and topical psoriasis therapy within 2 weeks before study.

Patients were randomized to receive placebo or oral baricitinib at 2, 4, 8 or 10 mg once daily for 12 weeks [71]. In this 12-week dose-ranging study, encouraging results in treatment were noticed [13]. The primary end point was Psoriasis Area and Severity Index (PASI) 75% (PASI-75) at 12 weeks. A 75% reduction in PASI was achieved by 43% patients treated with baricitinib 8 mg once daily and 54% treated with 10 mg versus placebo group (17%) [7]. Patients achieved significantly higher PASI75 response rates at week 12 compared with placebo. The majority (more than 81%) of the respondents maintained their scores through week 24 [45,71].

In conclusion, patients with moderate to severe psoriasis treated with baricitinib for 12 weeks obtained significant improvements in PASI-75 rates versus patients treated with placebo [71].

Adverse Effects of Baricitinib

There were no serious side effects observed for baricitinib, and this medicine was well tolerated during trial; however, changes in laboratory parameters were similar to those reported for tofacitinib. Baricitinib was observed to cause small dose-related decreases in neutrophil count and hemoglobin levels, as well as small increases in creatinine and lipoprotein levels [4,14,52,72,73]. Opportunistic infections were not observed in any treatment group [71].

1.6. Ruxolitinib—General Information and Clinical Trials

Ruxolitinib is a JAK1/JAK2 inhibitor that blocks signal transduction of multiple proinflammatory cytokines [69,72]. This JAKs inhibitor was used as a topical treatment.

The topical ruxolitinib cream was checked during three psoriasis clinical trials. In a phase 2 vehicle-controlled study in mild and moderate psoriasis, ruxolitinib reported PASI reduction, although no clear dose–response was observed [13].

During the next trial, a double-blind study, ruxolitinib in 1.0% or 0.5% cream used once per day or 1.5% cream twice per day was compared to two active comparators: calcipotriene 0.005% cream and betamethasone dipropionate 0.05% cream for 28 days [13,69]. Ruxolitinib achieved clinical efficacy and was non-inferior to active comparators. One percent ruxolitinib cream as well as 1.5% cream improved erythema, scaling, lesion thickness, erythema and reduced lesion area. It caused their composite lesion score to decrease by more than 50% compared with 32% for active comparators [69,72].

Finally, a third study conducted in 25 patients showed that epidermal hyperplasia was reduced with ruxolitinib in most patients [7]. Inclusion criteria in this study were: limited psoriasis (covering <20% of the body surface area) and age 18–65 years. Psoriatic lesions were rated on a scale of 0–4 for erythema, thickness and scaling. Disease activity in each patient was also scored by Physician's Global Assessment scale. The biopsies of pretreatment and posttreatment skin were compared with healthy skin. In these biopsies, histopathology, immunohistochemistry and mRNA expression were evaluated. Laboratory parameters were also measured: ruxolitinib concentrations in plasma, cytokine stimulated phosphorylated signal transducer and activator of transcription 3 phosphorylation (pSTAT3) levels in peripheral blood cells [71]. Topical ruxilitinib phosphate 1.0% or 1.5% cream was used once or twice daily for 28 days to 2–20% body surface area in five sequential groups of patients, each consisting of five patients [69,72]. After application of ruxolitinib phosphate cream 1.0% and 1.5%, there was significant improvement in lesion scores [72]. During the study, these were observed: decreased dermal inflammation, reduction of epidermal hyperplasia, reduction of dermal inflammation, downregulate transcription of Th1 and Th17 cytokines in psoriatic skin lesions and also reduction of CD3, CD11c, Ki67 and keratin 16 observed during immunohistochemical analysis. There were notable interconnections between clinical improvement and decreases in markers of Th17 lymphocyte activation, epidermal hyperplasia and dendritic-cell activation [4,45,69,72,74]. However, it was not a sustained improvement after discontinuation [54].

In conclusion of this study, topical ruxolitinib is pharmacologically active in patients with active psoriatic lesions and modulates proinflammatory cytokines [69,72].

1.7. Adverse Events of Ruxolitinib

During the double-blind study when ruxolitinib 1.0% or 0.5% cream once per day or 1.5% cream twice per day was compared to two active comparators, inhibition of phosphorylated STAT3 in peripheral blood cells was not observed, suggesting limited systemic exposure [7,14]. Systemic absorption was minimal, and there was no evidence of systemic toxicity [75]. Topical ruxolitinib was found to be well tolerated, safe, and efficacious in short-term treatment in a smaller cohort of patients [9].

During topical application in the 25 patients, there was no noticeable inhibition of pSTAT3 in peripheral blood cells observed. It was relevant to be consistent for low steady-state plasma concentrations of ruxolitinib [69,72].

1.8. Filgotinib—General Information and Clinical Trial

Filgotinib is an oral selective JAK1 inhibitor. The clinical studies of filgotinib in psoriatic arthritis patients and in other illnesses including rheumatoid arthritis, ankylosing spondylitis and ulcerative colitis are still undergoing and have not been confirmed for selling yet [76].

A randomized, double-blind, placebo-controlled phase II trial (EQUATOR) was conducted in active moderate-to-severe psoriasis arthritis. During these studies, evaluating the efficacy and safety of filgotinib in psoriatic arthritis was assessed [76].

The trial was conducted between 9 March and 27 September 2017. In this study, 191 adult patients from 25 cities in seven countries of Europe (Belgium, Bulgaria, Czech Republic, Estonia, Poland, Spain, and Ukraine) were screened. Of those, 131 patients were randomly divided into treatment regimens: 65 patients for filgotinib in dose 200 mg orally once a day and 66 patients for placebo orally once a day, for 16 weeks [75]. Inclusion criteria were: aged $\geq$18 years, active moderate-to-severe psoriatic arthritis, documented history or active of plaque psoriasis and an inadequate response or intolerance to at least one conventional synthetic disease-modifying anti-rheumatic drug (csDMARD) [76]. During the study, patients continued to take csDMAR= if they had received this treatment for at least 12 weeks before screening and had been taking at the same dose for at least 28 days before study [75].

The primary endpoint was proportionate to the patients who achieved 20% improvement in the American College of Rheumatology response criteria (ACR20) at week 16 [75]. Filgotinib showed better efficacy in the ACR20 and ACR50 rates at week 16 versus placebo. Filgotinib group achieved ACR20 in 80%, ACR50 in 55%, LDA (DAPSA $\leq$ 14) in 49%, and PASI75 in 45% of patients. The percentages of the placebo group were respectively 33%, 12%, 15%, and 15% [29,76]. The development in nail psoriasis at week 16 did not achieve statistical significance, probably because of the short study duration and relatively small amount of patients with nail psoriasis [75,76]. In total, 92% patients receiving filgotinib and 97% patients receiving placebo finished the study [75].

Adverse Events of Filgotinib

During the EQUATOR study, good tolerance of filgotinib was observed. The incidence of adverse events including infections that required treatment was similar in filgotinib group versus placebo group at 16 weeks (57% versus 59%). Most of adverse events were mild or moderate.

The most frequent adverse events were headache and nasopharyngitis (similar amount in both group of patients). There were no cases of thromboembolic events, malignances or opportunistic infections, and only one case of herpes zoster infection was observed. One serious treatment-emergent adverse event of pneumonia was reported in the filgotinib group. A decrease of platelets, and increases of hemoglobin, HDL and lymphocyte counts were observed in the filgotinib group [75,76].

1.9. Decernotinib—General Information and Clinical Trial

Decernotinib is the selective inhibitor of JAK3. In first evaluations, it was shown that it can modulate proinflammatory responses of autoimmune diseases such as rheumatoid arthritis.

During placebo-controlled monotherapy study, decernotinib used in doses 50–150 mg twice per day improved clinical signs of rheumatoid arthritis. Later, during two phase II studies, decernotinib was combined with methotreksat and also improved the symptoms of rheumatoid arthritis compared with placebo [4,46].

Adverse Events of Decernotinib

Different adverse effects were noticed during these researches: infections—two herpes zoster infections and one case of tuberculosis, neutropenia—in patients in the methotrexate study, increases of liver transaminase, creatin and lipid levels. The metabolite of decernotinib is a potent inhibitor of cytochrome P450, which is involved in metabolism of different drugs. This interaction can complicate the use of decernotinib [4,46].

2. Conclusions

The choice of treatment in psoriasis depends on the severity of the disease assessed on the available scales. The assessment considers the extent of the lesions, their locations and severity, the response to previously applied treatment and the impact on the quality of life of patients. Definitions of disease severity are mainly based on the criteria for including patients in randomized controlled trials. Although the classification of disease severity varies, mild psoriasis is generally characterized as a disease that can be treated locally. In moderate or severe psoriasis, an escalation of treatment using phototherapy or a systemic drug can be necessary [77]. From the available treatment options, in the first line are topical steroids, topical vitamin D analogues, retinoids, hydroxyurea and fumaric acid esters. During topical treatment, it is important to use creams with urea, salicylic acid, and cignolin. More advanced external treatment includes UVB or psoralen plus UVA phototherapy. Patients with severe psoriasis can be treated with systemic medications such as methotrexate, cyclosporine and acitretin [78]. Unfortunately, the effectiveness of these drugs is often insufficient and they can cause a variety of side effects. Currently, biologic drugs are an important therapeutic option. The decision to use biologic agents must be carefully considered, based on the clinic and the individual patient risk profile. The type of biologic for psoriasis treatment is chosen according to disease severity and comorbidities. A history of previous biologic treatment and its effectiveness are also important. The main indication for biologic treatment is "moderate-to-severe" psoriasis, but the practicing clinician needs to consider what the exact severity is before qualifying the patient for the treatment. The European Medicines Agency (EMA) guidelines refer to indications such as: failure of topical therapies to control the disease; body surface area (BSA) involvement >10% or PASI 10 to 20; thick lesions located in difficult-to-treat regions with BSA involvement <10% may also be considered; and category "moderate to severe" on the PGA (Physician's Global Assessment). The NICE recommendations for disease assessment state that both disease severity and impact are relevant and include the use of indexes such as PASI, PGA, patient assessment, enquiry about difficult-to-treat sites, NAPSI (Nails Psoriasis Severity Index), in which nails are the primary indication for systemic therapy, DLQI (Dermatology

Life Quality Index) and assessment of anxiety and depression [79,80]. In addition to the excellent therapeutic effects of biological drugs in psoriasis, there is more talk about the loss of efficacy and its causes. The main cause is the induction of an immune response directed against the foreign protein molecules. Consequently, antibodies directed against the drugs (ADA) are produced. The presence of ADA is associated with lower serum drug levels and loss of clinical efficacy. Furthermore, an increased incidence of ADA-related adverse drug reactions is observed [81]. The development of ADA in psoriasis is still uncertain, but it seems to be similar to the presence of ADA during biologic treatment in other autoimmune diseases such as Crohn's disease and rheumatoid arthritis. Strand et al. [82], in a systematic review based on data from published reports, found that 50% of patients receiving adalimumab and infliximab developed ADA. Certain factors may influence the immunogenic potential of the agents. These may include the molecular structure of the biologics, concomitant use of methotrexate or other immunosuppressive/anti-proliferative agents, dosage and regimen of the biologic administered and a history of ADA with previous biologic treatment. In addition, patient-related factors may include sex, ethnicity and comorbid conditions [82]. Previous studies indicate well-documented safety and tolerability of biological drugs used in psoriasis. General adverse events (AEs) of biologic treatment are similar. The most frequent (>10%) are various infections such as upper and lower respiratory tract infections, rhinitis, sinusitis, pharyngitis and nasopharyngitis. Serious AEs are rare (<1%) and may include sepsis, viral reactivation (VZV, HBV, HSV), tuberculosis reactivation and fungal infections. Compared to treatment of psoriasis with non-biologic therapy, biologic therapy has not been significantly associated with major adverse events such as cardiovascular events, malignancy, or death beyond what is anticipated in the overall psoriasis population. Other AEs associated with the liver, including severe hepatic reactions, hepatitis, cholestasis and acute liver dysfunction have been reported. Pancytopenia and aplastic anemia were observed rarely during TNF-α inhibitor treatment. In addition, several cutaneous adverse reactions have been associated with anti-TNF drugs. These include eczematous dermatitis, lupus-like skin reactions, leucocytoclastic vasculitis, lichen planus, lichen-planus-like eruptions and alopecia. The safety profile of anti–IL-12/23 has been reported from the results of large clinical trials, including PHOENIX 1, PHOENIX 2 and ACCEPT. The most common AEs were infections, while 0.7% of patients had a cardiac disorder and 0.7% had a serious infection. The most common adverse events that occurred during anti–IL-17A therapy were infections, injection site reactions, nausea and neutropenia [81]. The frequency of adverse effects during therapy with JAK inhibitors is similar to that of other biologic drugs. JAK inhibitors can inhibit the activity of many cytokines that play a role in the pathogenesis of psoriasis. Therefore, JAK inhibition may be associated with an increased risk of infections [83]. Studies to date do not indicate that JAK inhibitors are superior to recent biologic drugs in terms of efficacy. However, the efficacy observed for JAK inhibitors is better than for some currently used systemic therapies, such as some older biologic drugs such as etanercept [15]. JAK inhibitors, due to their lack of increased incidence of side effects compared to other biologic drugs, can be included in the psoriasis treatment algorithm because they are oral and less expensive than modern biologic drugs [15].

The expected results from the clinical trials about JAK inhibitors will be a major step toward extending the therapeutic spectrum of psoriasis by oral compounds. Currently, the number of registered studies on JAK inhibitors in psoriasis is rapidly growing [9,13]. The well-established efficacy of JAK inhibitors in inflammatory disorders, particularly rheumatoid arthritis and ulcerative colitis, suggests the potential of their positive effects in a myriad of inflammatory dermatoses as well [8]. More selective JAK inhibitors are currently in clinical trials [9]. Based on the experience with tofacitinib, numerous JAK inhibitors are tested as oral drugs or as topical formulation for psoriasis. Thus far, the efficacy of topical JAK inhibitors for psoriasis is not convincing [13]. Nevertheless, further studies are needed to evaluate long-term treatment effects with these drugs.

Author Contributions: S.S.-G.—manuscript writing, A.Z.-K.—manuscript writing, K.S.—manuscript writing, A.P.—manuscript writing. All authors have read and agreed to the published version of the manuscript.

Funding: This research received no external funding.

Institutional Review Board Statement: Not applicable.

Informed Consent Statement: Not applicable.

Data Availability Statement: Not applicable.

Conflicts of Interest: The authors declare no conflict of interest.

References

1. Di Meglio, P.; Villanova, F.; Nestle, F.O. Psoriasis. *Cold Spring Harb. Perspect. Med.* **2014**, *4*. [CrossRef]
2. Rapp, S.R.; Feldman, S.R.; Exum, M.L.; Fleischer, A.B., Jr.; Reboussin, D.M. Psoriasis causes as much disability as other major medical diseases. *J. Am. Acad. Dermatol.* **1999**, *41*, 401–407. [CrossRef]
3. Sbidian, E.; Chaimani, A.; Garcia-Doval, I.; Do, G.; Hua, C.; Mazaud, C.; Droitcourt, C.; Hughes, C.; Ingram, J.R.; Naldi, L.; et al. Systemic pharmacological treatments for chronic plaque psoriasis: A network meta-analysis. *Cochrane Database Syst. Rev.* **2017**, *12*, Cd011535. [CrossRef]
4. Virtanen, A.T.; Haikarainen, T.; Raivola, J.; Silvennoinem, O. Selective JAKinibs: Prospects in Inflammatory and Autoimmune Diseases. *BioDrugs* **2019**, *33*, 15. [CrossRef] [PubMed]
5. Gadina, M.; Schwartz, D.M.; O'Shea, J.J. Decernotinib: A Next-Generation Jakinib. *Arthritis Rheumatol.* **2016**, *68*, 31–34. [CrossRef]
6. Shuai, K.; Liu, B. Regulation of JAK-STAT signalling in the immune system. *Nat. Rev. Immunol.* **2003**, *3*, 900–911. [CrossRef] [PubMed]
7. Howell, M.D.; Kuo, F.I.; Smith, P.A. Targeting the Janus Kinase Family in Autoimmune Skin Diseases. *Front. Immunol.* **2019**, *10*, 2342. [CrossRef] [PubMed]
8. Huang, Y.W.; Tsai, T.F. Remission Duration and Long-Term Outcomes in Patients with Moderate-to-Severe Psoriasis Treated by Biologics or Tofacitinib in Controlled Clinical Trials: A 15-Year Single-Center Experience. *Dermatol. Ther.* **2019**, *9*, 553–569. [CrossRef]
9. Bechman, K.; Yates, M.; Galloway, J.B. The new entries in the therapeutic armamentarium: The small molecule JAK inhibitors. *Pharmacol. Res.* **2019**, *147*, 104392. [CrossRef]
10. Szilveszter, K.P.; Németh, T.; Mócsai, A. Tyrosine Kinases in Autoimmune and Inflammatory Skin Diseases. *Front. Immunol.* **2019**, *10*, 1862. [CrossRef]
11. Sonthalia, S.; Aggarwal, P. Oral Tofacitinib: Contemporary Appraisal of Its Role in Dermatology. *Indian Dermatol. Online J.* **2019**, *10*, 503–518. [CrossRef]
12. Leonard, W.J.; O'Shea, J.J. Jaks and STATs: Biological implications. *Annu. Rev. Immunol.* **1998**, *16*, 293–322. [CrossRef] [PubMed]
13. Solimani, F.; Meier, K.; Ghoreschi, K. Emerging Topical and Systemic JAK Inhibitors in Dermatology. *Front. Immunol.* **2019**, *10*, 2847. [CrossRef] [PubMed]
14. Cornejo, M.G.; Boggon, T.J.; Mercher, T. JAK3: A two-faced player in hematological disorders. *Int. J. Biochem. Cell Biol.* **2009**, *41*, 2376–2379. [CrossRef]
15. Kvist-Hansen, A.; Hansen, P.R.; Skov, L. Systemic Treatment of Psoriasis with JAK Inhibitors: A Review. *Dermatol. Ther.* **2020**, *10*, 29–42. [CrossRef]
16. Wang, H.; Feng, X.; Han, P.; Lei, Y.; Xia, Y.; Tian, D.; Yan, W. The JAK inhibitor tofacitinib ameliorates immune-mediated liver injury in mice. *Mol. Med. Rep.* **2019**, *20*, 4883–4892. [CrossRef] [PubMed]
17. Hsu, L.; Armstrong, A.W. JAK inhibitors: Treatment efficacy and safety profile in patients with psoriasis. *J. Immunol. Res.* **2014**, *2014*, 283617. [CrossRef]
18. Vainchenker, W.; Constantinescu, S.N. JAK/STAT signaling in hematological malignancies. *Oncogene* **2013**, *32*, 2601–2613. [CrossRef] [PubMed]
19. Seavey, M.M.; Dobrzanski, P. The many faces of Janus kinase. *Biochem. Pharmacol.* **2012**, *83*, 1136–1145. [CrossRef]
20. He, X.; Chen, X.; Zhang, H.; Xie, T.; Ye, X.Y. Selective Tyk2 inhibitors as potential therapeutic agents: A patent review (2015–2018). *Expert Opin. Ther. Pat.* **2019**, *29*, 137–149. [CrossRef]
21. Ghoreschi, K.; Laurence, A.; O'Shea, J.J. Janus kinases in immune cell signaling. *Immunol. Rev.* **2009**, *228*, 273–287. [CrossRef]
22. O'Sullivan, L.A.; Liongue, C.; Lewis, R.S.; Stephenson, S.E.; Ward, A.C. Cytokine receptor signaling through the Jak-Stat-Socs pathway in disease. *Mol. Immunol.* **2007**, *44*, 2497–2506. [CrossRef]
23. Perner, F.; Schnöder, T.M.; Ranjan, S.; Wolleschak, D.; Ebert, C.; Pils, M.C.; Frey, S.; Polanetzki, A.; Fahldieck, C.; Schönborn, U.; et al. Specificity of JAK-kinase inhibition determines impact on human and murine T-cell function. *Leukemia* **2016**, *30*, 991–995. [CrossRef]
24. Schwartz, D.M.; Kanno, Y.; Villarino, A.; Ward, M.; Gadina, M.; O'Shea, J.J. JAK inhibition as a therapeutic strategy for immune and inflammatory diseases. *Nat. Rev. Drug Discov.* **2017**, *17*, 78. [CrossRef] [PubMed]

25. Kim, J.; Tomalin, L.; Lee, J.; Fitz, L.J.; Berstein, G.; Correa-da Rosa, J.; Garcet, S.; Lowes, M.A.; Valdez, H.; Wolk, R.; et al. Reduction of Inflammatory and Cardiovascular Proteins in the Blood of Patients with Psoriasis: Differential Responses between Tofacitinib and Etanercept after 4 Weeks of Treatment. *J. Investig. Dermatol.* **2018**, *138*, 273–281. [CrossRef] [PubMed]
26. Singh, S.; Pradhan, D.; Puri, P.; Ramesh, V.; Aggarwal, S.; Nayek, A.; Jain, A.K. Genomic alterations driving psoriasis pathogenesis. *Gene* **2019**, *683*, 61–71. [CrossRef] [PubMed]
27. Eder, L.; Wu, Y.; Chandran, V.; Cook, R.; Gladman, D.D. Incidence and predictors for cardiovascular events in patients with psoriatic arthritis. *Ann. Rheum. Dis.* **2016**, *75*, 1680–1686. [CrossRef]
28. Sakkas, L.I.; Zafiriou, E.; Bogdanos, D.P. Mini Review: New Treatments in Psoriatic Arthritis. Focus on the IL-23/17 Axis. *Front. Pharmacol.* **2019**, *10*, 872. [CrossRef] [PubMed]
29. Elli, E.M.; Baratè, C.; Mendicino, F.; Palandri, F.; Palumbo, G.A. Mechanisms Underlying the Anti-inflammatory and Immunosuppressive Activity of Ruxolitinib. *Front. Oncol.* **2019**, *9*, 1186. [CrossRef]
30. US Food and Drug Administration. Xeljanz®Highlights of Prescribing Information. Available online: https://www.accessdata.fda.gov/drugsatfda_docs/label/2018/203214s018lbl.pdf (accessed on 4 December 2018).
31. Purohit, V.S.; Ports, W.C.; Wang, C.; Riley, S. Systemic Tofacitinib Concentrations in Adult Patients With Atopic Dermatitis Treated With 2% Tofacitinib Ointment and Application to Pediatric Study Planning. *J. Clin. Pharmacol.* **2019**, *59*, 811–820. [CrossRef]
32. Xie, R.; Deng, C.; Wang, Q.; Kanik, K.S.; Nicholas, T.; Menon, S. Population pharmacokinetics of tofacitinib in patients with psoriatic arthritis. *Int. J. Clin. Pharmacol. Ther.* **2019**, *57*, 464–473. [CrossRef] [PubMed]
33. US Department of Health and Human Services. Clinical Pharmacology and Biopharmaceutics Review(s). Application Number: 203214Orig1s000. 2011. Available online: https://www.accessdata.fda.gov/drugsatfda_docs/nda/2019/206089Orig1s000ClinPharmR.pdf (accessed on 10 January 2019).
34. Boyle, D.L.; Soma, K.; Hodge, J.; Kavanaugh, A.; Mandel, D.; Mease, P.; Shurmur, R.; Singhal, A.K.; Wei, N.; Rosengren, S.; et al. The JAK inhibitor tofacitinib suppresses synovial JAK1-STAT signalling in rheumatoid arthritis. *Ann. Rheum. Dis.* **2015**, *74*, 1311–1316. [CrossRef]
35. Gladman, D.; Rigby, W.; Azevedo, V.F.; Behrens, F.; Blanco, R.; Kaszuba, A.; Kudlacz, E.; Wang, C.; Menon, S.; Hendrikx, T.; et al. Tofacitinib for Psoriatic Arthritis in Patients with an Inadequate Response to TNF Inhibitors. *N. Engl. J. Med.* **2017**, *377*, 1525–1536. [CrossRef] [PubMed]
36. Nash, P.; Coates, L.C.; Fleischmann, R.; Papp, K.A.; Gomez-Reino, J.J.; Kanik, K.S.; Wang, C.; Wu, J.; Menon, S.; Hendrikx, T.; et al. Efficacy of Tofacitinib for the Treatment of Psoriatic Arthritis: Pooled Analysis of Two Phase 3 Studies. *Rheumatol. Ther.* **2018**, *5*, 567–582. [CrossRef]
37. Pouillon, L.; Bossuyt, P.; Peyrin-Biroulet, L. Tofacitinib Is the Right OCTAVE for Ulcerative Colitis. *Gastroenterology* **2017**, *153*, 862–864. [CrossRef] [PubMed]
38. Mease, P.; Hall, S.; FitzGerald, O.; Van der Heijde, D.; Merola, J.F.; Avila-Zapata, F.; Cieślak, D.; Graham, D.; Wang, C.; Menon, S.; et al. Tofacitinib or Adalimumab versus Placebo for Psoriatic Arthritis. *N. Engl. J. Med.* **2017**, *377*, 1537–1550. [CrossRef]
39. Ly, K.; Beck, K.M.; Smith, M.P.; Orbai, A.M.; Liao, W. Tofacitinib in the management of active psoriatic arthritis: Patient selection and perspectives. *Psoriasis* **2019**, *9*, 97–107. [CrossRef] [PubMed]
40. Dhillon, S. Tofacitinib: A Review in Rheumatoid Arthritis. *Drugs* **2017**, *77*, 1987–2001. [CrossRef]
41. Gladman, D.D.; Ang, M.; Su, L.; Tom, B.D.; Schentag, C.T.; Farewell, V.T. Cardiovascular morbidity in psoriatic arthritis. *Ann. Rheum. Dis.* **2009**, *68*, 1131–1135. [CrossRef]
42. Wolk, R.; Armstrong, E.J.; Hansen, P.R.; Thiers, B.; Lan, S.; Tallman, A.M.; Kaur, M.; Tatulych, S. Effect of tofacitinib on lipid levels and lipid-related parameters in patients with moderate to severe psoriasis. *J. Clin. Lipidol.* **2017**, *11*, 1243–1256. [CrossRef]
43. Krishnaswami, S.; Chow, V.; Boy, M.; Wang, C.; Chan, G. Pharmacokinetics of tofacitinib, a janus kinase inhibitor, in patients with impaired renal function and end-stage renal disease. *J. Clin. Pharmacol.* **2014**, *54*, 46–52. [CrossRef] [PubMed]
44. Bayart, C.B.; DeNiro, K.L.; Brichta, L.; Craiglow, B.G.; Sidbury, R. Topical Janus kinase inhibitors for the treatment of pediatric alopecia areata. *J. Am. Acad. Dermatol.* **2017**, *77*, 167–170. [CrossRef]
45. Desai, R.J.; Pawar, A.; Weinblatt, M.E.; Kim, S.C. Comparative Risk of Venous Thromboembolism in Rheumatoid Arthritis Patients Receiving Tofacitinib Versus Those Receiving Tumor Necrosis Factor Inhibitors: An Observational Cohort Study. *Arthritis Rheumatol.* **2019**, *71*, 892–900. [CrossRef]
46. Westhovens, R. Clinical efficacy of new JAK inhibitors under development. Just more of the same? *Rheumatology* **2019**, *58*, i27–i33. [CrossRef] [PubMed]
47. Mahadevan, U.; Dubinsky, M.C.; Su, C.; Lawendy, N.; Jones, T.V.; Marren, A.; Zhang, H.; Graham, D.; Clowse, M.E.B.; Feldman, S.R.; et al. Outcomes of Pregnancies With Maternal/Paternal Exposure in the Tofacitinib Safety Databases for Ulcerative Colitis. *Inflamm. Bowel Dis.* **2018**, *24*, 2494–2500. [CrossRef]
48. Fragoulis, G.E.; McInnes, I.B.; Siebert, S. JAK-inhibitors. New players in the field of immune-mediated diseases, beyond rheumatoid arthritis. *Rheumatology* **2019**, *58*, i43–i54. [CrossRef] [PubMed]
49. Callis Duffin, K.; Bushmakin, A.G.; Cappelleri, J.C.; Mallbris, L.; Mamolo, C. A multi-item Physician Global Assessment scale to assess psoriasis disease severity: Validation based on four phase III tofacitinib studies. *BMC Dermatol.* **2019**, *19*, 8. [CrossRef]
50. Colombel, J.F. Herpes Zoster in Patients Receiving JAK Inhibitors for Ulcerative Colitis: Mechanism, Epidemiology, Management, and Prevention. *Inflamm. Bowel Dis.* **2018**, *24*, 2173–2182. [CrossRef] [PubMed]

51. Winthrop, K.L.; Lebwohl, M.; Cohen, A.D.; Weinberg, J.M.; Tyring, S.K.; Rottinghaus, S.T.; Gupta, P.; Ito, K.; Tan, H.; Kaur, M.; et al. Herpes zoster in psoriasis patients treated with tofacitinib. *J. Am. Acad. Dermatol.* **2017**, *77*, 302–309. [CrossRef]
52. Papp, K.; Pariser, D.; Catlin, M.; Wierz, G.; Ball, G.; Akinlade, B.; Zeiher, B.; Krueger, J.G. A phase 2a randomized, double-blind, placebo-controlled, sequential dose-escalation study to evaluate the efficacy and safety of ASP015K, a novel Janus kinase inhibitor, in patients with moderate-to-severe psoriasis. *Br. J. Dermatol.* **2015**, *173*, 767–776. [CrossRef]
53. European Medicines Agency. Restrictions in Use of Xeljanz While EMA Reviews Risk of Blood Clots in Lungs. Available online: https://regulatory-access.parexel.com/news-and-press-releases/restrictions-in-use-of-xeljanz-while-ema-reviews-risk-of-blood-clots-in-lungs-prac-17-05-2019 (accessed on 24 September 2019).
54. Miller, I.M.; Skaaby, T.; Ellervik, C.; Jemec, G.B. Quantifying cardiovascular disease risk factors in patients with psoriasis: A meta-analysis. *Br. J. Dermatol.* **2013**, *169*, 1180–1187. [CrossRef] [PubMed]
55. Kitas, G.D.; Gabriel, S.E. Cardiovascular disease in rheumatoid arthritis: State of the art and future perspectives. *Ann. Rheum. Dis.* **2011**, *70*, 8–14. [CrossRef] [PubMed]
56. Toms, T.E.; Panoulas, V.F.; Kitas, G.D. Dyslipidaemia in rheumatological autoimmune diseases. *Open Cardiovasc. Med. J.* **2011**, *5*, 64–75. [CrossRef]
57. Hudgins, L.C.; Parker, T.S.; Levine, D.M.; Gordon, B.R.; Saal, S.D.; Jiang, X.C.; Seidman, C.E.; Tremaroli, J.D.; Lai, J.; Rubin, A.L. A single intravenous dose of endotoxin rapidly alters serum lipoproteins and lipid transfer proteins in normal volunteers. *J. Lipid Res.* **2003**, *44*, 1489–1498. [CrossRef]
58. Bachelez, H.; Van de Kerkhof, P.C.; Strohal, R.; Kubanov, A.; Valenzuela, F.; Lee, J.H.; Yakusevich, V.; Chimenti, S.; Papacharalambous, J.; Proulx, J.; et al. Tofacitinib versus etanercept or placebo in moderate-to-severe chronic plaque psoriasis: A phase 3 randomised non-inferiority trial. *Lancet* **2015**, *386*, 552–561. [CrossRef]
59. Samarasekera, E.J.; Neilson, J.M.; Warren, R.B.; Parnham, J.; Smith, C.H. Incidence of cardiovascular disease in individuals with psoriasis: A systematic review and meta-analysis. *J. Investig. Dermatol.* **2013**, *133*, 2340–2346. [CrossRef]
60. Ahlehoff, O.; Gislason, G.H.; Charlot, M.; Jørgensen, C.H.; Lindhardsen, J.; Olesen, J.B.; Abildstrøm, S.Z.; Skov, L.; Torp-Pedersen, C.; Hansen, P.R. Psoriasis is associated with clinically significant cardiovascular risk: A Danish nationwide cohort study. *J. Intern. Med.* **2011**, *270*, 147–157. [CrossRef] [PubMed]
61. Juneblad, K.; Rantapää-Dahlqvist, S.; Alenius, G.M. Disease Activity and Increased Risk of Cardiovascular Death among Patients with Psoriatic Arthritis. *J. Rheumatol.* **2016**, *43*, 2155–2161. [CrossRef]
62. Labitigan, M.; Bahče-Altuntas, A.; Kremer, J.M.; Reed, G.; Greenberg, J.D.; Jordan, N.; Putterman, C.; Broder, A. Higher rates and clustering of abnormal lipids, obesity, and diabetes mellitus in psoriatic arthritis compared with rheumatoid arthritis. *Arthritis Care Res.* **2014**, *66*, 600–607. [CrossRef]
63. Hansson, G.K. Inflammation, atherosclerosis, and coronary artery disease. *N. Engl. J. Med.* **2005**, *352*, 1685–1695. [CrossRef]
64. Charles-Schoeman, C.; Gonzalez-Gay, M.A.; Kaplan, I.; Boy, M.; Geier, J.; Luo, Z.; Zuckerman, A.; Riese, R. Effects of tofacitinib and other DMARDs on lipid profiles in rheumatoid arthritis: Implications for the rheumatologist. *Semin. Arthritis Rheum.* **2016**, *46*, 71–80. [CrossRef]
65. Wu, J.J.; Strober, B.E.; Hansen, P.R.; Ahlehoff, O.; Egeberg, A.; Qureshi, A.A.; Robertson, D.; Valdez, H.; Tan, H.; Wolk, R. Effects of tofacitinib on cardiovascular risk factors and cardiovascular outcomes based on phase III and long-term extension data in patients with plaque psoriasis. *J. Am. Acad. Dermatol.* **2016**, *75*, 897–905. [CrossRef] [PubMed]
66. Charles-Schoeman, C.; Wicker, P.; Gonzalez-Gay, M.A.; Boy, M.; Zuckerman, A.; Soma, K.; Geier, J.; Kwok, K.; Riese, R. Cardiovascular safety findings in patients with rheumatoid arthritis treated with tofacitinib, an oral Janus kinase inhibitor. *Semin. Arthritis Rheum.* **2016**, *46*, 261–271. [CrossRef] [PubMed]
67. Ogdie, A.; Yu, Y.; Haynes, K.; Love, T.J.; Maliha, S.; Jiang, Y.; Troxel, A.B.; Hennessy, S.; Kimmel, S.E.; Margolis, D.J.; et al. Risk of major cardiovascular events in patients with psoriatic arthritis, psoriasis and rheumatoid arthritis: A population-based cohort study. *Ann. Rheum. Dis.* **2015**, *74*, 326–332. [CrossRef]
68. Savage, L.J.; Wittmann, M.; McGonagle, D.; Helliwell, P.S. Ustekinumab in the Treatment of Psoriasis and Psoriatic Arthritis. *Rheumatol. Ther.* **2015**, *2*, 1–16. [CrossRef] [PubMed]
69. Punwani, N.; Burn, T.; Scherle, P.; Flores, R.; Shi, J.; Collier, P.; Hertel, D.; Haley, P.; Lo, Y.; Waeltz, P.; et al. Downmodulation of key inflammatory cell markers with a topical Janus kinase 1/2 inhibitor. *Br. J. Dermatol.* **2015**, *173*, 989–997. [CrossRef]
70. US Food and Drug Administration. Safety Trial Finds Risk of Blood Clots in the Lungs and Death with Higher Dose of Tofacitinib (Xeljanz, Xeljanz XR) in Rheumatoid Arthritis Patients; FDA to Investigate. Available online: https://www.fda.gov/drugs/drug-safety-and-availability/safety-trial-finds-risk-blood-clots-lungs-and-death-higher-dose-tofacitinib-xeljanz-xeljanz-xr (accessed on 15 April 2019).
71. Strober, B.; Buonanno, M.; Clark, J.D.; Kawabata, T.; Tan, H.; Wolk, R.; Valdez, H.; Langley, R.G.; Harness, J.; Menter, A.; et al. Effect of tofacitinib, a Janus kinase inhibitor, on haematological parameters during 12 weeks of psoriasis treatment. *Br. J. Dermatol.* **2013**, *169*, 992–999. [CrossRef]
72. Papp, K.A.; Menter, M.A.; Raman, M.; Disch, D.; Schlichting, D.E.; Gaich, C.; Macias, W.; Zhang, X.; Janes, J.M. A randomized phase 2b trial of baricitinib, an oral Janus kinase (JAK) 1/JAK2 inhibitor, in patients with moderate-to-severe psoriasis. *Br. J. Dermatol.* **2016**, *174*, 1266–1276. [CrossRef]

73. Bissonnette, R.; Luchi, M.; Fidelus-Gort, R.; Jackson, S.; Zhang, H.; Flores, R.; Newton, R.; Scherle, P.; Yeleswaram, S.; Chen, X.; et al. A randomized, double-blind, placebo-controlled, dose-escalation study of the safety and efficacy of INCB039110, an oral janus kinase 1 inhibitor, in patients with stable, chronic plaque psoriasis. *J. Dermatol. Treat.* **2016**, *27*, 332–338. [CrossRef]
74. Punwani, N.; Scherle, P.; Flores, R.; Shi, J.; Liang, J.; Yeleswaram, S.; Levy, R.; Williams, W.; Gottlieb, A. Preliminary clinical activity of a topical JAK1/2 inhibitor in the treatment of psoriasis. *J. Am. Acad. Dermatol.* **2012**, *67*, 658–664. [CrossRef]
75. Mease, P.; Coates, L.C.; Helliwell, P.S.; Stanislavchuk, M.; Rychlewska-Hanczewska, A.; Dudek, A.; Abi-Saab, W.; Tasset, C.; Meuleners, L.; Harrison, P.; et al. Efficacy and safety of filgotinib, a selective Janus kinase 1 inhibitor, in patients with active psoriatic arthritis (EQUATOR): Results from a randomised, placebo-controlled, phase 2 trial. *Lancet* **2018**, *392*, 2367–2377. [CrossRef]
76. Chen, M.; Dai, S.M. A novel treatment for psoriatic arthritis: Janus kinase inhibitors. *Chin. Med. J.* **2020**, *133*, 959–967. [CrossRef]
77. Smith, C.H.; Barker, J.N. Psoriasis and its management. *BMJ* **2006**, *333*, 380–384. [CrossRef] [PubMed]
78. Golbari, N.M.; Porter, M.L.; Kimball, A.B. Current guidelines for psoriasis treatment: A work in progress. *Cutis* **2018**, *101*, 10–12.
79. Abrouk, M.; Nakamura, M.; Zhu, T.H.; Farahnik, B.; Koo, J.; Bhutani, T. The impact of PASI 75 and PASI 90 on quality of life in moderate to severe psoriasis patients. *J. Dermatol. Treat.* **2017**, *28*, 488–491. [CrossRef]
80. Smith, C.H.; Yiu, Z.Z.N.; Bale, T.; Burden, A.D.; Coates, L.C.; Edwards, W.; MacMahon, E.; Mahil, S.K.; McGuire, A.; Murphy, R.; et al. British Association of Dermatologists guidelines for biologic therapy for psoriasis 2020: A rapid update. *Br. J. Dermatol.* **2020**, *183*, 628–637. [CrossRef] [PubMed]
81. Lockwood, S.J.; Prens, L.M.; Kimball, A.B. Adverse Reactions to Biologics in Psoriasis. *Curr. Probl. Dermatol.* **2018**, *53*, 1–14. [CrossRef]
82. Strand, V.; Balsa, A.; Al-Saleh, J.; Barile-Fabris, L.; Horiuchi, T.; Takeuchi, T.; Lula, S.; Hawes, C.; Kola, B.; Marshall, L. Immunogenicity of Biologics in Chronic Inflammatory Diseases: A Systematic Review. *BioDrugs* **2017**, *31*, 299–316. [CrossRef] [PubMed]
83. Bechman, K.; Subesinghe, S.; Norton, S.; Atzeni, F.; Galli, M.; Cope, A.P.; Winthrop, K.L.; Galloway, J.B. A systematic review and meta-analysis of infection risk with small molecule JAK inhibitors in rheumatoid arthritis. *Rheumatology* **2019**, *58*, 1755–1766. [CrossRef] [PubMed]

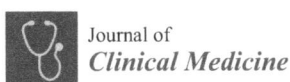

Review

Diagnosis and Intervention in Early Psoriatic Arthritis

Tomoyuki Hioki [1,2,*], Mayumi Komine [2,*] and Mamitaro Ohtsuki [2]

1. Department of Dermatology, Central Japan International Medical Center, Minokamo 505-8510, Japan
2. Department of Dermatology, Jichi Medical University, 3311-1 Yakushiji, Shimotsuke 329-0498, Japan; mamitaro@jichi.ac.jp
* Correspondence: m04067th@jichi.ac.jp (T.H.); mkomine12@jichi.ac.jp (M.K.)

Abstract: Psoriatic arthritis (PsA) is a chronic inflammatory disorder that affects approximately 20–30% of patients with psoriasis. PsA causes deformities and joint damage, impairing quality of life and causing long-term functional disability. Several recent studies demonstrated that early diagnosis and intervention for PsA prevents permanent invalidity. However, the clinical features of PsA vary and are shared with other differential diseases, such as reactive arthritis, osteoarthritis, and ankylosing spondylitis. The common and overlapping features among these diseases complicate the accurate early diagnosis and intervention of PsA. Therefore, this review focuses on the current knowledge of the diagnosis of early PsA and discusses the meaning of early intervention for early PsA.

Keywords: psoriatic arthritis; early diagnosis; treatment; early intervention

1. Introduction

Psoriatic arthritis (PsA) is a chronic inflammatory disorder that affects 14.0–22.7% of patients with psoriasis [1–3]. The incidence of PsA differs among counties: 22.7% in European psoriasis patients, 21.5% in South American patients, 19.5% in North American patients, 15.5% in African patients, and 14.0% in Asian patients with psoriasis [3]. A Japanese Society for Psoriatic Research survey revealed a 10.5% occurrence of PsA among newly visited psoriasis patients [4]. Its prevalence varies from 0.19% to 0.25% [5,6]. The main musculoskeletal manifestations of PsA are peripheral arthritis, spinal spondylitis, asymmetrical synovitis, enthesitis, and/or dactylitis [7]. In 1973, Moll and Wright proposed classifying PsA into five subgroups: (1) asymmetric oligoarthritis, (2) predominant distal interphalangeal joint involvement, (3) symmetric polyarthritis, (4) predominant axial involvement, and (5) arthritis mutilans [8].

PsA is a highly heterogeneous disease whose clinical features vary [9]. Its clinical features are also observed in other diseases, such as reactive arthritis, osteoarthritis, and ankylosing spondylitis [10]. The common and overlapping features of these diseases present challenges in the accurate diagnosis of PsA. The delayed diagnosis of PsA is associated with poor physical function and permanent invalidity [11,12]. There is increasing concern that early diagnosis and a rapid therapeutic intervention, such as biologics before the onset of structural damage, can inhibit joint damage and permanent invalidity [13]. Psoriasis patients without PsA reportedly show substantial signs of enthesophyte formation [14]. Early psoriatic arthritis (ePsA), which is defined as inflammatory joint symptoms and signs compatible with PsA of less than 24 months of duration [13], usually appears as enthesoarthritis with a consistent risk of evolving toward erosive and deforming arthritis in the first year of disease [15,16]. Several studies recently demonstrated that the early diagnosis and intervention of PsA prevent permanent invalidity.

This review focuses on the current knowledge regarding the diagnosis of ePsA and discusses the significance of its early intervention.

Citation: Hioki, T.; Komine, M.; Ohtsuki, M. Diagnosis and Intervention in Early Psoriatic Arthritis. *J. Clin. Med.* **2022**, *11*, 2051. https://doi.org/10.3390/jcm11072051

Academic Editor: Stamatis Gregoriou

Received: 18 February 2022
Accepted: 29 March 2022
Published: 6 April 2022

Publisher's Note: MDPI stays neutral with regard to jurisdictional claims in published maps and institutional affiliations.

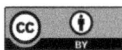

Copyright: © 2022 by the authors. Licensee MDPI, Basel, Switzerland. This article is an open access article distributed under the terms and conditions of the Creative Commons Attribution (CC BY) license (https://creativecommons.org/licenses/by/4.0/).

2. Recent Concept of PsA Onset

It is difficult to determine when PsA begins in individual patients. PsA is usually diagnosed when patients present with psoriasis skin lesions and rheumatoid factor (RF)-negative inflammatory arthritis. Recent literature argues that the pathophysiology of PsA starts at a much earlier time point several years prior to the diagnosis of PsA. The Delphi consensus study proposed three stages for such patients as follows: (1) individuals with psoriasis at increased risk for PsA; (2) individuals with psoriasis and asymptomatic synovio-entheseal imaging abnormalities; and (3) individuals with psoriasis and musculoskeletal symptoms not explained by other diagnoses [17].

2.1. Individuals with Psoriasis with Increased Risk for PsA

Patients with psoriasis are at a higher risk of developing PsA than healthy controls and at a higher risk of developing PsA than other patients [6,18,19]. Thus, there is a keen need to identify psoriasis patients at a higher risk of developing PsA to prevent progression to PsA, but knowledge of this is limited.

Some clinical features, such as nail pitting and scalp and genital involvement, are predictors of PsA in patients [20]. Others include obesity, the presence of arthralgia, severe psoriasis, a history of uveitis, nail psoriasis, scalp psoriasis, having a first-degree relative with PsA, and any associated gene (such as human leukocyte antigens [HLA]-B*08, HLA-B*27, HLA-B*38, and HLA-B*39) [6,21].

2.2. Individuals with Psoriasis and Asymptomatic Synovio-Entheseal Imaging Abnormalities

Recent studies revealed that, in some patients with psoriasis, even those without symptoms of arthritis such as joint swelling or pain, imaging analysis with magnetic resonance imaging (MRI) or ultrasonography (US) demonstrate abnormalities [22,23]. These modalities include MRI for axial disease, MRI for peripheral arthritis, US for peripheral arthritis, US for enthesis, and plain radiography for peripheral arthritis [24].

2.3. Individuals with Psoriasis and Musculoskeletal Symptoms Not Explained by Other Diagnoses

Some patients with psoriasis report heel pain, stiffness, and/or arthralgia, which are not explained by other diagnoses, and no imaging abnormalities [25]. Previous studies identified these patients as "prodromal PsA", "subclinical PsA", "psoriasis with arthralgia", "psoriasis with musculoskeletal symptoms", or "psoriasis with musculoskeletal symptoms without musculoskeletal signs".

The progression of these stages to PsA is shown in Figure 1.

More than 80% of PsA patients develop after the diagnosis of psoriasis (PsO), thus it is important to recognize PsO patients with increased risk to develop PsA. Nail psoriasis, scalp, and genital skin involvement are the risk factors to develop PsA in PsO patients. PsO patients with arthralgia (PsOAr) are also at higher risk to develop PsA. Almost 50% of PsO patients without articular symptoms show subclinical arthritis detected by imaging techniques. Among them, those who have active enthesitis detected by ultrasonography have higher risk to progress into PsA [27].

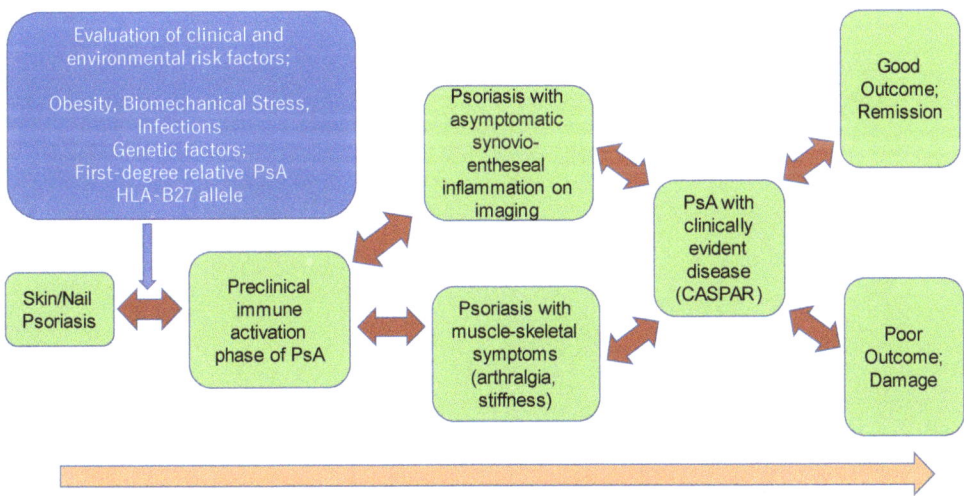

Figure 1. The natural clinical course of PsA, including its preclinical stages. Each stage can be reversed as represented by the two-way arrows. Adapted from Pennington and Fitzgerald [26], Frontiers in Medicine 2021 with permission.

3. Questionnaires

Questionnaires that include key questions about joint symptoms, morning stiffness, and function can aid the diagnosis of ePsA. Three representative questionnaires are available for screening patients with psoriasis and arthritis. First, the Psoriatic Arthritis Screening and Evaluation (PASE) questionnaire is an effective screening tool for detecting patients with PsA [28]. It reportedly has a sensitivity of 82% and a specificity of 73% [28]. Second, the Psoriasis and Arthritis Questionnaire (PAQ), first reported in 1997, can predict PsA in patients with psoriasis with a sensitivity of 85% and specificity of 88% [29]. A validation study of the PAQ showed a sensitivity of 60% and specificity of 62% [29]. The modified PAQ features improved sensitivity and specificity of 68.7% and 77.8%, respectively [29].

Third, the Toronto PsA screening questionnaire (ToPAS) evaluates the clinical features of patients with PsA [30]. Its inclusion of pictures of skin and nail lesions distinguishes it from other screening questionnaires. Although PASE and PAQ are limited for detecting arthritis in patients with psoriasis, the ToPAS can screen for PsA regardless of whether a patient has psoriasis [30]. Its sensitivity and specificity are reportedly 94% and 92% [30]. The higher sensitivity and specificity can help identify patients with PsA in various clinical settings.

The psoriasis epidemiology screening tool (PEST) was first presented in 2009 by Ibrahim et al. and developed on a primary care–based population of psoriasis patients [31]. It consisted of five simple questions and had a sensitivity and specificity of 92% and 78%, respectively [31]. The Early Arthritis for Psoriatic Patients (EARP) questionnaire, developed by Tinazzi et al. in 2012, consists of 10 simple questions and features a sensitivity and specificity of 91% and 85%, respectively [32].

The Screening Tool for Rheumatologic Investigation in Psoriatic Patients (STRIPP) tool was recently developed by Burlando et al. [33] The STRIPP is composed of six sections. The first section is about demographic data, such as age, sex, psoriasis onset, and the second part evaluates psoriasis with PASI and specific localization such as the nails, scalp, and genitalia. The third part concerns ongoing treatment. The fourth section is derived from the PASE with six questions, the fifth section is about uveitis and inflammatory bowel diseases, and the sixth section focuses on rheumatological evaluation with imaging and diagnosis. The sensitivity and specificity are 91.5% and 93.3%, respectively [33].

Several reports on the comparison of these psoriatic arthritis screening tools have been published, some revealed similar efficacy, and others, comparing EARP, PEST, PASE, and toPAS II, revealed that EARP showed the highest sensitivity, and ToPAS II showed highest specificity. However, these tools present relatively low specificity, allowing other causes of musculoskeletal pain to be evaluated as PsA. This is because PsA is a heterogeneous entity and developing a screening tool to identify PsA and exclude other causes of musculoskeletal pain is extremely difficult. Thus, we have to be aware that we might seeing patients with other musculoskeletal disease than PsA, even when they are screened by questionnaires [34–36].

Classification Criteria

Given the absence of a validated case definition of PsA, scientific and clinical research on PsA has been a major problem. However, an international group of rheumatologists proposed the Classification of Psoriatic Arthritis (CASPAR) criteria in 2006, which remain the current representative criteria based on the results of a large prospective study [37]. The CASPAR criteria were developed for use in clinical research and had a sensitivity and specificity of 91.4% and 98.7%, respectively, in patients with other forms of inflammatory arthritis. The high sensitivity and specificity suggest that it may also be used as a diagnostic criterion for PsA. Several studies have tested the sensitivity of CASPAR criteria for detecting early PsA. Classification criteria such as CASPAR are generally not useful for diagnostic purposes; however, their application for detecting ePsA remains to be established [37]. Since the initial development of CASPAR criteria, many studies have been conducted to establish its effectiveness as a criterium and also as a diagnostic tool, resulting in frequent use of CASPAR criteria in various clinical studies on PsA [38–40].

4. Biomarkers of ePsA

Biological markers (biomarkers) are objective and useful markers for the diagnosis and evaluation of alterations in physiological status [41]. To date, no disease-specific biomarkers have been identified for ePsA. PsA usually tests negative for rheumatoid factor, which differentiates it from rheumatoid arthritis (RA), the most common form of inflammatory arthritis [10]. However, many candidate biomarkers with potential utility in PsA have been reported [10], such as elevated erythrocyte sedimentation rate (ESR), C-reactive protein (CRP), and acute-phase serum amyloid A (A-SAA), all of which are nonspecific inflammatory markers that are also elevated in RA. Some cytokines are elevated in synovial fluids in PsA with polyarticular involvement compared to those with monoarticular involvement, such as interleukin (IL)-1, IL-12p40, interferon alpha, IL-15, and chemokine ligand 3, which could differentiate PsA patients with polyarticular involvement from those with oligoarticular involvement [10].

S100A8/S100A9 (calgranulin) levels are elevated in patients with high disease activity, which is decreased by treatment with methotrexate with a decreased number of swollen joints, the Richie articular index, and a disease activity score [42]. They are elevated in patients with >10 involved joints compared to those with <10 involved joints [43]. Vascular endothelial growth factor and angiopoetin-2 are angiogenic markers that predict joint damage in RA, and their levels are higher in PsA than in RA, which also predicts joint damage in PsA [43]. The radiographic progression of PsA patients correlates with the levels of macrophage colony-stimulating factor and receptor activator of nuclear factor kappa B ligand [44]. Baseline levels of A-SAA correlated with 1-year radiographic progression in patients with PsA. A-SAA levels correlate with the levels of matrix metalloproteinase (MMP)1, MMP3, MMP13, and tissue inhibitors of matrix metalloproteinases [45]. A-SAA is known to induce MMP production in synovial fibroblast-like cells [46], and MMP1 and MMP3 are reportedly associated with radiographic progression in patients with early RA [47], which suggests that they could also be early disease progression markers for PsA.

Some genetic markers indicate psoriasis and PsA as distinct populations. Many molecules have demonstrated differences in the prevalence of psoriasis and PsA, but most, even if involved in the pathophysiology, may not be involved in the pathogenesis, showing only very low correlation with the disease. HLA molecules are the only molecules that have been identified as risk factors for PsA [6,21].

Currently unidentified epigenetic markers can be used to distinguish psoriasis from PsA. IL-22 is one such candidate whose methylation levels in patients with cutaneous symptoms only and those with cutaneous and articular involvement changes [48].

5. Imaging Techniques

Imaging techniques are more sensitive than clinical examinations in the diagnosis of synovitis and enthesitis as well as the assessment of inflammatory activity in PsA. Incorporating imaging modalities in the assessment and early intervention of ePsA may be useful for preventing permanent invalidity. In early PsA, inflammatory changes occur in the soft tissue and bone marrow that cannot be detected using plain X-rays [9]. Ultrasonography and MRI are sensitive and useful tools for detecting inflammatory joint disease [49–51]. Ultrasonography is frequently used to evaluate arthritis. Recent studies by Zabotti et al. [52] revealed that psoriasis patients with arthralgia (PsOAr) are at higher risk to develop PsA, with higher positive sonographic findings of tenosynovitis, which was not correlated with development to PsA in longitudinal study. Sonographically determined active enthesitis was associated with disease progression to PsA.

Synovio-entheseal complex (SEC) has been shown the initial site of inflammation in PsA, where mechanistic stress occurs, which efficiently distinguishes PsA from RA. It has been revealed that up to half of asymptomatic psoriasis patients showed subclinical synovial or entheseal inflammation [27]. The most important findings suggestive of early PsA in ultrasonography is enthesitis of metacarpophalangeal (MP) joints, and proximal interphalangeal (PIP) joints of the hands [52]. The diagnosis of axial disease might require MRI, whereas enthesitis can be visualized using both MRI and ultrasound (US) [24]. Dynamic MRI may be a clinically useful measure of synovial inflammation. High-resolution peripheral quantitative computed tomography (HRpQ-CT) is a novel technique mainly used for the diagnosis and evaluation of disease progression [53]. High-resolution fluorine-18 fludeoxyglucose (^{18}F-FDG) positron emission tomography (PET)/CT imaging of the wrist and hand is feasible in RA or PsA patient cohorts and can provide quantifiable measures of disease activity [54,55]. In addition, it has been reported that ^{18}F-FDG PET/CT is a powerful tool for detecting subclinical arthritis in patients with psoriatic arthritis and/or psoriasis vulgaris [56].

6. Treatment of ePsA

The clinical signs and symptoms of ePsA often fluctuate, and the disease course is not simply in one direction; rather, it moves back and forth. Some sPsA patients rapidly progress to severe disease, whereas other ePsA patients develop clinical symptoms that disappear over time. Thus, our understanding is that some ePsA patients require early intervention to prevent the development of severe disease but others do not because their disease remains mild or spontaneously improves. If good markers were available to distinguish between patients with versus without severe ePsA severe disease, it would be easy to treat these patients. However, there are no such markers; therefore, we treat patients according to their current disease severity.

6.1. Nonsteroidal Anti-Inflammatory Drugs and Methotrexate

The first medications we tried for patients with ePsA were non-steroidal anti-inflammatory drugs (NSAIDs). Some patients are sufficiently treated with NSAIDs and the remaining mild disease or symptoms disappear during the disease course [57].

Other patients require more efficient treatment such as methotrexate (MTX) [57]. MTX is approved for use in severe psoriasis (which is often related to psoriatic arthritis) and rheumatoid arthritis (RA) by the U.S. Food and Drug Administration (FDA) and the European Medicines Agency (EMA), and frequently used to treat PsA, in spite of the lack of evidence with randomized controlled trials (RCTs). Pincus T et al. [58] discussed on MTX clinical trials on PsA and suggested that too high or too low dose of MTX use, insufficient stratification of patients, or insufficient statistical power to detect differences in old clinical trials caused the lack of evidence of MTX, and that the treatment advantage versus placebo without statistical significance ($p < 0.05$) does not necessarily mean the absence of clinical efficacy.

MTX was intensely used to treat PsA patients before biologics emerged, although it was not approved in Japan before March 2019 [59]. Adverse effects, including liver toxicity and hematopoiesis suppression, are disadvantages of this drug.

Leflunomide, a selective pyrimidine synthesis inhibitor with the property to inhibit T-cell activation and proliferation has also been shown to improve joint and skin symptoms of PsA (although with less efficacy in the skin) [57]. Leflunomide has been shown effective in several randomized double-blind placebo-controlled studies in PsA, but MTX has not [60,61].

The European League Against Rheumatism (EULAR) recommendation for the management of psoriatic arthritis recommends conventional synthetic disease-modifying antirheumatic drugs (csDMARDs) such as MTX or leflunomide for peripheral arthritis with polyarticular involvement, monoarthritis, or oligoarthritis with poor prognostic factors such as structural damage, high ESR and CRP levels, dactylitis, or nail involvement [57]. Biologic DMARDs (bDMARDs) are recommended when csDMARDs are ineffective.

6.2. Biologics

Tumor necrosis factor (TNF) antagonists are well established for the treatment of PsA [57]. To date, four anti-TNF agents, infliximab, adalimumab, and certolizumab-pegol, have been approved for the treatment of PsA by the Japanese authorities [62]. These agents effectively improve articular symptoms of peripheral and axial diseases, radiological findings, and skin and nail lesions [63].

Anti-IL-17 antibodies, including secukinumab, ixekizumab, and brodalumab, have proven effective at treating PsA with peripheral and axial involvement. The EULAR recommendation for the treatment of PsA recommends TNF inhibitors and IL-17 inhibitors for axial disease as the first choice because MTX and IL-23 are inferior [57]. On the other hand, IL-12/23 antibodies are effective for peripheral arthritis and are recommended at the same level as IL-17 and superior to TNF inhibitors for peripheral arthritis when the csDMARD efficacy is inadequate [57].

Anti-IL-23 antibodies including guselkumab, risankizumab, and tildrakizumab, have less efficacy for treating axial disease compared to anti-IL-17 antibodies and anti-TNF antibodies, maybe because IL-17-producing cells are independent on IL-23 stimulation in axial lesion, such as γδ T cells and mucosal-associated invariant cells [64]. Radiologic investigations, including MRI and HRpQ-CT, showed the absence of both erosive and bone anabolic damage, supporting the possibility of the arrest of progression of anabolic changes in PsA with secukinumab and ixekizumab.

Treatment of psoriasis and psoriatic arthritis with biologics have been shown to protect patients from systemic inflammatory comorbidities, such as cardiovascular diseases, diabetes, and abnormal lipid metabolism. It needs caution in that anti-IL-17 antibodies may cause newly onset or worsening of inflammatory bowel diseases [63].

6.3. Janus Kinase Inhibitors

Janus kinase (JAK) inhibitors were recently approved for the treatment of PsA in Japan. JAK inhibitors are classified as target-specific DMARDs (tsDMARDs). Owing to the adverse effects of this category of drugs, they are recommended for the treatment of PsA when bDMARDs are ineffective. The efficacy and safety of JAK inhibitors for PsA were recently discussed. Three JAK inhibitors–tofacitinib, baricitinib, and upadacitinib– have been approved for use in autoimmune diseases; of them, only tofacitinib has been approved for the treatment of PsA. Tofacitinib, an orally available JAK inhibitor, broadens the treatment options for PsA and other inflammatory conditions [65].

7. Early Intervention for ePsA

However, when to implement early intervention for PsA remains controversial. The open prospective exploratory Interception in Very Early PsA (IVEPSA) study showed that very early disease intervention with secukinumab, an IL-17A inhibitor, for PsA may lead to a comprehensive decline in skin symptoms [66]. The Tight Control Of inflammation in early Psoriatic Arthritis (TICOPA) study showed the effects in patients in the tight control group [67]. Moreover, trials to demonstrate the efficacy of targeted biologic therapies and DMARDs in early PsA will test the validity of early intervention as a strategy to alter the disease course [67].

Biologic treatment of psoriasis patients without psoriatic arthritis have reported to reduce the incidence of development of psoriatic arthritis [68]. Psoriasis patients without psoriatic arthritis may include those with increased risk, or with asymptomatic arthritis with imaging abnormalities, or with undiagnosed musculoskeletal symptoms as discussed in Section 2. It would be of importance to identify patients in need to be treated with bDMARDs to prevent the development of psoriatic arthritis, to avoid overtreatment.

However, the disease course of PsA is not simple, and various patients follow distinct disease courses with an ever-expanding and fluctuating disease course. Novel biomarkers that distinguish patients who need early intervention are needed to fully prevent disease progression in those with a poor prognosis.

7.1. Guidelines

The Group for Research and Assessement of Psoriasis and Psoriatic Arthritis (GRAPPA), European League Against Rheumatism (EULAR), American college of Rheumatology/National Psoriasis Foundation, and other national associations of dermatologists in each country including Japan, Great Britain, Germany, and so on, have published guidelines for treating psoriasis and psoriatic arthritis, and continue updating them to include the most recent advancements in treatment of psoriasis and psoriatic arthritis [69–72]. GRAPPA is a global research group for psoriasis and psoriatic arthritis, assessing both dermatological and musculoskeletal manifestations, while EULAR focuses on rheumatic diseases referring to dermatologists for significant skin disease but not recommendations for skin and nail manifestations. Each country has its own system of insurance and it is hard to establish a general recommendation to fit systems in all countries, and each country establishes its own guidelines referring to and modifying EULAR and/or GRAPPA. EULAR bases on Oxford Center for Evidence-Based Medicine: Levels of Evidence, and GRAPPA relies on newer Grading of Recommendations, Assessment, Development and Evaluation [73]. Both of them are based on a specific systematic literature review (SLR). GRAPPA mostly depends on randomized control trials. However, good RCTs are sometimes missing, especially for those medicines from old time, such as methotrexate (MTX). EULAR recommend MTX as a first line in treatment for PsA, based on experts' opinions, while GRAPPA dose not give rank to MTX, although it is included as one of potential DMARDs.

7.2. Costs

Although biologics are quite effective for the manifestation and health-related quality of life of PsA, they may increase the economic burden on health systems [74]. The total annual cost per patient ranged from US $10,924 to US $17,050, with purchasing power parity for PsA in five European countries [75]. It has also been reported that the introduction of biologics leads to a 3-fold to 5-fold increase in direct costs and, consequently, an increase in total costs [76].

The EULAR recommendation and Japanese guideline for the treatment of PsA do not recommend biologics as the first-choice treatment of PsA; rather, they recommend csDMARDs or MTX [57,76]. Biologics are highly efficient drugs for treating PsA, but their cost would burden the country's economy. In contrast, csDMARDs including MTX are inexpensive and effective drugs for the treatment of PsA and should be used before bDMARDs in these countries. However, the American College of Rheumatology/National

Psoriasis Foundation guidelines recommend biologics at the same level as csDMARDs due to the different insurance systems, mostly dependent on private insurance companies [77]. Each country adopts EULAR and GRAPPA recommendations, modifying them to fit its insurance system. Because recently developed biologics and targeted therapeutics cost tremendously, in some countries, the use of them are restricted to certain period of time. It would be necessary to develop guidelines to benefit both patients and social insurance systems effectively to continue providing good medical treatments.

Even with insurance, some patients cannot afford biologics for PsA treatment. There are certainly economic disparities in modern society in which many patients are not adequately treated because of economic reasons.

8. Conclusions

Despite tremendous advances in therapies and treatment strategies, there remains an unmet need to identify the optimal therapeutic approach for individual PsA patients. The diagnosis and intervention of ePsA are important to preventing disease progression, structural damage, and permanent invalidity. Therefore, standardized imaging techniques, validated scoring systems, and protocols are required. New imaging techniques such as US, MRI, and PET/CT have since been developed. Despite these developments, there is currently no gold standard technique to detect ePsA. Psoriatic arthritis is a heterogenous condition, which includes preclinical, subclinical, mild to severe disease, and these conditions may or may not progress to severer condition, depending on individual cases, which makes it difficult to establish a simple guidance to apply to all patients. Early intervention for PsA will probably inhibit inflammation and alter the disease course, and it is of importance to distinguish patients in need for early intervention not to overtreat mild disease patients and to save costs. However, an efficient tool to distinguish such patients in need and the evidence to support this is still lacking. Thus, further studies on the pathophysiology, diagnosis and intervention of ePsA are required.

Author Contributions: Conceptualization, T.H. and M.K.; writing—original draft preparation, T.H.; writing—review and editing, M.K.; supervision, M.O.; funding acquisition, M.O. All authors have read and agreed to the published version of the manuscript.

Funding: This research received no external funding.

Institutional Review Board Statement: Not applicable.

Informed Consent Statement: Not applicable.

Data Availability Statement: Not applicable.

Acknowledgments: We thank all the members of Psoriasis Outpatient Clinic at Department of Dermatology, Jichi Medical University for their cooperation in diagnosis and treatment of psoriasis patients.

Conflicts of Interest: The authors declare no conflict of interest.

References

1. Coates, L.C.; Helliwell, P.S. Psoriatic Arthritis: State of the Art Review. *Clin. Med.* **2017**, *17*, 65–70. [CrossRef]
2. Kaeley, G.S.; Eder, L.; Aydin, S.Z.; Gutierrez, M.; Bakewell, C. Enthesitis: A Hallmark of Psoriatic Arthritis. *Semin. Arthritis Rheum.* **2018**, *48*, 35–43. [CrossRef] [PubMed]
3. Alinaghi, F.; Calov, M.; Kristensen, L.E.; Gladman, D.D.; Coates, L.C.; Jullien, D.; Gottlieb, A.B.; Gisondi, P.; Wu, J.J.; Thyssen, J.P.; et al. Prevalence of Psoriatic Arthritis in Patients with Psoriasis: A Systematic Review and Meta-Analysis of Observational and Clinical Studies. *J. Am. Acad. Dermatol.* **2019**, *80*, 251–265. [CrossRef] [PubMed]
4. Yamamoto, T.; Ohtsuki, M.; Sano, S.; Igarashi, A.; Morita, A.; Okuyama, R.; Kawada, A.; Working Group of the Epidemiological Survey in the Japanese Society for Psoriasis Research. Epidemiological analysis of psoriatic arthritis patients in Japan. *J. Dermatol.* **2016**, *43*, 1193–1196. [CrossRef] [PubMed]
5. Ogdie, A.; Weiss, P. The Epidemiology of Psoriatic Arthritis. *Rheum. Dis. Clin. N. Am.* **2015**, *41*, 545–568. [CrossRef] [PubMed]
6. Ogdie, A.; Langan, S.; Love, T.; Haynes, K.; Shin, D.; Seminara, N.; Mehta, N.N.; Troxel, A.; Choi, H.; Gelfand, J.M. Prevalence and Treatment Patterns of Psoriatic Arthritis in the UK. *Rheumatology* **2013**, *52*, 568–575. [CrossRef] [PubMed]

7. Veale, D.J.; Fearon, U. What Makes Psoriatic and Rheumatoid Arthritis so Different? *RMD Open.* **2015**, *1*, e000025. [CrossRef] [PubMed]
8. Moll, J.M.H.; Wright, V. Psoriatic Arthritis. *Semin. Arthritis Rheum.* **1973**, *3*, 55–78. [CrossRef]
9. Butt, A.Q.; McArdle, A.; Gibson, D.S.; FitzGerald, O.; Pennington, S.R. Psoriatic Arthritis Under a Proteomic Spotlight: Application of Novel Technologies to Advance Diagnosis and Management. *Curr. Rheumatol. Rep.* **2015**, *17*, 35. [CrossRef] [PubMed]
10. McArdle, A.; Pennington, S.; FitzGerald, O. Clinical Features of Psoriatic Arthritis: A Comprehensive Review of Unmet Clinical Needs. *Clin. Rev. Allergy Immunol.* **2018**, *55*, 271–294. [CrossRef] [PubMed]
11. Tillett, W.; Jadon, D.; Shaddick, G.; Cavill, C.; Korendowych, E.; de Vries, C.S.; McHugh, N. Smoking and Delay to Diagnosis Are Associated with Poorer Functional Outcome in Psoriatic Arthritis. *Ann. Rheum. Dis.* **2013**, *72*, 1358–1361. [CrossRef] [PubMed]
12. Haroon, M.; Gallagher, P.; Fitzgerald, O. Diagnostic Delay of More Than 6 Months Contributes to Poor Radiographic and Functional Outcome in Psoriatic Arthritis. *Ann. Rheum. Dis.* **2015**, *74*, 1045–1050. [CrossRef]
13. Anandarajah, A. Imaging in Psoriatic Arthritis. *Clin. Rev. Allergy Immunol.* **2013**, *44*, 157–165. [CrossRef]
14. Simon, D.; Faustini, F.; Kleyer, A.; Haschka, J.; Englbrecht, M.; Kraus, S.; Hueber, A.J.; Kocijan, R.; Sticherling, M.; Schett, G.; et al. Analysis of Periarticular Bone Changes in Patients with Cutaneous Psoriasis Without Associated Psoriatic Arthritis. *Ann. Rheum. Dis.* **2016**, *75*, 660–666. [CrossRef] [PubMed]
15. Scarpa, R.; Cuocolo, A.; Peluso, R.; Atteno, M.; Gisonni, P.; Iervolino, S.; Di Minno, M.N.; Nicolai, E.; Salvatore, M.; del Puente, A. Early Psoriatic Arthritis: The Clinical Spectrum. *J. Rheumatol.* **2008**, *35*, 137–141.
16. McGonagle, D.; Ash, Z.; Dickie, L.; McDermott, M.; Aydin, S.Z. The Early Phase of Psoriatic Arthritis. *Ann. Rheum. Dis.* **2011**, *70*, i71–i76. [CrossRef]
17. Perez-Chada, L.M.; Haberman, R.H.; Chandran, V.; Rosen, C.F.; Ritchlin, C.; Eder, L.; Mease, P.; Reddy, S.; Ogdie, A.; Merola, J.F.; et al. Consensus Terminology for Preclinical Phases of Psoriatic Arthritis for Use in Research Studies: Results from a Delphi Consensus Study. *Nat. Rev. Rheumatol.* **2021**, *17*, 238–243. [CrossRef] [PubMed]
18. Gelfand, J.M.; Gladman, D.D.; Mease, P.J.; Smith, N.; Margolis, D.J.; Nijsten, T.; Stern, R.S.; Feldman, S.R.; Rolstad, T. Epidemiology of Psoriatic Arthritis in the Population of the United States. *J. Am. Acad. Dermatol.* **2005**, *53*, 573. [CrossRef]
19. Mease, P.J.; Gladman, D.D.; Papp, K.A.; Khraishi, M.M.; Thaçi, D.; Behrens, F.; Northington, R.; Fuiman, J.; Bananis, E.; Boggs, R.; et al. Prevalence of Rheumatologist-Diagnosed Psoriatic Arthritis in Patients with Psoriasis in European/North American Dermatology Clinics. *J. Am. Acad. Dermatol.* **2013**, *69*, 729–735. [CrossRef]
20. Paek, S.Y.; Thompson, J.M.; Qureshi, A.A.; Merola, J.F.; Husni, M.E. Comprehensive Assessment of the Psoriasis Patient (CAPP): A Report from the GRAPPA 2015 Annual Meeting. *J. Rheumatol.* **2016**, *43*, 961–964. [CrossRef]
21. Caso, F.; Costa, L.; Chimenti, M.S.; Navarini, L.; Punzi, L. Pathogenesis of Psoriatic Arthritis. *Crit. Rev. Immunol.* **2019**, *39*, 361–377. [CrossRef]
22. Hamdy, M.; Omar, G.; Elshereef, R.R.; Ellaban, A.S.; Amin, M. Early Detection of Spondyloarthropathy in Patients with Psoriasis by Using the Ultrasonography and Magnetic Resonance Image. *Eur. J. Rheumatol.* **2015**, *2*, 10–15. [CrossRef]
23. Offidani, A.; Cellini, A.; Valeri, G.; Giovagnoni, A. Subclinical Joint Involvement in Psoriasis: Magnetic Resonance Imaging and X-Ray Findings. *Acta Derm. Venereol.* **1998**, *78*, 463–465. [CrossRef]
24. Köhm, M.; Zerweck, L.; Ngyuen, P.H.; Burkhardt, H.; Behrens, F. Innovative Imaging Technique for Visualization of Vascularization and Established Methods for Detection of Musculoskeletal Inflammation in Psoriasis Patients. *Front. Med.* **2020**, *7*, 468. [CrossRef] [PubMed]
25. Eder, L.; Polachek, A.; Rosen, C.F.; Chandran, V.; Cook, R.; Gladman, D.D. The Development of Psoriatic Arthritis in Patients with Psoriasis Is Preceded by a Period of Nonspecific Musculoskeletal Symptoms: A Prospective Cohort Study. *Arthritis Rheumatol.* **2017**, *69*, 622–629. [CrossRef]
26. Pennington, S.R.; FitzGerald, O. Early Origins of Psoriatic Arthritis: Clinical, Genetic and Molecular Biomarkers of Progression From Psoriasis to Psoriatic Arthritis. *Front. Med.* **2021**, *8*, 723944. [CrossRef] [PubMed]
27. Zabotti, A.; Tinazzi, I.; Aydin, S.Z.; McGonagle, D. From Psoriasis to Psoriatic Arthritis: Insights from Imaging on the Transition to Psoriatic Arthritis and Implications for Arthritis Prevention. *Curr. Rheumatol. Rep.* **2020**, *22*, 24. [CrossRef] [PubMed]
28. Husni, M.E.; Meyer, K.H.; Cohen, D.S.; Mody, E.; Qureshi, A.A. The PASE Questionnaire: Pilot-Testing a Psoriatic Arthritis Screening and Evaluation Tool. *J. Am. Acad. Dermatol.* **2007**, *57*, 581–587. [CrossRef] [PubMed]
29. Alenius, G.M.; Stenberg, B.; Stenlund, H.; Lundblad, M.; Dahlqvist, S.R. Inflammatory Joint Manifestations Are Prevalent in Psoriasis: Prevalence Study of Joint and Axial Involvement in Psoriatic Patients, and Evaluation of a Psoriatic and Arthritic Questionnaire. *J. Rheumatol.* **2002**, *29*, 2577–2582.
30. Gladman, D.D.; Schentag, C.T.; Tom, B.D.; Chandran, V.; Brockbank, J.; Rosen, C.; Farewell, V.T. Development and Initial Validation of a Screening Questionnaire for Psoriatic Arthritis: The Toronto Psoriatic Arthritis Screen (ToPAS). *Ann. Rheum. Dis.* **2009**, *68*, 497–501. [CrossRef]
31. Ibrahim, G.H.; Buch, M.H.; Lawson, C.; Waxman, R.; Helliwell, P.S. Evaluation of an Existing Screening Tool for Psoriatic Arthritis in People with Psoriasis and the Development of a New Instrument: The Psoriasis Epidemiology Screening Tool (PEST) Questionnaire. *Clin. Exp. Rheumatol.* **2009**, *27*, 469–474.
32. Tinazzi, I.; Adami, S.; Zanolin, E.M.; Caimmi, C.; Confente, S.; Girolomoni, G.; Gisondi, P.; Biasi, D.; McGonagle, D. The Early Psoriatic Arthritis Screening Questionnaire: A Simple and Fast Method for the Identification of Arthritis in Patients with Psoriasis. *Rheumatology* **2012**, *51*, 2058–2063. [CrossRef] [PubMed]

33. Burlando, M.; Cozzani, E.; Schiavetti, I.; Cicchelli, S.; Repetto, M.; Rossotto, G.; Scaparro, E.; Parodi, A. The STRIPP Questionnaire (Screening Tool for Rheumatologic Investigation in Psoriatic Patients) as a New Tool for the Diagnosis of Early Psoriatic Arthritis. *G. Ital. Dermatol. Venereol.* **2020**, *155*, 294–298. [CrossRef] [PubMed]
34. Mease, P.J.; Gladman, D.D.; Helliwell, P.; Khraishi, M.M.; Fuiman, J.; Bananis, E.; Alvarez, D. Comparative performance of psoriatic arthritis screening tools in patients with psoriasis in European/North American dermatology clinics. *J. Am. Acad. Dermatol.* **2014**, *71*, 649–655. [CrossRef] [PubMed]
35. Mishra, S.; Kancharla, H.; Dogra, S.; Sharma, A. Comparison of four validated psoriatic arthritis screening tools in diagnosing psoriatic arthritis in patients with psoriasis (COMPAQ Study). *Br. J. Dermatol.* **2017**, *176*, 765–770. [CrossRef]
36. Coates, L.C.; Savage, L.; Waxman, R.; Moverley, A.R.; Worthington, S.; Helliwell, P.S. Comparison of screening questionnaires to identify psoriatic arthritis in a primary-care population: A cross-sectional study. *Br. J. Dermatol.* **2016**, *175*, 542–548. [CrossRef]
37. Taylor, W.; Gladman, D.; Helliwell, P.; Marchesoni, A.; Mease, P.; Mielants, H.; CASPAR Study Group. Classification Criteria for Psoriatic Arthritis: Development of New Criteria from a Large International Study. *Arthritis Rheum.* **2006**, *54*, 2665–2673. [CrossRef] [PubMed]
38. Zlatkovic-Svenda, M.; Kerimovic-Morina, D.; Stojanovic, R.M. Psoriatic arthritis classification criteria: Moll and Wright, ESSG and CASPAR—A comparative study. *Acta. Reumatol. Port.* **2013**, *38*, 172–178. [PubMed]
39. Congi, L.; Roussou, E. Clinical application of the CASPAR criteria for psoriatic arthritis compared to other existing criteria. *Clin. Exp. Rheumatol.* **2010**, *28*, 304–310. [PubMed]
40. Tillett, W.; Costa, L.; Jadon, D.; Wallis, D.; Cavill, C.; McHugh, J.; Korendowych, E.; McHugh, N. The ClASsification for Psoriatic ARthritis (CASPAR) criteria—A retrospective feasibility, sensitivity, and specificity study. *J. Rheumatol.* **2012**, *39*, 154–156. [CrossRef]
41. Gibson, D.S.; Rooney, M.E.; Finnegan, S.; Qiu, J.; Thompson, D.C.; Labaer, J.; Pennington, S.R.; Duncan, M.W. Biomarkers in Rheumatology, Now and in the Future. *Rheumatology* **2012**, *51*, 423–433. [CrossRef]
42. Kane, D.; Roth, J.; Frosch, M.; Vogl, T.; Bresnihan, B.; FitzGerald, O. Increased Perivascular Synovial Membrane Expression of Myeloid-Related Proteins in Psoriatic Arthritis. *Arthritis Rheum.* **2003**, *48*, 1676–1685. [CrossRef] [PubMed]
43. Aochi, S.; Tsuji, K.; Sakaguchi, M.; Huh, N.; Tsuda, T.; Yamanishi, K.; Komine, M.; Iwatsuki, K. Markedly Elevated Serum Levels of Calcium-Binding S100A8/A9 Proteins in Psoriatic Arthritis Are Due to Activated Monocytes/Macrophages. *J. Am. Acad. Dermatol.* **2011**, *64*, 879–887. [CrossRef]
44. Dalbeth, N.; Pool, B.; Smith, T.; Callon, K.E.; Lobo, M.; Taylor, W.J.; Jones, P.B.; Cornish, J.; McQueen, F.M. Circulating Mediators of Bone Remodeling in Psoriatic Arthritis: Implications for Disordered Osteoclastogenesis and Bone Erosion. *Arthritis Res. Ther.* **2010**, *12*, R164. [CrossRef]
45. Connolly, M.; Mullan, R.H.; McCormick, J.; Matthews, C.; Sullivan, O.; Kennedy, A.; FitzGerald, O.; Poole, A.R.; Bresnihan, B.; Veale, D.J.; et al. Acute-Phase Serum Amyloid a Regulates Tumor Necrosis Factor α and Matrix Turnover and Predicts Disease Progression in Patients with Inflammatory Arthritis Before and After Biologic Therapy. *Arthritis Rheum.* **2012**, *64*, 1035–1045. [CrossRef] [PubMed]
46. Ghasemi, S.; Sardari, K.; Mirshokraei, P.; Hassanpour, H. In Vitro Study of Matrix Metalloproteinases 1, 2, 9, 13 and Serum Amyloid A mRNAs Expression in Equine Fibroblast-Like Synoviocytes Treated with Doxycycline. *Can. J. Vet. Res.* **2018**, *82*, 82–88.
47. Green, M.J.; Gough, A.K.; Devlin, J.; Smith, J.; Astin, P.; Taylor, D.; Emery, P. Serum MMP-3 and MMP-1 and Progression of Joint Damage in Early Rheumatoid Arthritis. *Rheumatology* **2003**, *42*, 83–88. [CrossRef]
48. Pollock, R.A.; Zaman, L.; Chandran, V.; Gladman, D.D. Epigenome-Wide Analysis of Sperm Cells Identifies IL22 as a Possible Germ Line Risk Locus for Psoriatic Arthritis. *PLoS ONE.* **2019**, *14*, e0212043. [CrossRef]
49. Eshed, I.; Bollow, M.; McGonagle, D.G.; Tan, A.L.; Althoff, C.E.; Asbach, P.; Hermann, K.G. MRI of Enthesitis of the Appendicular Skeleton in Spondyloarthritis. *Ann. Rheum. Dis.* **2007**, *66*, 1553–1559. [CrossRef] [PubMed]
50. Delle Sedie, A.; Riente, L. Psoriatic Arthritis: What Ultrasound Can Provide Us. *Clin. Exp. Rheumatol.* **2015**, *33*, S60–S65. [PubMed]
51. Micu, M.C.; Fodor, D. Concepts in Monitoring Enthesitis in Patients with Spondylarthritis—The Role of Musculoskeletal Ultrasound. *Med. Ultrason.* **2016**, *18*, 82–89. [CrossRef] [PubMed]
52. Zabotti, A.; McGonagle, D.G.; Giovannini, I.; Errichetti, E.; Zuliani, F.; Zanetti, A.; Tinazzi, I.; De Lucia, O.; Batticciotto, A.; Idolazzi, L.; et al. Transition phase towards psoriatic arthritis: Clinical and ultrasonographic characterisation of psoriatic arthralgia. *RMD Open.* **2019**, *5*, e001067. [CrossRef] [PubMed]
53. Finzel, S.; Englbrecht, M.; Engelke, K.; Stach, C.; Schett, G. A Comparative Study of Periarticular Bone Lesions in Rheumatoid Arthritis and Psoriatic Arthritis. *Ann. Rheum. Dis.* **2011**, *70*, 122–127. [CrossRef]
54. Chaudhari, A.J.; Ferrero, A.; Godinez, F.; Yang, K.; Shelton, D.K.; Hunter, J.C.; Naguwa, S.M.; Boone, J.M.; Raychaudhuri, S.P.; Badawi, R.D. High-Resolution (18)F-FDG PET/CT for Assessing Disease Activity in Rheumatoid and Psoriatic Arthritis: Findings of a Prospective Pilot Study. *Br. J. Radiol.* **2016**, *89*, 20160138. [CrossRef]
55. Bains, S.; Reimert, M.; Win, A.Z.; Khan, S.; Aparici, C.M. A Patient with Psoriatic Arthritis Imaged with FDG-PET/CT Demonstrated an Unusual Imaging Pattern with Muscle and Fascia Involvement: A Case Report. *Nucl. Med. Mol. Imaging.* **2012**, *46*, 138–143. [CrossRef]
56. Takata, T.; Taniguchi, Y.; Ohnishi, T.; Kohsaki, S.; Nogami, M.; Nakajima, H.; Kumon, Y.; Terada, Y.; Ogawa, Y.; Tarutani, M.; et al. 18FDG PET/CT Is a Powerful Tool for Detecting Subclinical Arthritis in Patients with Psoriatic Arthritis and/or Psoriasis Vulgaris. *J. Dermatol. Sci.* **2011**, *64*, 144–147. [CrossRef] [PubMed]

57. Gossec, L.; Baraliakos, X.; Kerschbaumer, A.; de Wit, M.; McInnes, I.; Dougados, M.; Primdahl, J.; McGonagle, D.G.; Aletaha, D.; Balanescu, A.; et al. EULAR Recommendations for the Management of Psoriatic Arthritis with Pharmacological Therapies: 2019 Update. *Ann. Rheum. Dis.* **2020**, *79*, 700–712. [CrossRef]
58. Pincus, T.; Bergman, M.J.; Yazici, Y. Limitations of clinical trials in chronic diseases: Is the efficacy of methotrexate (MTX) underestimated in polyarticular psoriatic arthritis on the basis of limitations of clinical trials more than on limitations of MTX, as was seen in rheumatoid arthritis? *Clin. Exp. Rheumatol.* **2015**, *33*, S82–S93. [PubMed]
59. Ohtsuki, M.; Igarashi, A.; Campos, E.; Hirano, T.; Yoshii, N.; Hirose, T. Methotrexate as a Therapeutic Drug for Psoriasis: Utilization Pattern and Safety Measures in Japan. *Jpn. J. Dermatol.* **2019**, *129*, 1317–1328. [CrossRef]
60. Kaltwasser, J.P.; Nash, P.; Gladman, D.; Rosen, C.F.; Behrens, F.; Jones, P.; Wollenhaupt, J.; Falk, F.G.; Mease, P. Treatment of Psoriatic Arthritis Study Group. Efficacy and safety of leflunomide in the treatment of psoriatic arthritis and psoriasis: A multinational, double-blind, randomized, placebo-controlled clinical trial. *Arthritis Rheum.* **2004**, *50*, 1939–1950. [CrossRef]
61. Nash, P.; Thaçi, D.; Behrens, F.; Falk, F.; Kaltwasser, J.P. Leflunomide improves psoriasis in patients with psoriatic arthritis: An in-depth analysis of data from the TOPAS study. *Dermatology* **2006**, *212*, 238–249. [CrossRef] [PubMed]
62. Honma, M.; Hayashi, K. Psoriasis: Recent Progress in Molecular-Targeted Therapies. *J. Dermatol.* **2021**, *48*, 761–777. [CrossRef] [PubMed]
63. Kamata, M.; Tada, Y. Efficacy and Safety of Biologics for Psoriasis and Psoriatic Arthritis and Their Impact on Comorbidities: A Literature Review. *Int. J. Mol. Sci.* **2020**, *21*, 1690. [CrossRef]
64. Coulter, F.; Parrish, A.; Manning, D.; Kampmann, B.; Mendy, J.; Garand, M.; Lewinsohn, D.M.; Riley, E.M.; Sutherland, J.S. IL-17 Production from T Helper 17, Mucosal-Associated Invariant T, and Gammadelta Cells in Tuberculosis Infection and Disease. *Front. Immunol.* **2017**, *8*, 1252. [CrossRef] [PubMed]
65. Campanaro, F.; Batticciotto, A.; Zaffaroni, A.; Cappelli, A.; Donadini, M.P.; Squizzato, A. JAK Inhibitors and Psoriatic Arthritis: A Systematic Review and Meta-Analysis. *Autoimmun. Rev.* **2021**, *20*, 102902. [CrossRef]
66. Kampylafka, E.; Simon, D.; d'Oliveira, I.; Linz, C.; Lerchen, V.; Englbrecht, M.; Rech, J.; Kleyer, A.; Sticherling, M.; Schett, G.; et al. Disease Interception with Interleukin-17 Inhibition in High-Risk Psoriasis Patients with Subclinical Joint Inflammation-Data from the Prospective IVEPSA Study. *Arthritis Res. Ther.* **2019**, *21*, 178. [CrossRef]
67. Coates, L.C.; Moverley, A.R.; McParland, L.; Brown, S.; Navarro-Coy, N.; O'Dwyer, J.L.; Meads, D.M.; Emery, P.; Conaghan, P.G.; Helliwell, P.S. Effect of Tight Control of Inflammation in Early Psoriatic Arthritis (TICOPA): A UK Multicentre, Open-Label, Randomised Controlled Trial. *Lancet* **2015**, *386*, 2489–2498. [CrossRef]
68. Felquer, M.L.A.; LoGiudice, L.; Galimberti, M.L.; Rosa, J.; Mazzuoccolo, L.; Soriano, E.R. Treating the skin with biologics in patients with psoriasis decreases the incidence of psoriatic arthritis. *Ann. Rheum. Dis.* **2022**, *81*, 74–79. [CrossRef]
69. Smith, C.H.; Jabbar-Lopez, Z.K.; You, Z.Z.; Bale, T.; Burden, A.D.; Coates, L.C.; Cruickshank, M.; Hadoke, T.; MacMahon, E.; Murphy, R.; et al. British Association of Dermatologists guidelines for biologic therapy for psoriasis 2017. *Br. J. Dermatol.* **2017**, *177*, 628–636. [CrossRef]
70. Coates, L.C.; Kavanaugh, A.; Mease, P.J.; Soriano, E.R.; Laura Acosta-Felquer, M.; Armstrong, A.W.; Bautista-Molano, W.; Boehncke, W.H.; Campbell, W.; Cauli, A.; et al. Group for Research and Assessment of Psoriasis and Psoriatic Arthritis 2015 Treatment Recommendations for Psoriatic Arthritis. *Arthritis Rheumatol.* **2016**, *68*, 1060–1071. [CrossRef]
71. Coates, L.C.; Gossec, L.; Ramiro, S.; Mease, P.; van der Heijde, D.; Smolen, J.S.; Ritchlin, C.; Kavanaugh, A. New GRAPPA and EULAR recommendations for the management of psoriatic arthritis. *Rheumatology* **2017**, *56*, 1251–1253. [CrossRef] [PubMed]
72. Asahina, A.; Umezawa, Y.; Ohtsuki, M.; Okuyama, R.; Kato, N.; Kaneko, H.; Kameda, H.; Kishimoto, M.; Sano, S.; Tada, Y.; et al. Japanese guidelines for treatment of psoriatic arthritis 2019. *Jpn. J. Dermatol.* **2019**, *129*, 2675–2733. [CrossRef]
73. Coates, L.C.; Corp, N.; van der Windt, D.A.; Soriano, E.R.; Kavanaugh, A. GRAPPA Treatment Recommendations: An Update From the 2020 GRAPPA Annual Meeting. *J. Rheumatol.* **2021**, *97*, 65–66. [CrossRef] [PubMed]
74. Feldman, S.R.; Burudpakdee, C.; Gala, S.; Nanavaty, M.; Mallya, U.G. The Economic Burden of Psoriasis: A Systematic Literature Review. *Expert Rev. Pharmacoecon. Outcomes Res.* **2014**, *14*, 685–705. [CrossRef]
75. Burgos-Pol, R.; Martínez-Sesmero, J.M.; Ventura-Cerdá, J.M.; Elías, I.; Caloto, M.T.; Casado, M.Á. The Cost of Psoriasis and Psoriatic Arthritis in 5 European Countries: A Systematic Review. *Actas Dermo Sifiliogr.* **2016**, *107*, 577–590. [CrossRef] [PubMed]
76. Saeki, H.; Terui, T.; Morita, A.; Sano, S.; Imafuku, S.; Asahina, A.; Komine, M.; Etoh, T.; Igarashi, A.; Torii, H.; et al. Japanese guidance for use of biologics for psoriasis. Japanese Guidance for Use of Biologics for Psoriasis (The 2019 Version). *J. Dermatol.* **2020**, *47*, 201–222. [CrossRef] [PubMed]
77. Singh, J.A.; Guyatt, G.; Ogdie, A.; Gladman, D.D.; Deal, C.; Deodhar, A.; Dubreuil, M.; Dunham, J.; Husni, M.E.; Kenny, S.; et al. Special article: 2018 American College of Rheumatology/National Psoriasis Foundation Guideline for the Treatment Psoriatic Arthritis. *Arthritis Rheumatol.* **2019**, *71*, 5–32. [CrossRef] [PubMed]

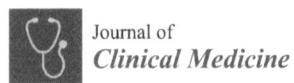

Review

Biologics for Psoriasis during the COVID-19 Pandemic

Koji Kamiya *, Mayumi Komine and Mamitaro Ohtsuki

Department of Dermatology, Jichi Medical University, 3311-1 Yakushiji, Shimotsuke, Tochigi 329-0498, Japan; mkomine12@jichi.ac.jp (M.K.); mamitaro@jichi.ac.jp (M.O.)
* Correspondence: m01023kk@jichi.ac.jp; Tel.: +81-285-58-7360

Abstract: Psoriasis is a chronic, immune-mediated inflammatory disease that predominantly affects the skin and joints. The recent therapeutic development for psoriasis has been remarkable and biologics have dramatically changed the treatment of psoriasis. In moderate-to-severe cases, systemic therapies are required to control their symptoms and biologics can provide greater efficacy when compared with other types of therapies. The coronavirus disease (COVID-19) pandemic has had a great impact on the lives of many people and has worsened substantially worldwide. During the ongoing COVID-19 pandemic, it still remains unclear whether biologics suppress the immune system and increase the risk of COVID-19. In this review, we have summarized the experience with biologics used for treating psoriasis during the COVID-19 pandemic. Biologics seem to be beneficial to COVID-19 infection. Shared decision-making that is based on updated information is highlighted in the time of COVID-19.

Keywords: psoriasis; COVID-19; SARS-CoV-2; systemic therapy; biologics

1. Introduction

Psoriasis is one of the most frequent chronic inflammatory skin diseases [1,2]. In the past decade, various molecular-targeted therapies have been developed, and these therapies have been approved for the treatment of psoriasis [3]. Molecular targeted therapies can be divided into two representative groups: biologics targeting cytokines and receptors involved in psoriasis pathomechanism, and small molecule inhibitors targeting intracellular signaling molecules. Biologics include tumor necrosis factor (TNF), interleukin (IL)-12/23, IL-23, and IL-17 inhibitors; and, small molecule inhibitors include phosphodiesterase-4 (PDE-4) and Janus-activated kinase (JAK) inhibitors. The exacerbation of psoriasis can cause systemic inflammation, leading to cardiovascular comorbidities [4,5]. In psoriatic arthritis (PsA), delays in diagnosis and treatment can cause irreversible joint destruction. Despite early treatment, some patients develop progressive damage and loss of function [6]. Therefore, effective systemic therapies should be considered in moderate-to-severe psoriasis, and biologics can provide significant symptomatic and functional improvement that cannot be achieved with other types of therapies.

Coronavirus disease (COVID-19) is caused by severe acute respiratory syndrome coronavirus 2 (SARS-CoV-2) [7]. The first case was identified in Wuhan, China, in December 2019. This new type of coronavirus has spread uncontrollably to many countries, and a global COVID-19 pandemic is ongoing. Personal protective measures, such as wearing masks, washing hands, alcohol disinfection, social distancing, and staying at home are recommended to prevent infection. In some areas, patients are unable to receive sufficient medical treatment and resources, leading to non-adherence to treatment regimens. Although patients with severe psoriasis require biologics to control disease severity, it is unclear whether biologics suppress the immune system and increase the risk of COVID-19 infection. The current situation may lead to dilemmas regarding the correct choice of treatment. During the COVID-19 pandemic, patients may discontinue treatment, owing to the fear of infection.

Hence, this review describes the effectiveness of biologics for psoriasis during COVID-19 and it discusses the risks and benefits of biologics in the era of the COVID-19 pandemic.

2. Risk Factors for the Exacerbation of Psoriasis and COVID-19

The risk factors for the development of psoriasis can be classified into extrinsic and intrinsic factors [8]. Extrinsic risk factors include mechanical stress, drugs, infection, and lifestyle. Vaccination can be also recognized as an extrinsic risk factor and influenza and adenovirus vaccines are often associated with the development of psoriasis [9–11]. In contrast, intrinsic risk factors include metabolic syndrome, obesity, diabetes mellitus (DM), dyslipidemia, hypertension, and mental stress [8]. Of these, mechanical stress, certain drugs, infection, and obesity are known to be associated with the exacerbation of psoriasis (Table 1) [12–17]. Certain drugs include β-blockers, lithium, anti-malarial drugs, interferons, imiquimod, terbinafine, and anti-programmed cell death-1 (PD-1) monoclonal antibodies [13,17]. Infections, such as streptococcal infection and human immunodeficiency virus (HIV) infection, are well-known risk factors for psoriasis [14,15]. Recently, it has been reported that rhinovirus and coronavirus are the most frequently detected pathogens in acute psoriasis flares after established respiratory virus infection [18]. There have been some case reports regarding the onset and exacerbation of psoriasis after COVID-19 infection [19–24].

Table 1. Risk factors for psoriasis and COVID-19.

Psoriasis	COVID-19
Mechanical stress	Cancer
β-blockers	Chronic kidney disease
Lithium	Chronic obstructive pulmonary disease
Anti-malarial drugs	Down syndrome
Interferons	Heart conditions
Imiquimod	Immunocompromised state
Terbinafine	Obesity
Anti-PD1 monoclonal antibodies	Pregnancy
Streptococcal infection	Sickle cell disease
HIV infection	Smoking
Obesity	Type 2 DM

In contrast, the increased risk of severe course of COVID-19 has not been fully elucidated. In 5700 patients hospitalized with COVID-19 in New York City, hypertension, obesity, and diabetes were the most common comorbidities [25]. As of 23 December 2020, the Centers for Disease Control and Prevention classified the following comorbidities as established risk factors for severe COVID-19: cancer, chronic kidney disease, chronic obstructive pulmonary disease, Down syndrome, heart conditions, immunocompromised state, obesity, pregnancy, sickle cell disease, smoking, and type 2 DM (Table 1) [26,27]. Psoriasis and COVID-19 share obesity as a risk factor for severe illness. However, it is unclear as to whether psoriasis is an important risk factor for severe COVID-19 infections. In a prospective study analyzing the dermatological comorbidity of 93 patients with COVID-19, 17 patients (11 men and six women) were positive for COVID-19 [28]. The most common diseases were superficial fungal infections (five cases, 25%), psoriasis (four cases, 20%), and viral skin diseases (three cases, 15%). In this study, psoriasis was among the most common dermatological diseases. It was speculated that the stress burden caused by the COVID-19 pandemic might have led to an increased number of visits to the outpatient clinic. A recent large epidemiological study showed the association between psoriasis and a higher risk of COVID-19 [29].

3. Biologics for Psoriasis

3.1. Biologics and COVID-19

Biologics for the treatment of psoriasis inhibit TNF, IL-12/23, IL-23, and IL-17 (Table 2). There are many case reports of psoriasis patients who presented with mild COVID-19 infections during biologic therapy and had favorable outcomes [30–38]; however, biologic therapy did not suppress the progression of COVID-19, which resulted in acute respiratory distress syndrome (ARDS) [39]. In COVID-19 patients, higher levels of TNF have been observed [40]. Moreover, the TNF levels were higher in intensive care unit (ICU) patients than in non-ICU patients [40]. SARS-CoV-2 enters host cells via the angiotensin-converting enzyme 2 (ACE2) receptor, which is expressed in various human organs [41]. TNF inhibition might be effective in reducing SARS-CoV-2 infection and the associated organ damage by decreasing TNF-converting enzyme-dependent shedding of the ACE2 ectodomain (Figure 1) [42]. IL-17 appears to be associated with hypercytokinemia in COVID-19 infections. In a patient with severe COVID-19, there was an increased concentration of highly proinflammatory CCR6+ T-helper (Th) 17 cells in the peripheral blood [43]. It is speculated that, in the cytokine storm, the upregulation of IL-17A and possibly IL-17F is mostly responsible for the pathogenesis of COVID-19 and ARDS [44]. IL-17 inhibition might be effective in controlling the cytokine storm due to the correlation between disease severity and the levels of IL-17 and other Th17 cell-related proinflammatory cytokines [45]. In contrast, the role of IL-23 in the pathogenesis of COVID-19 still remains unknown.

Table 2. Biologics for psoriasis.

Classification	Target Molecule	Agent
TNF-inhibitor	TNF	Adalimumab Certolizumab pegol Etanercept Infliximab
IL-12/23 inhibitor	IL-12/23 p40 subunit	Ustekinumab
IL-23 inhibitor	IL-23 p19 subunit	Guselkumab Risankizumab Tildrakizumab
IL-17 inhibitor	IL-17A	Ixekizumab Secukinumab
	IL-17 receptor A	Brodalumab

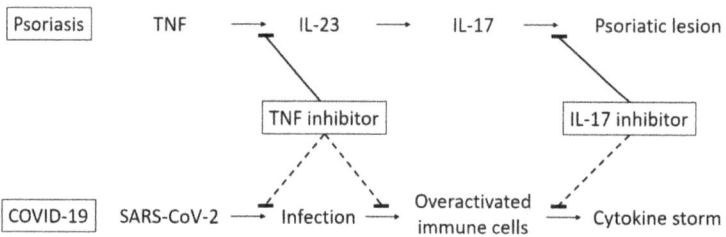

Figure 1. Biologics for psoriasis and COVID-19. Tumor necrosis factor (TNF) inhibitors and interleukin (IL)-17 inhibitors have the potential to prevent the infection of severe acute respiratory syndrome coronavirus 2 (SARS-CoV-2) and the cytokine storm of COVID-19.

3.2. At the Beginning of the COVID-19 Pandemic

It has been shown that psoriasis is independently associated with a small, but increased, risk of serious infection, which leads to hospitalization and associated significant morbidity and/or mortality [46]. At the beginning of the COVID-19 pandemic, it was not known whether this was the most appropriate time to commence immunosuppressive therapy in patients with psoriasis [47]. It was suggested that, in areas of high infection rate or outbreaks, treatment with cyclosporine, methotrexate, and TNF inhibitors should be carefully considered, because these drugs have potency to cause immunosuppression [47]. However, immunosuppressive monotherapy, target therapy, and the absence of significant comorbidities could be associated with a lower risk, and a case-by-case assessment seems to be more appropriate than stopping ongoing therapy or reducing therapy in patients with severe psoriasis [48]. Treatment protocols should be prioritized and individualized based on disease severity, other medical conditions, and viral invasiveness [49]. From a rheumatologic point of view, it was suggested to evaluate not only the infectious profile of immunosuppressants, but also the underlying inflammatory nature of psoriatic disease itself, especially if severe and/or associated with articular involvement [50].

At the beginning of the COVID-19 pandemic, there was concern about immunosuppressive or immunomodulating effects that might lead to more susceptible to COVID-19 infections in patients who received biologic therapies [51]. In the pre-coronavirus era, the respiratory infection rates of biologics were similar to those with placebo in phase III trials, and the treatment continuation of biologics was decided based on these data [51]. It has been suggested that patients with psoriasis can continue their treatment during the COVID-19 outbreak, preventing disease flares, because immunosuppressive and immunomodulatory drugs may have the potency to control the cytokine storm that is associated with a poorer outcome in these patients [52]. With due care, biologics for the treatment of psoriasis should not be discontinued during the COVID-19 pandemic [53]. In a retrospective observational study, no hospitalization or death was observed in 980 patients with chronic plaque psoriasis treated with biologics [54]. The limitations of this study include the large difference in sample size between patients and the general population and the very low number of hospitalizations and deaths in the patient group. However, others have suggested that biologic and immunosuppressive therapies in COVID-19 patients should be discontinued and to carefully weigh the risks and benefits of these therapies [55].

Several studies have analyzed the discontinuation of biologics. In a multicenter retrospective study that was conducted during the peak of COVID-19 cases in Canada, 2095 patients received biologic therapy for psoriasis, and the total number of patients who temporarily discontinued their therapy due to COVID-19-related concerns was 23 (1.1%) [56]. In a prospective study that was conducted during the lockdown in Italy, 178 patients were observed, of which 11 (6%) discontinued their therapy due to the lack of safety in continuing [57]. A telephone survey was also conducted during the Italian lockdown period [58]. When 226 patients with negative COVID-19 results were interviewed, 27.9% (63/226) described a worsening of the disease, with 19% (43/226) correlating this to drug withdrawal. The rate of discontinuation varied in different areas [59], possibly due to the regional status of COVID-19 and concerns regarding the increased risk of infection.

3.3. During the COVID-19 Pandemic

In a retrospective Italian multicenter observational study, there were no cases of deaths from COVID-related disease in patients with chronic plaque psoriasis treated with biologics [60]. In addition, there was no significant increased risk of hospitalization associated with COVID-related interstitial pneumonia. These observations have been confirmed in other studies [61–69]. PsoProtect (Psoriasis Patient Registry for Outcomes, Therapy and Epidemiology of Covid-19 infecTion) is an international web-based registry (www.psoprotect.org) for healthcare providers to report outcomes of COVID-19 in individuals with psoriasis [70]. Based on this registry, the factors that were associated with adverse COVID-19 outcomes were analyzed [71]. A total of 374 patients with confirmed or suspected COVID-19 infection were registered by clinicians from 25 countries. Most of the patients (71%, 267/374) received a biologic therapy, rather than a non-biological systemic agent (18%, 67/374) or no systemic therapy (10%, 36/374). In this registry, 348 patients (93%) fully recovered from COVID-19, 77 (21%) were hospitalized, and nine (2%) died. An increased hospitalization risk was associated with older age, male sex, non-white ethnicity, and comorbid chronic lung disease. Biologics were associated with a lower risk of COVID-19-related hospitalization than non-biologic systemic therapies. Therefore, biologics for the treatment of psoriasis may not be associated with severe COVID-19. Moreover, in a study of a global electronic medical record database, including more than 53 million patient records, the combination of TNF and methotrexate did not increase the risk of hospitalization [72]. In contrast, it was unclear whether biologics are associated with an increased risk of SARS-CoV-2 infection [61,66,69,73]. However, patients with immune-mediated inflammatory diseases, including psoriasis treated with cytokine inhibitors, had reduced susceptibility to SARS-CoV-2 infection when compared with patients not receiving cytokine inhibitors, as well as the general population [74].

PSO-BIO-COVID is an observational, multicentric study, supported by the Italian Society of Dermatology (SIDeMaST), which aimed at evaluating the impact of SARS-CoV-2 infection on the management of patients with psoriasis in Italy during the first year of the pandemic [75]. Patients with moderate-to-severe chronic plaque psoriasis, aged >18 years, and receiving any biological agent as of 22 February 2020, were enrolled. Of the 12,807 patients with psoriasis, 328 patients (2.6%) stopped treatment during the observation period without consulting their dermatologist, mainly because of the fear of high contagious risk; and, 233 (1.8%) interrupted their therapy after consulting their dermatologist, mainly because of suspected infection or contact with SARS-CoV-2. Therapy continuation during the COVID-19 emergency seems to strictly depend on the quality of information that patients acquire, and only knowledge of epidemiology and preventive measures of COVID-19 prevents biologics discontinuation [76].

3.4. Adherence to Treatment

During the COVID-19 pandemic, there has been many restrictions. In some areas, the suspension of all outpatient services was mandated, including clinics for psoriasis patients, and dermatologists had to adapt to provide more counseling to support patients, detect unmet needs, find ways to reassure patients about their disease, and keep them safe at home [77]. The adherence of patients with psoriasis that were treated with systemic therapies was analyzed in an observational single-institution study [78]. A total of 237 patients with psoriasis were interviewed by telephone. In this study, most patients (76.4%) continued to take their medication. However, patients with more than three comorbidities were over six times more likely to not adhere to their treatment. Age, type of treatment, or any particular type of comorbidity did not appear to influence the therapeutic routine. The drug discontinuation seemed to be mainly due to concerns regarding the potential for COVID-19 infection. During the COVID-19 pandemic national lockdown, a multicenter study revealed that treatment safety concerns were significantly more common in patients that were treated with biologics. Of these patients, 40.7% either agreed or strongly agreed to have experienced an increased risk of COVID-19 infection, as compared to 21.3% in the conventional systemic therapy group and 10.9% in the topical therapy group [79]. In a web-based survey in China, 926 questionnaires were collected regarding outdoor activity restriction and income loss [80]. Outdoor activity restriction was positively associated with the exacerbation of psoriasis, stress, and symptoms of anxiety and depression in a dose-response manner, but was not associated with non-adherence. Similarly, income loss was associated with the exacerbation of psoriasis, stress, and symptoms of anxiety and depression. In contrast, income loss was significantly associated with non-adherence to treatment, but it was not associated with healthcare utilization. Non-adherence behavior and perceived stress were independently associated with both income loss and exacerbation of psoriasis. This survey also investigated the association between nonadherence to treatment and patient-reported outcomes of psoriasis [81]. In total, 634 (68.5%) patients reported nonadherence to treatment, and patients that were treated with systemic therapy and topical therapy showed worse adherence than those treated with biologic therapy.

Non-adherence to treatment was significantly associated with deterioration of psoriasis, perceived stress, and symptoms of anxiety and depression.

During the COVID-19 pandemic, telemedicine has been one of the most effective strategies for mental health and education of patients, contributing to adherence to treatment. In Taiwan, telemedicine was legally granted by an amendment to Taiwan's Physician Act in 2018, and its telemedicine service is anticipated to help, not only under-served regions, but also in situations with the COVID-19 pandemic [82]. In Italy, Brunasso et al. started a teledermatology service using telephone and email when lockdown imposed the closure of non-urgent outpatient clinics on 9 March 2020 [83]. Remote consultations included triage for COVID-19 suspected symptoms, an email check of clinical pictures and laboratory examinations, advice for topical and systemic therapy continuation or discontinuation/switch, and rescheduling of the next appointment. This service was effective in preventing an unnecessary worsening of severe chronic skin diseases and poor outcomes due to the withdrawal of current therapy. Furthermore, this service provided an important advantage for female physicians who also took care of their children during lockdown when the schools closed. The limitations of personal dermatological care of patients with skin diseases can be partially compensated by an extension of teledermatology as a convenient and safe method [84].

4. Conclusions

In this review, we summarized the risks and benefits of biologics for the treatment of psoriasis during the COVID-19 pandemic. Biologics seem to be beneficial to COVID-19 infection. Vaccines using mRNA technology are expected to prevent the onset and exacerbation of COVID-19 infections. The Psoriasis Group of the Spanish Academy of Dermatology and Venereology and National Psoriasis Foundation developed a series of recommendations and guidance on the management of psoriasis during the COVID-19 pandemic [85–87]. Biologics for psoriasis are not a contraindication to COVID-19 mRNA vaccines, and it is recommended that patients with psoriasis should receive COVID-19 mRNA vaccines. There is no evidence that vaccines affect the onset and severity of psoriasis. Registry data should be collected to inform whether COVID-19 vaccines affect the clinical outcomes of psoriasis. During the ongoing pandemic, shared decision-making between clinicians and patients is required based on updated information. This may also change the provision of medical care in the post-COVID-19 era.

Author Contributions: Conceptualization, K.K., M.K., and M.O.; data curation, K.K.; writing—original draft preparation, K.K.; writing—review and editing, K.K., M.K., and M.O.; supervision, M.O.; project administration, M.O. All authors have read and agreed to the published version of the manuscript.

Funding: This research received no external funding.

Institutional Review Board Statement: Not applicable.

Informed Consent Statement: Not applicable.

Conflicts of Interest: The authors declare no conflict of interest.

References

1. Nestle, F.O.; Kaplan, D.H.; Barker, J. Psoriasis. *N. Engl. J. Med.* **2009**, *361*, 496–509. [CrossRef] [PubMed]
2. Boehncke, W.H.; Schon, M.P. Psoriasis. *Lancet* **2015**, *386*, 983–994. [CrossRef]
3. Honma, M.; Hayashi, K. Psoriasis: Recent progress in molecular-targeted therapies. *J. Dermatol.* **2021**. [CrossRef] [PubMed]
4. Caiazzo, G.; Fabbrocini, G.; Di Caprio, R.; Raimondo, A.; Scala, E.; Balato, N.; Balato, A. Psoriasis, cardiovascular events, and biologics: Lights and shadows. *Front. Immunol.* **2018**, *9*, 1668. [CrossRef]
5. Sajja, A.P.; Joshi, A.A.; Teague, H.L.; Dey, A.K.; Mehta, N.N. Potential immunological links between psoriasis and cardiovascular disease. *Front. Immunol.* **2018**, *9*, 1234. [CrossRef]
6. Kane, D.; Stafford, L.; Bresnihan, B.; FitzGerald, O. A prospective, clinical and radiological study of early psoriatic arthritis: An early synovitis clinic experience. *Rheumatology* **2003**, *42*, 1460–1468. [CrossRef]
7. Hu, B.; Guo, H.; Zhou, P.; Shi, Z.L. Characteristics of SARS-CoV-2 and COVID-19. *Nat. Rev. Microbiol.* **2020**. [CrossRef]

8. Kamiya, K.; Kishimoto, M.; Sugai, J.; Komine, M.; Ohtsuki, M. Risk factors for the development of psoriasis. *Int. J. Mol. Sci.* **2019**, *20*. [CrossRef]
9. Gunes, A.T.; Fetil, E.; Akarsu, S.; Ozbagcivan, O.; Babayeva, L. Possible triggering effect of influenza vaccination on psoriasis. *J. Immunol. Res.* **2015**, *2015*, 258430. [CrossRef]
10. Sbidian, E.; Eftekahri, P.; Viguier, M.; Laroche, L.; Chosidow, O.; Gosselin, P.; Trouche, F.; Bonnet, N.; Arfi, C.; Tubach, F.; et al. National survey of psoriasis flares after 2009 monovalent H1N1/seasonal vaccines. *Dermatology* **2014**, *229*, 130–135. [CrossRef]
11. Choudhry, A.; Mathena, J.; Albano, J.D.; Yacovone, M.; Collins, L. Safety evaluation of adenovirus type 4 and type 7 vaccine live, oral in military recruits. *Vaccine* **2016**, *34*, 4558–4564. [CrossRef]
12. Weiss, G.; Shemer, A.; Trau, H. The koebner phenomenon: Review of the literature. *J. Eur. Acad. Dermatol. Venereol.* **2002**, *16*, 241–248. [CrossRef]
13. Balak, D.M.; Hajdarbegovic, E. Drug-induced psoriasis: Clinical perspectives. *Psoriasis* **2017**, *7*, 87–94. [CrossRef]
14. Telfer, N.R.; Chalmers, R.J.; Whale, K.; Colman, G. The role of streptococcal infection in the initiation of guttate psoriasis. *Arch. Dermatol.* **1992**, *128*, 39–42. [CrossRef]
15. Mallon, E.; Bunker, C.B. HIV-associated psoriasis. *AIDS Patient Care STDS* **2000**, *14*, 239–246. [CrossRef] [PubMed]
16. Armstrong, A.W.; Harskamp, C.T.; Armstrong, E.J. The association between psoriasis and obesity: A systematic review and meta-analysis of observational studies. *Nutr. Diabetes.* **2012**, *2*, e54. [CrossRef] [PubMed]
17. Bonigen, J.; Raynaud-Donzel, C.; Hureaux, J.; Kramkimel, N.; Blom, A.; Jeudy, G.; Breton, A.-L.; Hubiche, T.; Bedane, C.; Legoupil, D.; et al. Anti-PD1-induced psoriasis: A study of 21 patients. *J. Eur. Acad. Dermatol. Venereol.* **2017**, *31*, e254–e257. [CrossRef] [PubMed]
18. Sbidian, E.; Madrange, M.; Viguier, M.; Salmona, M.; Duchatelet, S.; Hovnanian, A.; Smahi, A.; Le Goff, J.; Bachele, H. Respiratory virus infection triggers acute psoriasis flares across different clinical subtypes and genetic backgrounds. *Br. J. Dermatol.* **2019**, *181*, 1304–1306. [CrossRef] [PubMed]
19. Kutlu, O.; Metin, A. A case of exacerbation of psoriasis after oseltamivir and hydroxychloroquine in a patient with COVID-19: Will cases of psoriasis increase after COVID-19 pandemic? *Derm. Ther.* **2020**, *33*, e13383. [CrossRef] [PubMed]
20. Mathieu, R.J.; Cobb, C.B.C.; Telang, G.H.; Firoz, E.F. New-onset pustular psoriasis in the setting of severe acute respiratory syndrome coronavirus 2 infection causing coronavirus disease 2019. *JAAD Case Rep.* **2020**, *6*, 1360–1362. [CrossRef]
21. Novelli, L.; Motta, F.; Ceribelli, A.; Guidelli, G.M.; Luciano, N.; Isailovic, N.; Vecellio, M.; Caprioli, M.; Clementi, N.; Clementi, M.; et al. A case of psoriatic arthritis triggered by SARS-CoV-2 infection. *Rheumatology* **2021**, *60*, e21–e23. [CrossRef] [PubMed]
22. Shahidi Dadras, M.; Diab, R.; Ahadi, M.; Abdollahimajd, F. Generalized pustular psoriasis following COVID-19. *Dermatol. Ther.* **2020**, e14595. [CrossRef]
23. Gananandan, K.; Sacks, B.; Ewing, I. Guttate psoriasis secondary to COVID-19. *BMJ Case Rep.* **2020**, *13*. [CrossRef] [PubMed]
24. Shakoei, S.; Ghanadan, A.; Hamzelou, S. Pustular psoriasis exacerbated by COVID-19 in a patient with the history of psoriasis. *Dermatol. Ther.* **2020**, *33*, e14462. [CrossRef] [PubMed]
25. Richardson, S.; Hirsch, J.S.; Narasimhan, M.; Crawford, J.M.; McGinn, T.; Davidson, K.W.; Barnaby, D.P.; Becker, L.B.; Chelico, J.D.; Cohen, S.L.; et al. Presenting Characteristics, Comorbidities, and Outcomes Among 5700 Patients Hospitalized With COVID-19 in the New York City Area. *JAMA* **2020**, *323*, 2052–2059. [CrossRef]
26. Centers for Disease Control and Prevention. Coronavirus Disease 2019 (COVID-19): Who is at Increased Risk for Severe Illness?—People of Any Age with Underlying Medical Conditions. Available online: https://www.cdc.gov/coronavirus/2019-ncov/need-extra-precautions/people-with-medical-conditions.html (accessed on 15 January 2021).
27. Centers for Disease Control and Prevention. Coronavirus Disease 2019 (COVID-19): Evidence used to update the list of underlying medical conditions that increase a person's risk of severe illness from COVID-19. Available online: https://www.cdc.gov/coronavirus/2019-ncov/need-extra-precautions/evidence-table.html (accessed on 15 January 2021).
28. Kutlu, O.; Metin, A. Dermatological diseases presented before COVID-19: Are patients with psoriasis and superficial fungal infections more vulnerable to the COVID-19? *Dermatol. Ther.* **2020**, *33*, e13509. [CrossRef] [PubMed]
29. Patrick, M.T.; Zhang, H.; Wasikowski, R.; Prens, E.P.; Weidinger, S.; Gudjonsson, J.E.; Elder, J.T.; He, K.; Tsoi, L.C. Associations between COVID-19 and skin conditions identified through epidemiology and genomic studies. *J. Allergy. Clin. Immunol.* **2021**. [CrossRef]
30. Messina, F.; Piaserico, S. SARS-CoV-2 infection in a psoriatic patient treated with IL-23 inhibitor. *J. Eur. Acad. Dermatol. Venereol.* **2020**, *34*, e254–e255. [CrossRef]
31. Mugheddu, C.; Dell'Antonia, M.; Sanna, S.; Agosta, D.; Atzori, L.; Rongioletti, F. Successful guselkumab treatment in a psoriatic patient affected with Cornelia de Lange syndrome, and prosecution during the COVID-19 pandemic. *Dermatol. Ther.* **2020**, *33*, e13433. [CrossRef]
32. Balestri, R.; Rech, G.; Girardelli, C.R. SARS-CoV-2 infection in a psoriatic patient treated with IL-17 inhibitor. *J. Eur. Acad. Dermatol. Venereol.* **2020**, *34*, e357–e358. [CrossRef]
33. Conti, A.; Lasagni, C.; Bigi, L.; Pellacani, G. Evolution of COVID-19 infection in four psoriatic patients treated with biological drugs. *J. Eur. Acad. Dermatol. Venereol.* **2020**, *34*, e360–e361. [CrossRef]
34. Benhadou, F.; Del Marmol, V. Improvement of SARS-CoV-2 symptoms following Guselkumab injection in a psoriatic patient. *J. Eur. Acad. Dermatol. Venereol.* **2020**, *34*, e363–e364. [CrossRef] [PubMed]
35. Di Lernia, V.; Bombonato, C.; Motolese, A. COVID-19 in an elderly patient treated with secukinumab. *Dermatol. Ther.* **2020**, *33*, e13580. [CrossRef]

36. Brownstone, N.D.; Thibodeaux, Q.G.; Reddy, V.D.; Myers, B.A.; Chan, S.Y.; Bhutani, T.; Liao, W. Novel Coronavirus Disease (COVID-19) and Biologic Therapy for Psoriasis: Successful Recovery in Two Patients After Infection with Severe Acute Respiratory Syndrome Coronavirus 2 (SARS-CoV-2). *Dermatol. Ther.* **2020**, *10*, 881–885. [CrossRef] [PubMed]
37. Valenti, M.; Facheris, P.; Pavia, G.; Gargiulo, L.; Borroni, R.G.; Costanzo, A.; Narcisi, A. Non-complicated evolution of COVID-19 infection in a patient with psoriasis and psoriatic arthritis during treatment with adalimumab. *Dermatol. Ther.* **2020**, *33*, 13708. [CrossRef]
38. Ward, M.; Gooderham, M. Asymptomatic SARS-CoV2 infection in a patient receiving risankizumab, an inhibitor of interleukin 23. *JAAD Case Rep.* **2021**, *7*, 60. [CrossRef] [PubMed]
39. Foti, R.; Amato, G.; Visalli, E. SARS-CoV-2 infection in a psoriatic arthritis patient treated with IL-17 inhibitor. *Med. Hypotheses* **2020**, *144*, 110040. [CrossRef]
40. Huang, C.; Wang, Y.; Li, X.; Ren, L.; Zhao, J.; Hu, Y.; Zhang, L.; Fan, G.; Xu, J.; Gu, X.; et al. Clinical features of patients infected with 2019 novel coronavirus in Wuhan, China. *Lancet* **2020**, *395*, 497–506. [CrossRef]
41. Ni, W.; Yang, X.; Yang, D.; Bao, J.; Li, R.; Xiao, Y.; Hou, C.; Wang, H.; Liu, J.; Yang, D.; et al. Role of angiotensin-converting enzyme 2 (ACE2) in COVID-19. *Crit. Care* **2020**, *24*, 1–10. [CrossRef] [PubMed]
42. Fu, Y.; Cheng, Y.; Wu, Y. Understanding SARS-CoV-2-mediated inflammatory responses: From mechanisms to potential therapeutic tools. *Virol. Sin.* **2020**, *35*, 266–271. [CrossRef]
43. Xu, Z.; Shi, L.; Wang, Y.; Zhang, J.; Huang, L.; Zhang, C.; Liu, S.; Zhao, P.; Liu, H.; Zhu, L.; et al. Pathological findings of COVID-19 associated with acute respiratory distress syndrome. *Lancet Respir. Med.* **2020**, *8*, 420–422. [CrossRef]
44. Shibabaw, T. Inflammatory cytokine: IL-17A signaling pathway in patients present with COVID-19 and current treatment strategy. *J. Inflamm. Res.* **2020**, *13*, 673–680. [CrossRef] [PubMed]
45. Pacha, O.; Sallman, M.A.; Evans, S.E. COVID-19: A case for inhibiting IL-17? *Nat. Rev. Immunol.* **2020**, *20*, 345–346. [CrossRef]
46. Yiu, Z.; Parisi, R.; Lunt, M.; Warren, R.; Griffiths, C.; Langan, S.; Ashcroft, D. Risk of hospitalization and death due to infection in people with psoriasis: A population-based cohort study using the Clinical Practice Research Datalink. *Br. J. Dermatol.* **2021**, *184*, 78–86. [CrossRef] [PubMed]
47. Conforti, C.; Giuffrida, R.; Dianzani, C.; Di Meo, N.; Zalaudek, I. COVID-19 and psoriasis: Is it time to limit treatment with immunosuppressants? A call for action. *Dermatol. Ther.* **2020**, *33*, e13298. [CrossRef]
48. Di Lernia, V. Antipsoriatic treatments during COVID-19 outbreak. *Dermatol. Ther.* **2020**, *33*, e13345. [CrossRef]
49. Abdelmaksoud, A.; Goldust, M.; Vestita, M. Comment on "COVID-19 and psoriasis: Is it time to limit treatment with immunosuppressants? A call for action". *Dermatol. Ther.* **2020**, *33*, e13360. [CrossRef]
50. Coletto, L.A.; Favalli, E.G.; Caporali, R. Psoriasis and psoriatic arthritis: How to manage immunosuppressants in COVID-19 days. *Dermatol. Ther.* **2020**, *33*, e13415. [CrossRef]
51. Lebwohl, M.; Rivera-Oyola, R.; Murrell, D.F. Should biologics for psoriasis be interrupted in the era of COVID-19? *J. Am. Acad. Dermatol.* **2020**, *82*, 1217–1218. [CrossRef]
52. Torres, T.; Puig, L. Managing cutaneous immune-Mediated diseases during the COVID-19 pandemic. *Am. J. Clin. Dermatol.* **2020**, *21*, 307–311. [CrossRef] [PubMed]
53. Amerio, P.; Prignano, F.; Giuliani, F.; Gualdi, G. COVID-19 and psoriasis: Should we fear for patients treated with biologics? *Dermatol. Ther.* **2020**, *33*, e13434. [CrossRef]
54. Gisondi, P.; Zaza, G.; Del Giglio, M.; Rossi, M.; Iacono, V.; Girolomoni, G. Risk of hospitalization and death from COVID-19 infection in patients with chronic plaque psoriasis receiving a biologic treatment and renal transplant recipients in maintenance immunosuppressive treatment. *J. Am. Acad. Dermatol.* **2020**, *83*, 285–287. [CrossRef] [PubMed]
55. Conforti, C.; Giuffrida, R.; Dianzani, C.; Di Meo, N.; Zalaudek, I. Biologic therapy for psoriasis during the COVID-19 outbreak: The choice is to weigh risks and benefits. *Dermatol. Ther.* **2020**, *33*, e13490. [CrossRef]
56. Georgakopoulos, J.R.; Mufti, A.; Vender, R.; Yeung, J. Treatment discontinuation and rate of disease transmission in psoriasis patients receiving biologic therapy during the COVID-19 pandemic: A Canadian multicenter retrospective study. *J. Am. Acad. Dermatol.* **2020**, *83*, 1212–1214. [CrossRef]
57. Sacchelli, L.; Evangelista, V.; Di Altobrando, A.; Lacava, R.; Rucci, P.; Rosa, S.; Patrizi, A.; Bardazzi, F. How infodemic during the COVID-19 outbreak influenced common clinical practice in an Outpatient Service of Severe Psoriasis. *Dermatol. Ther.* **2020**, *33*, 14065. [CrossRef] [PubMed]
58. Pirro, F.; Caldarola, G.; Chiricozzi, A.; Tambone, S.; Mariani, M.; Calabrese, L.; D'Urso, D.F.; De Simone, C.; Peris, K. The impact of COVID-19 pandemic in a cohort of Italian psoriatic patients treated with biological therapies. *J. Dermatol. Treat.* **2020**, 1–5. [CrossRef]
59. Camela, E.; Fabbrocini, G.; Cinelli, E.; Lauro, W.; Megna, M. Biologic therapies, psoriasis, and COVID-19: Our experience at the psoriasis unit of the university of naples federico II. *Dermatology* **2020**, *1*, 1–2. [CrossRef]
60. Gisondi, P.; Facheris, P.; Dapavo, P.; Piaserico, S.; Conti, A.; Naldi, L.; Cazzaniga, S.; Malagoli, P.; Costanzo, A. The impact of the COVID-19 pandemic on patients with chronic plaque psoriasis being treated with biological therapy: The Northern Italy experience. *Br. J. Dermatol.* **2020**, *183*, 373–374. [CrossRef]
61. Damiani, G.; Pacifico, A.; Bragazzi, N.L.; Malagoli, P. Biologics increase the risk of SARS-CoV-2 infection and hospitalization, but not ICU admission and death: Real-life data from a large cohort during red-zone declaration. *Dermatol. Ther.* **2020**, *33*, e13475. [CrossRef]

62. Piaserico, S.; Gisondi, P.; Cazzaniga, S.; Naldi, L. Lack of evidence for an increased risk of severe COVID-19 in psoriasis patients on biologics: A cohort study from northeast Italy. *Am. J. Clin. Dermatol.* **2020**, *21*, 749–751. [CrossRef]
63. Gisondi, P.; Piaserico, S.; Naldi, L.; Dapavo, P.; Conti, A.; Malagoli, P.; Marzano, A.V.; Bardazzi, F.; Gasperini, M.; Cazzaniga, S.; et al. Incidence rates of hospitalization and death from COVID-19 in patients with psoriasis receiving biological treatment: A Northern Italy experience. *J. Allergy Clin. Immunol.* **2021**, *147*, 558–560.e1. [CrossRef]
64. Ciechanowicz, P.; Dopytalska, K.; Mikucka-Wituszyńska, A.; Dźwigała, M.; Wiszniewski, K.; Herniczek, W.; Szymańska, E.; Walecka, I. The prevalence of SARS-CoV-2 infection and the severity of the course of COVID-19 in patients with psoriasis treated with biologic therapy. *J. Dermatol. Treat.* **2020**, 1–4. [CrossRef] [PubMed]
65. Polat, A.K.; Topal, I.O.; Karadag, A.S.; Aksoy, H.; Aksu, A.E.K.; Ozkur, E.; Akbulut, T.O.; Demir, F.T.; Engin, B.; Uzuncakmak, T.K.; et al. The impact of COVID-19 in patients with psoriasis: A multicenter study in Istanbul. *Dermatol. Ther.* **2021**, *34*, e14691. [CrossRef]
66. Fougerousse, A.; Perrussel, M.; Bécherel, P.; Begon, E.; Pallure, V.; Zaraa, I.; Chaby, G.; Parier, J.; Kemula, M.; Mery-Bossard, L.; et al. Systemic or biologic treatment in psoriasis patients does not increase the risk of a severe form of COVID-19. *J. Eur. Acad. Dermatol. Venereol.* **2020**, *34*, e676–e679. [CrossRef]
67. Fulgencio-Barbarin, J.; Puerta-Pena, M.; Ortiz-Romero, P.; Garcia-Donoso, C.; Rivera-Diaz, R. COVID-19 and systemic therapies in psoriasis: Experience of a tertiary hospital in Madrid. *Int. J. Dermatol.* **2020**. [CrossRef]
68. Baniandrés-Rodríguez, O.; Vilar-Alejo, J.; Rivera, R.; Carrascosa, J.M.; Daudén, E.; Herrera-Acosta, E.; Sahuquillo-Torralba, A.; Gómez-García, F.J.; Nieto-Benito, L.M.; de la Cueva, P.; et al. Incidence of severe COVID-19 outcomes in psoriatic patients treated with systemic therapies during the pandemic: A Biobadaderm cohort analysis. *J. Am. Acad. Dermatol.* **2021**, *84*, 513–517. [CrossRef]
69. Polat Ekinci, A.; Pehlivan, G.; Gokalp, M.O. Surveillance of psoriatic patients on biologic treatment during the COVID-19 pandemic: A single-center experience. *Dermatol. Ther.* **2020**, e14700. [CrossRef]
70. Mahil, S.; Yiu, Z.; Mason, K.; Dand, N.; Coker, B.; Wall, D.; Fletcher, G.; Bosma, A.; Capon, F.; Iversen, L.; et al. Global reporting of cases of COVID-19 in psoriasis and atopic dermatitis: An opportunity to inform care during a pandemic. *Br. J. Dermatol.* **2020**, *183*, 404–406. [CrossRef] [PubMed]
71. Mahil, S.K.; Dand, N.; Mason, K.J.; Yiu, Z.Z.; Tsakok, T.; Meynell, F.; Coker, B.; McAteer, H.; Moorhead, L.; MacKenzie, T.; et al. Factors associated with adverse COVID-19 outcomes in patients with psoriasis—Insights from a global registry–based study. *J. Allergy Clin. Immunol.* **2021**, *147*, 60–71. [CrossRef] [PubMed]
72. Yousaf, A.; Gayam, S.; Feldman, S.; Zinn, Z.; Kolodney, M. Clinical outcomes of COVID-19 in patients taking tumor necrosis factor inhibitors or methotrexate: A multicenter research network study. *J. Am. Acad. Dermatol.* **2021**, *84*, 70–75. [CrossRef]
73. Brazzelli, V.; Isoletta, E.; Barak, O.; Barruscotti, S.; Vassallo, C.; Giorgini, C.; Michelerio, A.; Tomasini, C.F.; Musella, V.; Klersy, C. Does therapy with biological drugs influence COVID-19 infection? Observational monocentric prevalence study on the clinical and epidemiological data of psoriatic patients treated with biological drugs or with topical drugs alone. *Dermatol. Ther.* **2020**, *33*, e14516. [CrossRef] [PubMed]
74. Simon, D.; Tascilar, K.; Krönke, G.; Kleyer, A.; Zaiss, M.M.; Heppt, F.; Meder, C.; Atreya, R.; Klenske, E.; Dietrich, P.; et al. Patients with immune-mediated inflammatory diseases receiving cytokine inhibitors have low prevalence of SARS-CoV-2 seroconversion. *Nat. Commun.* **2020**, *11*, 1–7. [CrossRef] [PubMed]
75. Talamonti, M.; Galluzzo, M.; Chiricozzi, A.; Quaglino, P.; Fabbrocini, G.; Gisondi, P.; Marzano, A.; Potenza, C.; Conti, A.; Parodi, A.; et al. Management of biological therapies for chronic plaque psoriasis during COVID-19 emergency in Italy. *J. Eur. Acad. Dermatol. Venereol.* **2020**, *34*, e770–e772. [CrossRef]
76. Bragazzi, N.L.; Riccò, M.; Pacifico, A.; Malagoli, P.; Kridin, K.; Pigatto, P.; Damiani, G. COVID-19 knowledge prevents biologics discontinuation: Data from an Italian multicenter survey during RED-ZONE declaration. *Dermatol. Ther.* **2020**, *33*, e13508. [CrossRef] [PubMed]
77. Atzori, L.; Mugheddu, C.; Addis, G.; Sanna, S.; Satta, R.; Ferreli, C.; Atzori, M.; Montesu, M.; Rongioletti, F. Psoriasis health care in the time of the coronavirus pandemic: Insights from dedicated centers in Sardinia (Italy). *J. Eur. Acad. Dermatol. Venereol.* **2020**, *34*, 247. [CrossRef]
78. Vakirlis, E.; Bakirtzi, K.; Papadimitriou, I.; Vrani, F.; Sideris, N.; Lallas, A.; Ioannides, D.; Sotiriou, E. Treatment adherence in psoriatic patients during COVID-19 pandemic: Real-world data from a tertiary hospital in Greece. *J. Eur. Acad. Dermatol. Venereol.* **2020**, *34*, e673–e675. [CrossRef]
79. Rob, F.; Hugo, J.; Tivadar, S.; Boháč, P.; Gkalpakiotis, S.; Vargová, N.; Arenbergerová, M.; Hercogová, J. Compliance, safety concerns and anxiety in patients treated with biologics for psoriasis during the COVID-19 pandemic national lockdown: A multicenter study in the Czech Republic. *J. Eur. Acad. Dermatol. Venereol.* **2020**, *34*, e682–e684. [CrossRef]
80. Kuang, Y.; Shen, M.; Wang, Q.; Xiao, Y.; Lv, C.; Luo, Y.; Zhu, W.; Chen, X. Association of outdoor activity restriction and income loss with patient-reported outcomes of psoriasis during the COVID-19 pandemic: A web-based survey. *J. Am. Acad. Dermatol.* **2020**, *83*, 670–672. [CrossRef]
81. Wang, Q.; Luo, Y.; Lv, C.; Zheng, X.; Zhu, W.; Chen, X.; Shen, M.; Kuang, Y. Nonadherence to Treatment and Patient-Reported Outcomes of Psoriasis During the COVID-19 Epidemic: A Web-Based Survey. *Patient Preference Adherence* **2020**, *14*, 1403–1409. [CrossRef]

82. Lee, C.-H.; Huang, C.-C.; Huang, J.-T.; Wang, C.-C.; Fan, S.; Wang, P.-S.; Lan, K.-C. Live-interactive teledermatology program in Taiwan: One-year experience serving a district hospital in rural Taitung County. *J. Formos. Med Assoc.* **2021**, *120*, 422–428. [CrossRef]
83. Brunasso, A.M.G.; Massone, C. Teledermatologic monitoring for chronic cutaneous autoimmune diseases with smartworking during COVID-19 emergency in a tertiary center in Italy. *Dermatol. Ther.* **2020**, *33*, e13495. [CrossRef] [PubMed]
84. Elsner, P. Teledermatology in the times of COVID-19—A systematic review. *J. Dtsch. Dermatol. Ges.* **2020**, *18*, 841–845. [CrossRef] [PubMed]
85. Belinchon, I.; Puig, L.; Ferrandiz, L.; de la Cueva, P.; Carrascosa, J.M.; on behalf of the Grupo de Psoriasis de la AEDV. Managing Psoriasis Consultations During the COVID-19 Pandemic: Recommendations from the psoriasis group of the spanish academy of dermatology and venereology (AEDV). *Actas Dermosifiliogr.* **2020**, *111*, 802–804. [CrossRef] [PubMed]
86. Gelfand, J.M.; Armstrong, A.W.; Bell, S.; Anesi, G.L.; Blauvelt, A.; Calabrese, C.; Dommasch, E.D.; Feldman, S.R.; Gladman, D.; Kircik, L.; et al. National Psoriasis Foundation COVID-19 Task Force Guidance for Management of Psoriatic Disease During the Pandemic: Version 1. *J. Am. Acad. Dermatol.* **2020**, *83*, 1704–1716. [CrossRef]
87. Gelfand, J.M.; Armstrong, A.W.; Bell, S.; Anesi, G.L.; Blauvelt, A.; Calabrese, C.; Dommasch, E.D.; Feldman, S.R.; Gladman, D.; Kircik, L.; et al. National Psoriasis Foundation COVID-19 Task Force guidance for management of psoriatic disease during the pandemic: Version 2—Advances in psoriatic disease management, COVID-19 vaccines, and COVID-19 treatments. *J. Am. Acad. Dermatol.* **2021**. [CrossRef]

Review

Efficacy and Safety of Different Formulations of Calcipotriol/Betamethasone Dipropionate in Psoriasis: Gel, Foam, and Ointment

Lidia Rudnicka [1,*], Małgorzata Olszewska [1], Mohamad Goldust [2], Anna Waśkiel-Burnat [1], Olga Warszawik-Hendzel [1], Przemysław Dorożyński [3], Jadwiga Turło [3] and Adriana Rakowska [1]

[1] Department of Dermatology, Medical University of Warsaw, 02-008 Warsaw, Poland; malgorzata.olszewska@wum.edu.pl (M.O.); anna.waskiel@wum.edu.pl (A.W.-B.); olga.warszawik-hendzel@wum.edu.pl (O.W.-H.); adriana.rakowska@wum.edu.pl (A.R.)
[2] Department of Dermatology, University Medical Center of the Johannes Gutenberg University, 55122 Mainz, Germany; drmgjgoldust@gmail.com
[3] Department of Drug Technology and Pharmaceutical Biotechnology, Medical University of Warsaw, 02-097 Warsaw, Poland; pdorozynski@wum.edu.pl (P.D.); jadwiga.turlo@wum.edu.pl (J.T.)
* Correspondence: lidia.rudnicka@dermatolodzy.com.pl; Tel.: +48-225021324; Fax: +48-228242200

Abstract: Preparations containing calcipotriol combined with betamethasone dipropionate (in the forms of ointment, gel, and foam) are available for the topical treatment of psoriasis. This review summarizes the differences in the efficacy and safety of these formulations, as well as the preferences of patients with various forms of psoriasis (plaque, scalp, and nail psoriasis). It has been documented that foams provide higher bioavailability, resulting in increased efficacy in plaque psoriasis compared to ointments and gels. Gels or foams are preferred by patients for their different practical qualities (e.g., gels for "easy application", and foams for "immediate relief"). The available data indicate that ointments may be the most effective formulation in nail psoriasis, and gels are preferred by patients with scalp psoriasis because of their cosmetic features. Treatment with a foam formulation is associated with a lower number of medical appointments compared to treatment with an ointment and with a lower probability of developing indications for systemic treatment. The safety profiles of foams, ointments, and gels are comparable, with the most common adverse effect being pruritus at the application site (in 5.8% of the patients). A long-term proactive maintenance therapy markedly reduces the number of relapses and is likely to close the gap between topical and systemic treatment in psoriasis.

Keywords: calcipotriol; betamethasone dipropionate; long-term treatment; nail psoriasis; proactive treatment; psoriasis; topical therapy; treatment; scalp psoriasis; vitamin D3 derivatives

1. Introduction

Preparations containing calcipotriol combined with betamethasone (in the form of betamethasone dipropionate) are available for the topical treatment of mild psoriasis [1,2]. The topical formulations of calcipotriol with betamethasone available in most countries are ointments, gels, and foams [3–6]. The specific properties of the these preparations may not be comprehensible to every clinical practitioner.

The aim of this article is to review the similarities and differences between these three formulations. In this article, we use the terms "foam" and "foam containing calcipotriol with betamethasone" interchangeably as equivalent to "foam containing calcipotriol with betamethasone dipropionate", the terms "ointment" and "ointment containing calcipotriol with betamethasone" as equivalent to "ointment containing calcipotriol with betamethasone dipropionate", and the terms "gel" or "gel containing calcipotriol with betamethasone" as equivalent to "gel containing calcipotriol with betamethasone dipropionate". All data refer to the approved calcitriol/betamethasone dipropionate concentration of 0.005%/0.064%.

As of 2021, the concentration of active ingredients is identical in all formulations across all countries. The literature search for this article was performed until 31 January 2021 in PubMed and Scopus, using the search terms "calcipotriol" and "betamethasone" with "ointment" or "gel" or "foam". All search results were analyzed in detail.

2. Pharmacodynamics of Calcipotriol/Betamethasone Dipropionate

Calcipotriol, a synthetic vitamin D3 analogue, has a similar mode of action to calcitriol—changing the expression of genes responsive to vitamin D. It binds to the retinoid X receptor and influences cell differentiation and growth regulation, immune functions, and the balance of calcium and phosphorus in the body [7]. It also has a reductive effect on the hyperproliferation of keratinocytes, normalizes their differentiation, and reduces the pro-inflammatory cytokine level, which induces anti-inflammatory and immunomodulatory effects [7,8].

Betamethasone dipropionate belongs to the group of synthetic fluorinated glucocorticoids that exhibit anti-inflammatory and immunosuppressive effects by binding to glucocorticoid cytosolic receptors and then translocating to the nucleus where they regulate the transcription of numerous genes responsible for the immune response. It limits inflammatory infiltration, erythema, and edema, inhibits cell hyperproliferation, and improves the differentiation of keratinocytes in psoriasis [8,9].

Pharmacodynamic studies showed the anti-inflammatory and immunoregulatory synergy of the combination of calcipotriol and betamethasone dipropionate with respect to the effects of these active substances administered individually [10]. The effectiveness of calcipotriol/betamethasone dipropionate mixtures is related to a synergy of action of the two substances. Calcipotriol affects keratinocyte differentiation, while betamethasone influences inflammatory processes and minimizes skin irritation (e.g., pruritus) after calcipotriol application [11].

The mechanism of calcipotriol/betamethasoneantipsoriatic activity has remained only partially known for a long time. However, in the last decade, a number of publications have started to discuss the immune background of psoriasis and the influence of T cells, B cells, dendric cells, as well as cytokines in its pathogenesis [12–15]. A novel approach to the investigation of the mechanism of action of therapeutics applied in psoriasis treatment has been proposed. Recently, Satake et al. [16] have investigated the synergistic effects of drug substances in combination therapy with Cal/BS for dermatitis-like psoriasis. They investigated the basic immune mechanisms in a mouse model of imiquimod-induced psoriasis. Cal/BS combination appeared effective in inhibiting the effects induced by imiquimod in comparison with a monotherapy with calcipotriol or betamethasone. The authors emphasized that Cal/BS synergistically induced $CD8^+$ regulatory T cells and improved the balance between $CD8^+$ or $CD4^+$ regulatory T cells and pro-inflammatory $CCR6^+$ $\gamma\delta$ T17 lymphocytes in the lymph nodes. The data indicated that the synergistic antipsoriatic effect of Cal/BS was based on a reduction of the imbalance between regulatory $CD8^+$ or $CD4^+$ T cells and pro-inflammatory $CCR6^+$ $\gamma\delta$ T17 cells.

Calcipotriol is stable in alkaline solutions with pH above 8, whereas betamethasone dipropionate requires an acidic environment with pH between 4 and 6. Therefore, the presence of both substances in an aqueous environment leads to interactions and to their decomposition [8]. For this reason, the treatment of psoriasis with calcipotriol and betamethasone dipropionate was initially carried out by applying them separately twice a day or sequentially [10]. The development of a formulation type of fixed dose combinations created the possibility of the simultaneous application of calcipotriol and betamethasone dipropionate, increasing their effectiveness and convenience of use, as well as patients' compliance [17]. The treatment is safe, systemic exposure after topical administration of calcipotriol and betamethasone dipropionate is low, and the absorption of the substances after application to healthy skin does not exceed 1%. In patients with psoriasis, the blood levels of the drugs were below the quantification level after 4 to 8 weeks of treatment [7].

3. Supersaturated Foam Formulation of Calcipotriol/Betamethasone

Dermal and transdermal drug delivery is a continuous challenge for pharmaceutical technology. A number of various strategies of drug delivery across the skin barrier have been tested through the decades. A rich set of methods has also been proposed and tested for psoriasis treatment, e.g., laser-assisted drug delivery, foam formulations, nanoparticles, ethosomes, niomes [18]. Among these methods, the application of supersaturated solutions is widely accepted for the treatment with calcipotriol/betamethasone formulations [19]. The penetration of the skin by active substances after topical application is directly proportional to their concentration. Low solubility in the vehicle is a limitation for the majority of active substances in topical preparations. The chemical potential of a substance may be "artificially" increased above its solubility by using supersaturated solutions, which gives the opportunity to improve its delivery. Supersaturated solutions are thermodynamically unstable but they may be temporarily stabilized during treatment.

Supersaturation, involving the increased concentration of a substance above its vehicle solubility threshold, was introduced for foams containing calcipotriol and betamethasone [19,20]. A supersaturated solution is formed on the skin surface ex tempore after the application of the preparation through immediate propellant evaporation. According to the information in the Summary of Product Characteristics (SmPC) of commercial foam formulations containing calcipotriol/betamethasone, the following main excipients are present: white petrolatum, polyoxypropylene stearyl ether, liquid paraffin, butane, and dimethyl ether. According to their role in foam formulations, these substances may be divided into two groups, i.e., lipid anhydrous bases for calcipotriol/betamethasone and volatile solvents, which also act as propellants. The non-aqueous environment protects the active substances from decomposition due to their pH sensitivity. The processes occurring after foam application are shown in Figure 1. After application, butane and dimethyl ether, whose boiling points are below 0 °C, quickly evaporate, leaving a supersaturated solution of calcipotriol/betamethasone in a lipid basis on the surface of the skin. A study presented by Lind et al. [19] showed that the propellant concentration within the foam was reduced to below 2% within 30 s. Microscopy, Raman imaging, and X-ray powder diffraction (XRPD) studies confirmed that the active substances do not recrystallize in foam formulations for at least 18 h, and probably much longer. In contrast, crystals were observed immediately after the application of a standard ointment formulation. Research on the penetration of calcipotriol and betamethasone dipropionate through pig ear skin confirmed a statistically significant increase in active substance concentrations in comparison with the concentrations reached when using an ointment. From a practical point of view, the occlusive properties of the supersaturated layer are very important. They increase the hydration of the stratum corneum by inhibiting water evaporation, which improves skin permeability.

Both in vitro and in vivo research showed the superiority in active substances' speed of penetration and concentration reached when using foams compared to gels or ointments [19].

The outcomes obtained with the use of foams support the view of an increasing number of dermatologists that foams leading to supersaturation of calcipotriol and betamethasone will change dermatology and clinical practice as regards the treatment of psoriasis [21,22].

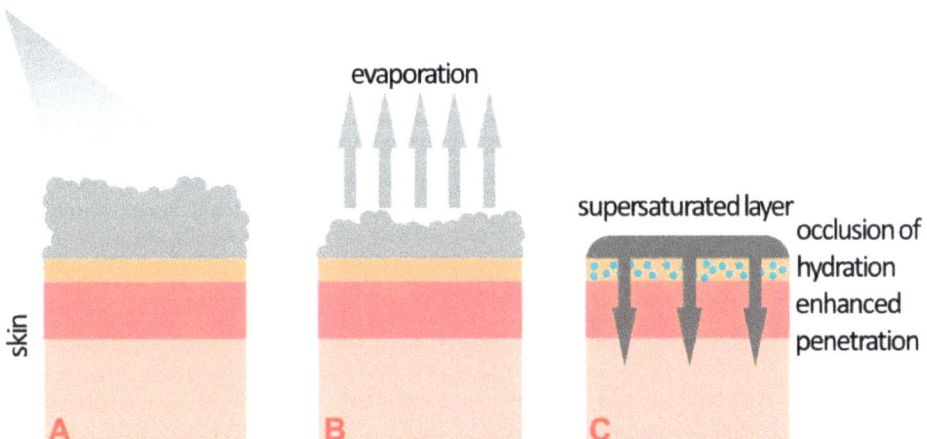

Figure 1. Illustration of the formation of a supersaturated layer on the skin after the administration of a calcipotriol/betamethasone foam. (**A**) Foam application, (**B**) solvent evaporation, (**C**) formation of a supersaturated layer.

4. Comparison of Foam and Ointment

A double-blind multicenter phase II study [23] compared the effectiveness and safety of two preparations containing calcipotriol and betamethasone dipropionate—a foam and an ointment. The study included a total of 376 patients. The primary endpoint to evaluate the formulations' effectiveness was the percentage of patients whose skin lesions regressed or almost completely regressed as confirmed by Physicians Global Assessment (PGA) analysis after 4 weeks. The number of patients in whom therapeutic success was achieved was significantly higher in the group who had used the foam formulation compared to the group who had used the ointment (54.6% and 43.0%, respectively, $p = 0.025$). Moreover, assessment with the mPASI method (modification of the Psoriasis Area and Severity Index, which excludes the hairy scalp on which no foam/ointment was applied) demonstrated a statistically significant advantage of foam over ointment at both assessed time points (1 week and 4 weeks). The authors concluded that the effectiveness of the foam formulation was markedly higher than that of the ointment, with a comparable safety profile.

The standard vasoconstriction test for the evaluation of glucocorticoid effects was used to compare the activities of a foam containing calcipotriol and betamethasone and an ointment containing betamethasone (no calcipotriol). The degree of vasoconstriction obtained with the foam was (median) 2.00 points, while that achieved with the ointment containing betamethasone but without calcipotriol was 1.75 points, with the difference being statistically insignificant ($p = 0.30$) [24].

An analysis of the cost effectiveness of foams and ointments containing calcipotriol and betamethasone was conducted in Sweden [25]. A relatively complex organizational regimen involved the application of a foam or an ointment prior to systemic treatment. A significantly higher effectiveness of the foam was observed in comparison with the ointment. The use of foam was associated with a lower number of medical consultations and a lower percentage of patients for whom systemic treatment was necessary.

5. Comparison of Foam and Gel

A 12-week PSO-ABLE phase III study [26] was conducted to compare the therapeutic effectiveness and safety of a foam containing calcipotriol and betamethasone and a gel containing the same amount of active substances. The study included 463 patients. The average baseline BSA was 7.1 ± 5.7 in the group of patients using the foam and 7.0 ± 5.5 in the group who used the gel. The primary endpoint of effectiveness assessment was the percentage of patients in whom therapeutic success was achieved. Therapeutic success was defined according to the PGA scale (0–4) as "no lesions" in case of patients with mild lesions at baseline and "no lesions" or "almost no lesions" in patients with moderate or severe psoriasis at baseline. On the basis of the above definition, the effectiveness of the foam was characterized as markedly higher compared to that of the gel. The percentages of patients in whom therapeutic success was achieved ("no" or "almost no" psoriatic lesions) were 38.3% and 19.6% after 4 weeks for the foam and gel groups, respectively, while after 8 weeks, the respective percentages were 44.5% and 22.5%. The study also showed that, after 4 weeks, therapeutic success was achieved in a significantly higher percentage of patients using the foam, whereas it required 8 weeks in patients using the gel. A similar difference was observed when analyzing the effectiveness with mPASI. During the study, the patients used on average 98.6 g of foam and 164.3 g of gel (after 4 and 8 weeks, respectively). They used 236.4 g of foam and 193.1 g of gel over 12 weeks.

The secondary endpoints of effectiveness were the percentage of patients achieving at least 75% of modified PASI (mPASI75) reduction and the time to treatment success. A significant advantage of the foam was demonstrated also for those parameters. The authors emphasized that the median time for achieving the standard index of improvement of mPASI75 was 4 weeks for the foam and 12 weeks for the gel.

A phase III clinical trial also assessed the influence of using foam and gel formulations on patients' quality of life [27]. The following scales were used in the assessment: Health-Related Quality of Life (HRQoL), including the Dermatology Life Quality Index (DLQI), the EuroQoL-5D-5L-PSO (EQ-5D), and the Psoriasis QoL (PQoL-12). Moreover, the researchers evaluated such variables as pruritus, sleep deprivation triggered by pruritus, and the influence of the disease on the working life. The study included 463 patients with plaque psoriasis with BSA of 2 to 30%. In this group, 185 patients applied a foam, 188 used a gel formulation, 47 used a foam vehicle without active substances, and 43 used a gel vehicle. DLQI 0 or 1 were obtained by considerably more patients using the foam rather than the gel at week 4 (45.7% vs 32.4%, respectively; $p = 0.013$) and at week 12 (60.5% vs 44.1%, respectively; $p = 0.003$). The foam was also more effective as regards other parameters concerning the quality of life, including EQ-5D (0.09 vs 0.03; $p < 0.001$) and PQoL-12 (-2.23 vs -2.07; $p = 0.029$), and in terms of the influence on pruritus, pruritus-related sleep deprivation, and work impairment.

Another phase III clinical trial [28] evaluated the preferences of patients concerning the vehicle. The authors compared a foam containing calcipotriol with a gel containing the same active substance. "The previous treatment" was the reference point. It was a prospective multicenter study (NCT02310646). The foam was used once daily for 7 days and then was substituted by the gel or the opposite. The study included 213 patients. For some parameters, the patients claimed they preferred the foam, e.g., because of immediate relief, the soothing quality of the preparation, or the feeling of alleviating the condition. As regards the gel, the patients indicated its easy application or easy spreading.

6. Special Locations

The efficacy of gel, ointment, and foam formulations was not extensively studied in special locations which are difficult to treat. Some studies were conducted on the efficacy of calcipotriol/betamethasone in nail psoriasis.

Rigopoulos et al. [29] treated 22 patients with nail psoriasis (114 nails) with an ointment once daily for 12 weeks. An average improvement of 72% was observed in the nail psoriasis severity index (NAPSI). Saki et al. [30] investigated 16 patients with nail psoriasis treated with an ointment formulation for 6 months and observed a mean improvement of 55.5% in the NAPSI.

In a study performed by Gregoriou et al. [31], a calcipotriol/betamethasone foam was applied once daily on the proximal nail fold and hyponychium. The mean total NAPSI was reduced by 44%. Case reports also indicated the possible efficacy of a gel formulation monotherapy in nail psoriasis [32].

There were no head-to-head studies, but indirect data may indicate that the ointment formulation is more effective in nail psoriasis compared to foam.

The effect of a calcipotriol/betamethasone gel and foam in scalp psoriasis was extensively studied [33–38]. No head-to-head studies are available to evaluate the relative efficacy or safety of different formulations for scalp psoriasis. A 2017 Cochrane review of topical treatment options in scalp psoriasis indicated the presence of overall moderate-quality evidence confirming that the two-compound combination was only of small benefit over the formulation containing only the corticosteroid and that both therapies were similarly safe in short-term therapy. It was also concluded that there was overall moderate-quality evidence confirming that the two-compound combination was more effective and safer than vitamin D alone in short-term therapy [39]. Differences in the methodology of various short-term studies (4–8 weeks) performed in adult patients with scalp psoriasis limit the possibility of comparing the efficacy of these two formulations. The ointment formulation was not studied in isolated scalp psoriasis in clinical trials. A small case series indicated the possibility of significant efficacy [40]. However, difficulty in washing the ointment out of the hair may be a limiting factor [40].

A long-term study of a calcipotriol/betamethasone gel in adult patients performed by Saraceno et al. [36] indicated that maintenance therapy with twice-weekly applications versus on-demand treatment was more effective and was associated with a lower rate of relapse. The treatment was considered cosmetically acceptable by 79% of the patients [23].

Scalp psoriasis in adolescents was not extensively studied. An analysis of data from phase 2 studies was performed to evaluate the efficacy of a foam formulation in scalp psoriasis in adults and adolescents from the age of 12 years. An improvement was observed in PGA classification at week 4 in 73.6% of the adolescents and it was higher compared to that reached in the adults [38]. There are no studies focusing on the possible application of betamethasone/calcipotriol in patients with intertriginous or genital psoriasis. However, expert opinions indicate that a short course of treatment is likely to have a good efficacy and safety profile [41]. The comparison of the pharmaceutic properties may indicate a preference for foam over ointment or gel.

7. Adverse Effects

The safety profile of foams was compared to that of ointments by Koo et al. [23] and to that of gels by Paul et al. [26]. The available safety data related to foams have recently been collected and analyzed by Amat-Samaranch and Puig [42]. The data showed that that the safety profiles of foams, ointments, and gels were comparable, with adverse effects observed in more than 1% of patients being application site pruritus (5.8%), skin atrophy (1.9%), folliculitis (1.9%), skin burning sensation (1.4%), skin depigmentation (1.4%), and erythema (1.0%).

8. Calcipotriol/Betamethasone Foam as a Formulation Bridging the Gap between Topical and Systemic Treatment in Psoriasis

A study published in December 2020 evaluating foam containing calcipotriol with betamethasone indicated the latter as a drug that might influence the costs of the biologic treatment of patients with the moderate-to-severe disease [43]. The authors indicated that biologic treatment was effective as a monotherapy in numerous patients suffering from psoriasis, while in some patients a change in treatment was necessary. The study aimed to analyze possible cost savings resulting from the use of a foam formulation combined with a systemic biologic treatment compared to a monotherapy treatment. The study included 30 patients. It was a 16-week, open-label, single-arm study of adjunctive therapy with a foam containing calcipotriol and betamethasone in patients who had been treated with etanercept or adalimumab for more than 24 weeks, without obtaining a satisfactory treatment response. The analysis involved the assessment of the affected body surface area (BSA), a general evaluation of disease severity performed by a doctor (PGA), BSA × PGA, NPF Treat to Target, and the probability of changing a biologic drug by the attending physician. Simultaneously, the authors analyzed the cost of treatment. Notably, the abundance of results obtained in the study showed that the probability of switching the biologic drug into another (potentially more expensive) decreased from 90.0% at baseline to 7.1% after 16 weeks of research which included 4 weeks of treatment with the topical drug applied once daily, followed by 12 weeks of maintenance/proactive therapy. The National Psoriasis FoundationTreat to Target status was achieved by over 75% of the patients by 4 weeks. The pharmacoeconomic assessment revealed that the adjuvant use of foam was more cost-effective compared to switching biologic drugs. In conclusion, the authors indicated that adjuvant therapy with calcipotriol and betamethasone dipropionate in a foam formulation may result not only in considerable clinical benefits but also in potential cost savings.

A recent meta-analysis was performed to compare literature data referring to the effectiveness of a treatment with a foam containing calcipotriol and betamethasone compared to that of classic methods for the systemic treatment of psoriasis [44]. The time to therapeutic effect for each of the analyzed drugs was the reference point. Patients treated with a foam containing calcipotriol and betamethasone were characterized by a significantly better response assessed with the PASI75 scale compared to patients administered apremilast, methotrexate, and acitretin, and by a similar response compared to patients administered fumaric acid esters. Despite numerous methodological limitations of such analysis of literature data, the presented material reflects the questions frequently asked by dermatologists nowadays.

A similar presumption was the basis of a publication which analyzed the treatment costs of a foam containing calcipotriol and betamethasone and of systemic treatment [45]. The authors compared short-term costs and treatment effectiveness. The analysis comprised methotrexate, acitretin, fumaric acid esters, and apremilast. The authors assumed the perspective of the payer, which included the drug, medical appointments, and treatment monitoring as treatment costs. The lowest cost per responder (CPR) was generated by foam in all countries. It was calculated as the standard time necessary for achieving clinical response. The cost of treatment with foam was 190–359 Euros lower than that with methotrexate, apremilast, and acitretin. On the basis of the data in this publication, it may be concluded that in cases in which topical treatment is possible and clinically indicated, a foam with calcipotriol and betamethasone may constitute an attractive alternative for the short-term treatment of patients with psoriasis on the border of clinical indications for systemic treatment.

Bagel et al. [46] investigated whether patients who did not respond to systemic treatment with apremilast as monotherapy might be successfully treated for psoriasis (treatment effectiveness defined as PASI75) if a foam containing calcipotriol and betamethasone was introduced. The authors demonstrated that the majority of patients with partial response to treatment at week 8 might achieve PASI75 at week 12 with the combination therapy in topical foam and maintain PASI75 until week 16 with a systemic drug as monotherapy. It may indicate that even a short-term addition of foam containing calcipotriol to systemic treatment leads to an improvement and the maintenance of good response to the same drug, without the necessity of changing drugs in systemic treatment (Table 1).

Table 1. Major differences between calcipotriol/betamethasone foam, ointment, and gel.

Differences between Calcipotriol/Betamethasone Gel, Foam, and Ointment
• higher bioavailability of foam compared to ointment [19] • higher clinical efficacy of foam compared to ointment and gel documented in clinical trials [22–24,26,27] • higher efficacy of foam compared to gel as regards relieving pruritus [27] • higher efficacy of foam compared to gel in relieving pruritus-related sleep disorders [27] • higher efficacy of foam compared to gel as regards the influence on the quality of life [27] • gel or foam are preferred by patients for their different practical qualities (e.g., gel for "easy application" and foam for "immediate relief") [28] • lower number of medical appointments with foam compared to ointment [25] • lower probability of developing indications for systemic treatment or for switching to a different systemic treatment with foam in comparison with ointment [25,47], maintenance therapy markedly reduces the number of relapses (approved for foam, not for ointment or gel) • ointment appears to be more effective compared to foam in nail psoriasis (no head-to-head data) [30,31,48] • the efficacy of foam and gel in scalp psoriasis was studied with inequivalent methodologies; gel is cosmetically acceptable by 79% of patients [36,38]

9. Proactive Maintenance Treatment

The chronic course of psoriasis and the tendency towards rapid relapses after topical treatment constitute a significant problem in the treatment of psoriasis. Topical corticoid treatments are approved for no more than 4–8 weeks, leaving the patient and physician with limited possibilities for treatment continuation. According to the registered posology regimen, the possibility of using a foam with calcipotriol and betamethasone as a proactive treatment for up to 52 weeks opens a new avenue for the long-term therapy of psoriasis.

A phase III clinical trial (NCT02899962) described by Lebwohl et al. [49] and Stein Gold et al. [50] in 2020 collected positive results. It involved the assessment of the safety and effectiveness of a calcipotriol and betamethasone foam used twice weekly for 52 weeks as a proactive maintenance therapy aiming to prevent a relapse or achieve the longest possible clinical remission time. This idea is based on the long-term application of the foam to healthy-appearing areas following the resolution of skin lesions.

In this context, it is worth emphasizing that the clinical regression of lesions is not equivalent to the resolution of the inflammatory process in the skin. A study conducted with the use of noninvasive skin imaging techniques indicated that an inflammation persisted in the skin despite achieving the apparent regression of skin lesions [51]. It was also demonstrated that the post-treatment dermoscopic picture of skin lesions allowed the determination of prognosis regarding the recurrence of cutaneous lesions in psoriasis [52]. The subclinical presence of an ongoing inflammatory process in the skin of patients with psoriasis explains the tendency towards rapid recurrences of psoriatic skin lesions in a significant proportion of patients treated with conventional 4–8 week courses of calcipotriol and betamethasone ointments or gels. This phenomenon identified in recent years has become one of the most important presumptions as regards the development of proactive psoriasis treatments which would offer a chance to prolong the remission time after topical treatment.

The phase III clinical trial which was mentioned above [49] included 650 patients, with 521 being randomized to the proactive phase of maintenance therapy. The time to first relapse was the primary endpoint. A total of 251 randomized patients (46.1%) completed the study. The median of the time to first relapse was 56 days (in a group of patients undergoing proactive treatment) and 30 days (control group), which indicated that the time to first relapse was 87% longer in patients treated proactively. In total, the patients in the proactive treatment group had additional 41 days of remission over 52 weeks compared to the control group of patients in whom subsequent treatment cycles were introduced according to previous clinical practice, i.e., after a clinical relapse ($p < 0.001$). The number of relapses during 52 weeks was 3.1 (study group), which was 35% lower than in the control group (4.8). Moreover, the tendency towards rebounds was lower compared to that at baseline (PASI $\geq$ 125%). The safety profile was comparable for both therapeutic methods.

In 2020, Kircik et al. [47] summarized available scientific evidence and literature data in a review article. Data analysis indicated that foams (but not other pharmaceutical formulations) containing calcipotriol and betamethasone have such a high anti-psoriatic effectiveness that, in some psoriasis patients, the decision to implement systemic treatment might be unnecessary.

10. Conclusions

Calcipotriol/betamethasone foams show significantly higher efficacy compared to ointment and gel formulations in the treatment of plaque psoriasis. The higher clinical efficacy may be attributed to the supersaturation technique which was used for the production of the foam formulations. Gels and ointments have shown some benefits in the topical treatment of scalp and nail psoriasis, respectively. The available data indicate that the foam formulation may close the gap between topical and systemic therapy in plaque psoriasis, particularly when applied as a long-term proactive maintenance treatment.

Author Contributions: Conceptualization, L.R. and M.O.; methodology, A.R. and A.W.-B., validation, L.R., M.O., M.G., A.W.-B., O.W.-H., P.D., J.T., and A.R., formal analysis, all; resources (published data): all, data curation all; writing—original draft preparation, L.R. and M.O.; writing—all, visualization, L.R., P.D.; supervision, L.R.; project administration, L.R. and M.O.; funding acquisition, none. All authors have read and agreed to the published version of the manuscript.

Funding: This research received no external funding. The article was neither inspired nor supported by any company.

Institutional Review Board Statement: Not applicable.

Informed Consent Statement: Not applicable.

Conflicts of Interest: This article was neither inspired nor supported by any company. No company had any role in the design of the study, in the collection of data, analyses, or interpretation, in the writing of the manuscript, or in the decision to publish. Potential conflicts of interest: L.R.—member of advisory boards—Janssen Pharmaceutical Companies, L'Oreal, Leo, Lilly, Pfizer, Sanofi, Novartis, UCB, Timber Pharma; invited speaker—Eli Lilly, Leo, Abbvie, L'Oreal, Lilly, Pierre Fabre; M.O.— invited speaker—Axxon, Leo, medac; A.W.-B.— invited speaker — Pierre Fabre; M.G., A.R., O.W.-H., P.D. and J.T.—no conflicts of interest.

References

1. Elmets, C.A.; Korman, N.J.; Prater, E.F.; Wong, E.B.; Rupani, R.N.; Kivelevitch, D.; Armstrong, A.W.; Connor, C.; Cordoro, K.M.; Davis, D.M.R.; et al. Joint AAD-NPF Guidelines of care for the management and treatment of psoriasis with topical therapy and alternative medicine modalities for psoriasis severity measures. *J. Am. Acad. Dermatol.* **2021**, *84*, 432–470. [CrossRef]
2. Carrascosa, J.M.; Theng, C.; Thaci, D. Spotlight on Topical Long-Term Management of Plaque Psoriasis. *Clin. Cosmet. Investig. Dermatol.* **2020**, *13*, 495–498. [CrossRef]
3. Reich, A.; Adamski, Z.; Chodorowska, G.; Kaszuba, A.; Krasowska, D.; Lesiak, A.; Maj, J.; Narbutt, J.; Osmola-Mańkowska, A.J.; Owczarczyk-Saczonek, A.; et al. Psoriasis. Diagnostic and therapeutic recommendations of the Polish Dermatological Society. Part 1. *Dermatol. Rev. Przegląd Dermatol.* **2020**, *107*, 92–108. [CrossRef]
4. Chiricozzi, A.; Pimpinelli, N.; Ricceri, F.; Bagnoni, G.; Bartoli, L.; Bellini, M.; Brandini, L.; Caproni, M.; Castelli, A.; Fimiani, M.; et al. Treatment of psoriasis with topical agents: Recommendations from a Tuscany Consensus. *Dermatol. Ther.* **2017**, *30*. [CrossRef]
5. Thaci, D.; de la Cueva, P.; Pink, A.E.; Jalili, A.; Segaert, S.; Hjuler, K.F.; Calzavara-Pinton, P. General practice recommendations for the topical treatment of psoriasis: A modified-Delphi approach. *BJGP Open* **2020**, *4*. [CrossRef]
6. Kleyn, E.C.; Morsman, E.; Griffin, L.; Wu, J.J.; Cm van de Kerkhof, P.; Gulliver, W.; van der Walt, J.M.; Iversen, L. Review of international psoriasis guidelines for the treatment of psoriasis: Recommendations for topical corticosteroid treatments. *J. Dermatolog. Treat.* **2019**, *30*, 311–319. [CrossRef] [PubMed]
7. McCormack, P.L. Spotlight on calcipotriene/betamethasone dipropionate in psoriasis vulgaris of the trunk, limbs, and scalp. *Am. J. Clin. Dermatol.* **2011**, *12*, 421–424. [CrossRef] [PubMed]

8. McCormack, P.L. Calcipotriol/betamethasone dipropionate: A review of its use in the treatment of psoriasis vulgaris of the trunk, limbs and scalp. *Drugs* **2011**, *71*, 709–730. [CrossRef] [PubMed]
9. Stein Gold, L.; Bagel, J.; Allenby, K.; Sidgiddi, S. Betamethasone dipropionate spray 0.05% alleviates troublesome symptoms of plaque psoriasis. *Cutis* **2020**, *105*, 97–102.e101.
10. Patel, N.U.; Felix, K.; Reimer, D.; Feldman, S.R. Calcipotriene/betamethasone dipropionate for the treatment of psoriasis vulgaris: An evidence-based review. *Clin. Cosmet. Investig. Dermatol.* **2017**, *10*, 385–391. [CrossRef]
11. Traulsen, J. Bioavailability of betamethasone dipropionate when combined with calcipotriol. *Int. J. Dermatol.* **2004**, *43*, 611–617. [CrossRef]
12. Grän, F.; Kerstan, A.; Serfling, E.; Goebeler, M.; Muhammad, K. Current Developments in the Immunology of Psoriasis. *Yale J. Biol. Med.* **2020**, *93*, 97–110.
13. Ogawa, K.; Okada, Y. The current landscape of psoriasis genetics in 2020. *J. Dermatol. Sci.* **2020**, *99*, 2–8. [CrossRef]
14. Baliwag, J.; Barnes, D.H.; Johnston, A. Cytokines in psoriasis. *Cytokine* **2015**, *73*, 342–350. [CrossRef]
15. Lowes, M.A.; Suárez-Fariñas, M.; Krueger, J.G. Immunology of psoriasis. *Annu. Rev. Immunol.* **2014**, *32*, 227–255. [CrossRef]
16. Satake, K.; Amano, T.; Okamoto, T. Calcipotriol and betamethasone dipropionate synergistically enhances the balance between regulatory and proinflammatory T cells in a murine psoriasis model. *Sci. Rep.* **2019**, *9*, 16322. [CrossRef] [PubMed]
17. Kuehl, B.; Shear, N.H. The Evolution of Topical Formulations in Psoriasis. *Skin Ther. Lett.* **2018**, *23*, 5–9.
18. Wollina, U.; Tirant, M.; Vojvodic, A.; Lotti, T. Treatment of Psoriasis: Novel Approaches to Topical Delivery. *Open Access Maced. J. Med. Sci.* **2019**, *7*, 3018–3025. [CrossRef] [PubMed]
19. Lind, M.; Nielsen, K.T.; Schefe, L.H.; Nørremark, K.; Eriksson, A.H.; Norsgaard, H.; Pedersen, B.T.; Petersson, K. Supersaturation of Calcipotriene and Betamethasone Dipropionate in a Novel Aerosol Foam Formulation for Topical Treatment of Psoriasis Provides Enhanced Bioavailability of the Active Ingredients. *Dermatol. Ther. (Heidelb)* **2016**, *6*, 413–425. [CrossRef]
20. Paul, C.; Bang, B.; Lebwohl, M. Fixed combination calcipotriol plus betamethasone dipropionate aerosol foam in the treatment of psoriasis vulgaris: Rationale for development and clinical profile. *Expert Opin. Pharmacother.* **2017**, *18*, 115–121. [CrossRef]
21. Puig, L.; Carretero, G. Update on Topical Treatments for Psoriasis: The Role of Calcipotriol Plus Betamethasone Dipropionate Aerosol Foam. *Actas Dermosifiliogr.* **2019**, *110*, 115–123. [CrossRef]
22. Megna, M.; Cinelli, E.; Camela, E.; Fabbrocini, G. Calcipotriol/betamethasone dipropionate formulations for psoriasis: An overview of the options and efficacy data. *Expert Rev. Clin. Immunol.* **2020**, *16*, 599–620. [CrossRef] [PubMed]
23. Koo, J.; Tyring, S.; Werschler, W.P.; Bruce, S.; Olesen, M.; Villumsen, J.; Bagel, J. Superior efficacy of calcipotriene and betamethasone dipropionate aerosol foam versus ointment in patients with psoriasis vulgaris–A randomized phase II study. *J. Dermatolog. Treat.* **2016**, *27*, 120–127. [CrossRef] [PubMed]
24. Queille-Roussel, C.; Bang, B.; Clonier, F.; Lacour, J.P. Enhanced vasoconstrictor potency of the fixed combination calcipotriol plus betamethasone dipropionate in an innovative aerosol foam formulation vs. other corticosteroid psoriasis treatments. *J. Eur. Acad. Dermatol. Venereol.* **2016**, *30*, 1951–1956. [CrossRef]
25. Duvetorp, A.; Levin, L.A.; Engerstedt Mattsson, E.; Ryttig, L. A Cost-utility Analysis of Calcipotriol/Betamethasone Dipropionate Aerosol Foam versus Ointment for the Topical Treatment of Psoriasis Vulgaris in Sweden. *Acta Derm. Venereol.* **2019**, *99*, 393–399. [CrossRef] [PubMed]
26. Paul, C.; Stein Gold, L.; Cambazard, F.; Kalb, R.E.; Lowson, D.; Bang, B.; Griffiths, C.E. Calcipotriol plus betamethasone dipropionate aerosol foam provides superior efficacy vs. gel in patients with psoriasis vulgaris: Randomized, controlled PSO-ABLE study. *J. Eur. Acad. Dermatol. Venereol.* **2017**, *31*, 119–126. [CrossRef]
27. Griffiths, C.E.; Stein Gold, L.; Cambazard, F.; Kalb, R.E.; Lowson, D.; Moller, A.; Paul, C. Greater improvement in quality of life outcomes in patients using fixed-combination calcipotriol plus betamethasone dipropionate aerosol foam versus gel: Results from the PSO-ABLE study. *Eur. J. Dermatol.* **2018**, *28*, 356–363. [CrossRef] [PubMed]
28. Hong, C.H.; Papp, K.A.; Lophaven, K.W.; Skallerup, P.; Philipp, S. Patients with psoriasis have different preferences for topical therapy, highlighting the importance of individualized treatment approaches: Randomized phase IIIb PSO-INSIGHTFUL study. *J. Eur. Acad. Dermatol. Venereol.* **2017**, *31*, 1876–1883. [CrossRef]
29. Rigopoulos, D.; Gregoriou, S.; Daniel Iii, C.R.; Belyayeva, H.; Larios, G.; Verra, P.; Stamou, C.; Kontochristopoulos, G.; Avgerinou, G.; Katsambas, A. Treatment of nail psoriasis with a two-compound formulation of calcipotriol plus betamethasone dipropionate ointment. *Dermatology* **2009**, *218*, 338–341. [CrossRef] [PubMed]
30. Saki, N.; Hosseinpoor, S.; Heiran, A.; Mohammadi, A.; Zeraatpishe, M. Comparing the Efficacy of Triamcinolone Acetonide Iontophoresis versus Topical Calcipotriol/Betamethasone Dipropionate in Treating Nail Psoriasis: A Bilateral Controlled Clinical Trial. *Dermatol. Res. Pract.* **2018**, *2018*, 2637691. [CrossRef]
31. Gregoriou, S.; Sidiropoulou, P.; Tsimpidakis, A.; Rompoti, N.; Tsironi, T.; Panagakis, P.; Polydorou, D.; Kostakis, P.; Rigopoulos, D. Treatment of nail psoriasis with calcipotriol/betamethasone dipropionate foam versus pulse dye laser: An unblinded, intra-patient, left-to-right prospective study. *J. Eur. Acad. Dermatol. Venereol.* **2020**, *34*, e519–e520. [CrossRef] [PubMed]
32. Takama, H.; Ando, Y.; Yanagishita, T.; Ohshima, Y.; Akiyama, M.; Watanabe, D. Two cases of refractory nail psoriasis successfully treated with calcipotriol plus betamethasone dipropionate gel. *J. Dermatol.* **2020**, *47*, e211–e213. [CrossRef] [PubMed]

33. Liu, L.; Zhang, C.; Wang, J.; Chen, K.; Ding, Y.; Yan, G.; Lu, Q.; Li, W.; Fang, H.; Cheng, H.; et al. Comparison of safety and efficacy between calcipotriol plus betamethasone dipropionate gel and calcipotriol scalp solution as long-term treatment for scalp psoriasis in Chinese patients: A national, multicentre, prospective, randomized, active-controlled phase 4 trial. *Eur. J. Dermatol.* **2020**, *30*, 580–590. [CrossRef] [PubMed]
34. Gual, A.; Pau-Charles, I.; Molin, S. Topical treatment for scalp psoriasis: Comparison of patient preference, quality of life and efficacy for non-alcoholic mometasone emulsion versus calcipotriol/betamethasone gel in daily clinical practice. *J. Dermatolog. Treat.* **2016**, *27*, 228–234. [CrossRef] [PubMed]
35. Ma, L.; Yang, Q.; Yang, H.; Wang, G.; Zheng, M.; Hao, F.; Gu, J.; Sun, Q.; Cui, P.; Ge, M.; et al. Calcipotriol plus betamethasone dipropionate gel compared with calcipotriol scalp solution in the treatment of scalp psoriasis: A randomized, controlled trial investigating efficacy and safety in a Chinese population. *Int. J. Dermatol.* **2016**, *55*, 106–113. [CrossRef]
36. Saraceno, R.; Camplone, G.; D'Agostino, M.; De Simone, C.; Di Cesare, A.; Filosa, G.; Frascione, P.; Gabellini, M.; Lunghi, F.; Mazzotta, A.; et al. Efficacy and maintenance strategies of two-compound formulation calcipotriol and betamethasone dipropionate gel (Xamiol(R) gel) in the treatment of scalp psoriasis: Results from a study in 885 patients. *J. Dermatolog. Treat.* **2014**, *25*, 30–33. [CrossRef]
37. Bottomley, J.M.; Taylor, R.S.; Ryttov, J. The effectiveness of two-compound formulation calcipotriol and betamethasone dipropionate gel in the treatment of moderately severe scalp psoriasis: A systematic review of direct and indirect evidence. *Curr. Med. Res. Opin.* **2011**, *27*, 251–268. [CrossRef]
38. Petersen, B.; Lebwohl, M. Treating Scalp Psoriasis with Calcipotriene/Betamethasone Dipropionate Fixed-dose Combination Cutaneous Foam: Review of Phase 2 Data. *J. Drugs Dermatol.* **2020**, *19*, 784–786. [CrossRef]
39. Schlager, J.G.; Rosumeck, S.; Werner, R.N.; Jacobs, A.; Schmitt, J.; Schlager, C.; Nast, A. Topical treatments for scalp psoriasis: Summary of a Cochrane Systematic Review. *Br. J. Dermatol.* **2017**, *176*, 604–614. [CrossRef]
40. Downs, A.M. Dovobet ointment under occlusion overnight for troublesome scalp psoriasis. *Acta Derm. Venereol.* **2006**, *86*, 57–58. [CrossRef]
41. Beck, K.M.; Yang, E.J.; Sanchez, I.M.; Liao, W. Treatment of Genital Psoriasis: A Systematic Review. *Dermatol. Ther.* **2018**, *8*, 509–525. [CrossRef]
42. Amat-Samaranch, V.; Puig, L. Safety of calcipotriene and betamethasone dipropionate foam for the treatment of psoriasis. *Expert Opin. Drug Saf.* **2020**, *19*, 423–432. [CrossRef]
43. Bagel, J.; Nelson, E.; Zapata, J.; Hetzel, A. Adjunctive Use of Calcipotriene/Betamethasone Dipropionate Foam in a Real-World Setting Curtails the Cost of Biologics Without Reducing Efficacy in Psoriasis. *Dermatol. Ther. (Heidelb)* **2020**, *10*, 1383–1396. [CrossRef]
44. Bewley, A.P.; Shear, N.H.; Calzavara-Pinton, P.G.; Hansen, J.B.; Nyeland, M.E.; Signorovitch, J. Calcipotriol plus betamethasone dipropionate aerosol foam vs. apremilast, methotrexate, acitretin or fumaric acid esters for the treatment of plaque psoriasis: A matching-adjusted indirect comparison. *J. Eur. Acad. Dermatol. Venereol.* **2019**, *33*, 1107–1115. [CrossRef] [PubMed]
45. Balak, D.M.W.; Carrascosa, J.M.; Gregoriou, S.; Calzavara-Pinton, P.; Bewley, A.; Antunes, J.; Nyeland, M.E.; Viola, M.G.; Sawyer, L.M.; Becla, L. Cost per PASI-75 responder of calcipotriol plus betamethasone dipropionate cutaneous foam versus nonbiologic systemic therapies for the treatment of plaque psoriasis in seven European countries. *J. Dermatolog. Treat.* **2020**, 1–8. [CrossRef]
46. Bagel, J.; Nelson, E.; Riley, C.; Hetzel, A. Apremilast with Add-On Calcipotriene/Betamethasone Dipropionate for Treating Moderate to Severe Plaque Psoriasis. *J. Drugs Dermatol.* **2020**, *19*, 1149–1155. [CrossRef] [PubMed]
47. Kircik, L.; Stein Gold, L.; Teng, J.; Moore, A.; Cantrell, W.; Alonso-Llamazares, J.; Koo, J. Fixed Combination Calcipotriene and Betamethasone Dipropionate (Cal/BD) Foam for Beyond-Mild Psoriasis: A Possible Alternative to Systemic Medication. *J. Drugs Dermatol.* **2020**, *19*, 723–732. [CrossRef] [PubMed]
48. Park, J.M.; Cho, H.H.; Kim, W.J.; Mun, J.H.; Song, M.; Kim, H.S.; Ko, H.C.; Kim, B.S.; Kim, M.B. Efficacy and Safety of Calcipotriol/Betamethasone Dipropionate Ointment for the Treatment of Trachyonychia: An Open-Label Study. *Ann. Dermatol.* **2015**, *27*, 371–375. [CrossRef]
49. Lebwohl, M.; Kircik, L.; Lacour, J.P.; Liljedahl, M.; Lynde, M.; Morch, M.H.; Papp, K.A.; Perrot, J.L.; Gold, L.S.; Takhar, A.; et al. Twice-weekly topical calcipotriene/betamethasone dipropionate foam as proactive management of plaque psoriasis increases time in remission and is well tolerated over 52 weeks (PSO-LONG trial). *J. Am. Acad. Dermatol.* **2020**. [CrossRef] [PubMed]
50. Stein Gold, L.; Alonso-Llamazares, J.; Lacour, J.P.; Warren, R.B.; Tyring, S.K.; Kircik, L.; Yamauchi, P.; Lebwohl, M.; Investigators, P.-L.T. PSO-LONG: Design of a Novel, 12-Month Clinical Trial of Topical, Proactive Maintenance with Twice-Weekly Cal/BD Foam in Psoriasis. *Adv. Ther.* **2020**, *37*, 4730–4753. [CrossRef] [PubMed]
51. Grajdeanu, I.A.; Statescu, L.; Vata, D.; Popescu, I.A.; Porumb-Andrese, E.; Patrascu, A.I.; Taranu, T.; Crisan, M.; Solovastru, L.G. Imaging techniques in the diagnosis and monitoring of psoriasis. *Exp. Ther. Med.* **2019**, *18*, 4974–4980. [CrossRef] [PubMed]
52. Errichetti, E.; Croatto, M.; Arnoldo, L.; Stinco, G. Plaque-Type Psoriasis Treated with Calcipotriene Plus Betamethasone Dipropionate Aerosol Foam: A Prospective Study on Clinical and Dermoscopic Predictor Factors in Response Achievement and Retention. *Dermatol. Ther. (Heidelb)* **2020**, *10*, 757–767. [CrossRef] [PubMed]

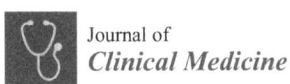

Article

Implementation of the Treat-to-Target Concept in Evaluation of Psoriatic Arthritis Patients

Tal Gazitt [1,2,*,†], Muhanad Abu Elhija [1,†], Amir Haddad [1], Idit Lavi [3], Muna Elias [1] and Devy Zisman [1,4]

1. Rheumatology Unit, Carmel Medical Center, Haifa 3436212, Israel; Mahanedab@clalit.org.il (M.A.E.); haddadamir@yahoo.com (A.H.); munael@clalit.org.il (M.E.); devyzisman@gmail.com (D.Z.)
2. Division of Rheumatology, Department of Medicine, University of Washington Medical Center, Seattle, WA 98195, USA
3. Department of Community Medicine and Epidemiology, Carmel Medical Center, Haifa 3436212, Israel; lavi_idit@clalit.org.il
4. The Ruth and Bruce Rappaport Faculty of Medicine, Technion, Haifa 3525433, Israel
* Correspondence: tgazitt@gmail.com or talgaz@clalit.org.il; Tel.: +972-4-8250486; Fax: +972-4-8260213
† Both authors contributed equally to the writing of this manuscript.

Abstract: Background: The treat-to-target approach was recently adopted for psoriatic arthritis (PsA) management. Objective: To assess the implementation of the "treat-to-target" (T2T) concept in daily management of PsA by use of composite scores of disease activity versus clinical judgement alone. Methods: A total of 117 PsA patients from a longitudinal PsA cohort were enrolled consecutively in the study during each patient's first clinic visit during 2016–2017. Clinic notes from the treating rheumatologist were reviewed by an independent rheumatologist, noting clinical impression of disease activity, treatment changes based on clinical judgement, and rationale. Treatment changes were then compared to the use of formal disease activity parameters in Minimal Disease Activity (MDA) and Disease Activity Index for Psoriatic Arthritis (DAPSA) composite measures. All associations were assessed using the chi-square test or the Mann–Whitney test, as appropriate. Results: The 117 PsA patient cohort consisted of 65.5% women, mean age 58.4 ± 13.6 years. Clinical judgement of treating rheumatologist concorded with MDA and DAPSA in 76 (65.5%) and 74 (64.9%) patients, respectively. Agreement between clinical judgement and composite measure criteria did not correlate with patient age, sex, alcohol/tobacco use, or treatment regimens chosen. Disagreement between physician assessment and MDA occurred in 40 (34.5%) cases: in 30 cases, the MDA status was overestimated due to disregard of patient reported outcomes (PRO), while underestimation of MDA status occurred in 25% of cases with treatment changes made in patients with a single active joint or enthesis. Underestimation of disease activity using DAPSA occurred in 22 cases and could be attributed to disregarding tender joint count, patient pain visual analogue scale and C-reactive protein level. Conclusion: In our cohort, agreement between clinical impression and formal composite measure utilization for implementation of T2T strategy occurred in 65% of patients. Discordance resulted from physicians' overlooking PRO and emphasizing objective findings when using clinical judgement alone.

Keywords: psoriatic arthritis; assessment; disease activity; composite disease activity measures; patient-reported outcomes

1. Introduction

In many areas of medicine, it has been shown that following a predefined treatment goal, termed the treat-to-target (T2T) approach, is more helpful in reducing complications and organ damage than treatment based on clinical judgement alone [1,2]. This approach was adopted in the management of rheumatic diseases [3–6].

Psoriatic arthritis (PsA) belongs to seronegative spondyloarthropathies, a group of rheumatic diseases that have common genetic associations and share certain clinical features aside from peripheral arthritis, such as spondylitis, enthesitis, dactylitis, uveitis,

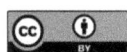

and inflammatory bowel disease. PsA is associated with significant morbidity due to progressive joint damage, reducing patients' health-related quality of life and functional capacity, compared to psoriasis patients or healthy controls [7,8]. Maintaining sustained minimal disease activity is of importance in PsA, as it is associated with low progression of radiologic joint damage over time [9].

The Group for Research and Assessment of Psoriasis and Psoriatic Arthritis (GRAPPA) published recommendations for PsA management with six overarching goals of therapy, including achievement of the lowest possible level of disease activity in all disease domains—arthritis, enthesitis, dactylitis, axial, skin, and nail involvement—in order to optimize functional status, prevent structural damage, and improve quality of life and well-being [10]. Given the multifaceted nature of PsA, it was noted that patients should be evaluated regularly and have treatment adjusted as needed in order to achieve these goals, with the current accepted main treatment target being remission or low disease activity to reduce inflammatory burden [11–14]. As no specific disease activity measure has been endorsed to date in the management of PsA, it is recommended to assess disease activity by using any one of the several disease activity measures addressing different domains of disease, including patient-reported outcomes (PRO) [11–13].

Currently, several valid composite measures exist for assessing disease activity in PsA [15], such as the PsA Disease Activity Score (PASDAS) [16,17], the Composite Disease Activity Index in PsA (CPDAI) [18], Minimal Disease Activity (MDA) [19–21], and the Disease Activity Index for Psoriatic Arthritis (DAPSA) score [22–24]. While these composite measures are being increasingly used in clinical research and observational studies [21,25–28], the relative concordance between their respective parameters and the parameters used by physicians in assessing disease activity in daily clinical practice is unknown.

The objective of our study was thus to assess the real-life implementation of the T2T concept in daily clinical practice using clinical impression vs. formal composite disease activity measure utilization, using MDA and DAPSA.

2. Methods

2.1. Study Population

PsA patients that fulfilled the Classificiation for Psoriatic Arthritis (CASPAR) criteria who were ≥ 18 years of age, who also agreed to participate in a longitudinal observational cohort study, were followed in a combined rheumatology–dermatology clinic at 6–12 month intervals, according to a standardized protocol that includes collection of clinical and laboratory data regarding patient demographics, self-reported formal disability status (i.e., receiving a living stipend from the Israeli National Social Security System due to formal recognition of disability from patient's rheumatologic illness), clinical data with emphasis on skin, joints, entheses, and dactylitis involvement as well as PRO, laboratory data including markers of inflammation, and medication use. Each enrolled patient's first clinic visit during 2016–2017 was included in this study. All patients were assessed by one of two rheumatologists (D.Z and A.H).

A third rheumatologist (M.A.H) was assigned to retrospectively review the clinic visit notes for all patient visits included in the cohort. Data extracted from each protocol visit note included patient demographics; alcohol and tobacco use; duration of PsA and psoriasis; and clinical manifestation, including 68 tender joint count (TJC), 66 swollen joint count (SJC), 16 enthesial and 20 dactylitis counts, skin involvement (Psoriasis Area and Severity Index, (PASI) or total body surface area (BSA)), patient PRO (patient visual analogue scale (VAS), patient global disease activity VAS (PtGA), and Health Assessment Questionnaire (HAQ)), C-reactive protein (CRP) levels, medication use, physician global assessment on a 0–10 numerical scale, and treatment changes and rationale recorded by the treating physician.

The evaluating rheumatologist (M.A.H) then calculated the MDA and DAPSA scores based on the data included in the clinic visit notes, reviewed treatment changes, and determined the concordance between clinical judgement and formal disease activity scores in assessing disease activity and need for treatment change.

MDA evaluated in this study is a valid composite disease activity measure representative of the multifaceted domains of psoriatic disease, including peripheral arthritis (tender and swollen joints) and enthesis and skin involvement. It also includes three categories of PRO: patient pain VAS, PtGA, and HAQ. MDA status is achieved when any five of the seven criteria are met, while patients are said to have very low disease activity, which could represent a state of remission, if all seven criteria are fulfilled [19]. Unlike MDA, which is a binary tool signifying active/inactive disease, the DAPSA, an additional valid composite disease activity measure used in this study, is a continuous measure of disease activity and has several cut-off values: remission (0–4), low (5–14), moderate (15–28), and high disease activity (>28). The DAPSA score includes peripheral arthritis involvement, CRP level, and two PRO categories (patient VAS and PtGA) [22–24].

In this study, proper implementation of T2T strategy for tight disease activity control was defined as the physician's alteration of treatment regimen based on clinical judgement whenever the physician noted that patients were not in low disease activity or remission, or the physician's recorded rationale for forgoing treatment alteration based on medication side effects, patient comorbidities, pregnancy, patient preferences, etc., in comparison with the formal use of MDA and DAPSA as validated composite measures as the target for disease management.

In our analysis, two cutoff values for the MDA score were used to analyze T2T adherence: MDA < 5 signifying active disease and MDA $\geq$ 5 signifying low disease activity or remission. For the purpose of T2T analysis using DAPSA, two different cutoff possibilities for the DAPSA score were evaluated—one in which remission and low disease activity levels were grouped together (DAPSA score $\leq$ 14) vs. moderate to high disease activity grouped together (DAPSA score > 14).

2.2. Statistical Analysis

Continuous data are presented as mean $\pm$ standard deviation (SD), while categorical variables are presented as numbers and percentages. The associations between proper T2T concept implementation and categorical and continuous variables were assessed by chi-square test or Mann–Whitney test, as appropriate. The association between physician's assessment at each clinic visit with each of the MDA or DAPSA parameters was evaluated using chi-square test or Fisher's exact test for small samples, as appropriate.

All data were analyzed using SPSS, version 24 (IBM SPSS Statistics for Windows, version 24.0, 2016, Armonk, NY, USA). All tests were two sided; p values of <0.05 were considered statistically significant.

All patients signed informed consent according to the declaration of Helsinki agreeing to participate in this PsA longitudinal cohort. The study was approved by the Institutional Review Board (IRB, also known as the Helsinki Committee) of Carmel Hospital (CMC 0044-11).

3. Results

3.1. Study Population Characteristics

A total of 117 consecutive patient visits of 117 different patients were evaluated; one patient visit was excluded from the analysis due to a lack of complete data in calculating MDA, and three patient visits were excluded from the analysis due to a lack of complete data in calculating DAPSA. The mean patient age was 58.4 $\pm$ 13.6 years, 74 (63.8%) of whom were women, with a mean age of 42.7 $\pm$ 13.0 years at PsA onset and 32.0 $\pm$ 16.3 years for psoriasis (Table 1). Most patients had at least one major comorbidity (84/116, 72.4%) chief among which was cardiovascular disease (63/116, 54.3%). A concurrent diagnosis of fibromyalgia syndrome (FMS) was present in 6/116 (5.2%) patients, and 16/116 (13.8%) had osteoarthritis (OA). Despite most patients having significant comorbidities, only 15/116 (12.9%) of patients self-reported formal recognition of disability status. Predominant PsA patterns were polyarthritis in 55/116 (47.0%), oligoarthritis in 36/116 (31.0%), axial involvement as a sole disease manifestation in 3/116 (2.6 %), dactylitis in 13/116 (11.2 %) and enthesitis in 64/116 (55.2%). The average PASI score was 2.0 ± 3.5. In none of the visits was a validated disease activity score used by the treating physician, and treatment changes were based on the physician's clinical impression of disease activity.

Table 1. Study population characteristics.

Parameter		T2T Implemented * N = 76	T2T Not Implemented * N = 40	Total N = 116	p Value
Age Mean (±SD)	Age at baseline	57.7 ± 12.5	59.9 ± 15.5	58.4 ± 13.6	NS
	Age at onset of PsO	31.0 ± 15.2	33.6 ± 18.4	32.0 ± 16.3	NS
	Age at diagnosis of PsO	34.0 ± 15.4	38.3 ± 17.3	35.5 ± 16.1	NS
	Age at PsA onset	42.2 ± 12.1	43.9 ± 14.2	42.7 ± 13.0	NS
	Age at diagnosis PsA	45.2 ± 12.1	47.1 ± 13.6	45.8 ± 12.8	NS
Sex	Female	47 / 61.80%	27 / 67.50%	74 / 63.80%	NS
Ethnicity	Jewish	70 / 92.10%	36 / 90%	106 / 91.40%	NS
	Arabs	4 / 5.30%	4 / 10.00%	8 / 6.90%	NS
Smoking	Ever	18 / 23.70%	6 / 15.00%	24 / 20.70%	NS
Alcohol use	Ever	27 / 35.50%	10 / 25.00%	37 / 31.90%	NS
Comorbidities	Overall	56 / 73.70%	28 / 70.00%	84 / 72.40%	NS
	Cardiovascular	44 / 57.90%	19 / 47.50%	63 / 54.30%	NS
	Hypertension	13 / 17.10%	7 / 17.50%	20 / 17.20%	NS
	Diabetes mellitus	13 / 17.10%	11 / 27.50%	24 / 20.70%	NS
	Hyperlipidemia	34 / 44.70%	13 / 30.20%	47 / 40.50%	NS
	Osteoarthritis	10 / 13.20%	6 / 15.00%	16 / 13.80%	NS
	Fibromyalgia	4 / 5.30%	2 / 5.00%	6 / 5.20%	NS

Table 1. Cont.

Parameter		T2T Implemented * N = 76	T2T Not Implemented * N = 40	Total N = 116	p Value
Clinical parameters No. patients, % (Mean ± SD)	Tender joints	42, 55.3%	22, 55.0%	64, 55.2%	NS
		(4.3 ± 6.9)	(2.9 ± 4.7)	(3.8 ± 6.6)	
	Swollen joints	44, 57.9%	30, 75.0%	74, 63.8%	NS
		(2.9 ± 4.7)	(1.4 ± 2.7)	(2.4 ± 4.2)	
	Dactylitis	9, 11.8%	4, 10.0%	13, 11.2%	NS
		(0.2 ± 0.6)	(0.1 ± 0.4)	(0.2 ± 0.5)	
	Enthesitis	40, 52.6%	24, 60%	64, 55.2%	NS
		(3.5 ± 5.4)	(3.1 ± 5.4)	(3.4 ± 5.4)	
	PASI	35, 46.1%	28, 70.0%	63, 54.3%	NS
		(2.4 ± 4.0)	(1.2 ± 2.1)	(2.0 ± 3.5)	
Assessment questionnaires	Patient pain VAS	21, 27.6%	11, 27.5%	32, 27.6%	NS
		(4.5, ± 3.1)	(4.4 ± 3.4)	(4.5 ± 3.2)	
	PtGA	25, 32.9%	13, 32.5%	38, 32.8%	NS
		(4.2 ± 2.7)	(4.5 ± 3.3)	(4.3 ± 3.1)	
	HAQ	30, 39.5%	17, 42.5%	47, 40.5%	NS
		(0.9 ± 0.8)	(0.8 ± 0.7)	(0.9 ± 0.7)	
Medications	Methotrexate	29	15	44	NS
		38.20%	37.50%	37.90%	
	Cyclosporine	1	1	2	NS
		1.30%	2.50%	1.70%	
	Sulfasalazine	5	0	5	NS
		6.60%	0.00%	4.30%	
	Hydroxychloroquine	0	0	0	-
		0.00%	0.00%	0.00%	
	Leflunomide	4	2	6	NS
		5.30%	5.00%	5.20%	
	Apremilast	10	3	13	NS
		13.20%	7.50%	11.20%	
	Golimumab	7	2	9	NS
		9.20%	5.00%	7.80%	
	Infliximab	3	1	4	NS
		3.90%	2.50%	3.40%	
	Adalimumab	10	8	18	NS
		13.20%	20.00%	15.50%	
	Etanercept	15	11	26	NS
		19.70%	27.50%	22.40%	
	Ustekinumab	5	3	8	NS
		6.60%	7.50%	6.90%	

Table 1. Cont.

Parameter	T2T Implemented * N = 76	T2T Not Implemented * N = 40	Total N = 116	p Value
Secukinumab	10 / 13.20%	7 / 17.50%	17 / 14.70%	NS
Corticosteroids	5 / 6.60%	1 / 2.50%	6 / 5.20%	NS
cDMARDs	38 / 50.00%	17 / 42.50%	55 / 47.40%	NS
bDMARDs	52 / 68.40%	33 / 82.50%	85 / 73.30%	NS

Abbreviations: b/c DMARDs = biologic/conventional disease-modifying anti-rheumatic drugs, HAQ = Health Assessment Questionnaire, N = number of patients, NS = not significant, PASI = Psoriasis Area and Severity Index, PsA = psoriatic arthritis, PsO = psoriasis, PtGA = Patient Global Assessment of Disease Activity, SD = standard deviation, T2T = Treat to Target, VAS = Visual Analogue Scale. * Treat to Target (T2T) implemented or not implemented based on comparison of clinical judgement to validated minimal disease activity (MDA) score.

3.2. T2T Implementation Using MDA and DAPSA Scores versus Clinical Judgement

After reviewing patient visit notes, the independent assessing rheumatologist concluded that agreement between implementation of T2T strategy using clinical judgement versus using MDA criteria occurred only in 76/116 (65.5%) cases, and was not affected by patient age, sex, alcohol or tobacco use, as well as the various treatment regimens ((conventional synthetic disease modifying anti-rheumatic drugs (csDMARD) versus biologic DMARD (bDMARD)) (Table 1). Physician assessment of disease activity did not correlate with the MDA score in assessment of 40 (34.5%) patients (Table 2). In 30/40 (75.0%) of cases, the patients' MDA status was overestimated, so patients were considered in MDA due to disregard of the PRO categories of the MDA score, including 29 patients reporting a high VAS pain score, 22 patients reporting a high PtGA, and 25 patients reporting a high HAQ score (Table 3). Conversely, patient achievement of MDA status was underestimated in 10/40 (25.0%) of cases in which treatment changes were made by the treating physician based on a single involved joint/enthesis, in discordance with the MDA composite measure criteria in which inflammation in a single joint/enthesis is still considered low disease activity/remission (Table 3). Similarly, the independent assessing rheumatologist concluded that concordance between implementation of T2T strategy using clinical judgement versus using DAPSA criteria occurred in 74/114 (64.9%) of patients (Table 2), with underestimation of disease activity on the part of the treating physician occurring in 22/40 (55.0%) patients due to the overlooking of subjective findings (tender joint count, and patient VAS) as well as the CRP level (Table 3). Overestimation of disease activity occurred in 18/40 cases with no specific component of the DAPSA composite measure being overlooked in this type of inaccurate physician impression in a statistically significant manner (Table 3).

Table 2. The degree of concordance between treatment decision. Based on clinical judgment to validated MDA and DAPSA scores.

	Physician Impression and Decision				
	No Active Disease No Treatment Changes	Active Disease Treatment Changed	Active Disease No Treatment Changes	Active Disease No Treatment Changes Due to Physician/Patient Decision (Noted in Chart)	Total Number of Patients
MDA < 5	30 56.6% Incorrect clinical decision (Underestimation)	40 83.3% Correct clinical decision	2 100.0% Incorrect clinical decision (Overestimation)	11 83.3% Correct clinical decision	83 71.3%
MDA ≥ 5 (Remission)	23 43.4% Correct clinical decision	8 16.7% Incorrect clinical decision (Overestimation)	0 0.0% Correct clinical decision	2 16.7% Correct clinical decision	33 28.7%
Total	53 100.0%	48 100.0%	2 100.0%	13 100.0%	116 100.0%
DAPSA > 14 (Active disease)	21 40.4% Incorrect clinical decision (Underestimation)	30 62.5% Correct clinical decision	1 50.0% Incorrect clinical decision (Underestimation)	10 83.3% Correct clinical decision	62 54.4%
DAPSA ≤ 14 (Low disease activity to Remission)	31 59.6% Correct clinical decision	18 37.5% Incorrect clinical decision (Overestimation)	1 50.0% Correct clinical decision	2 16.7% Correct clinical decision	52 45.6%
Total	52 100.0%	48 100.0%	2 100.0%	12 100.0%	114 100.0%

T2T implemented—blue; T2T not implemented—red; Abbreviations: MDA = Minimal Disease Activity; Abbreviations: DAPSA = Disease Activity Index for Psoriatic Arthritis.

Table 3. Factors influencing discordance between physician clinical impression and individual MDA and DAPSA score components.

	Underestimation * MDA < 5 30 Patients (%)	Overestimation # MDA ≥ 5 10 Patients (%)	p-Value	Overestimation # DAPSA ≤ 14 18 Patients (%)	Underestimation * DAPSA > 14 21 + 1 Patients (%)	p-Value
TJC	16 (53.3%)	2 (20.0%)	NS	0.6 ± 0.9	4.0 ± 7.4	0.03
SJC	8 (26.7%)	2 (20.0%)	NS	0.8 ± 1.0	1.5 ± 2.8	NS
PASI	8 (20.7%)	4 (40.0%)	NS	N/A	N/A	N/A
Tender entheseal points	15 (50.0%)	1 (10.0%)	0.03	N/A	N/A	N/A
Patient pain VAS	29 (96.7%)	0 (0.0%)	<0.0001	1.9 ± 32.0	7.1 ± 2.0	<0.0001
PtGA, n (%)	25 (83.3%)	2 (20.0%)	0.001	3 (16.7%)	7 (31.8%)	NS
HAQ	22 (73.3%)	1 (10.0%)	0.001	N/A	N/A	N/A
CRP	N/A	N/A	N/A	2.2 ± 2.7	5.2 ± 5.6	0.02

Abbreviations: CRP = C-reactive protein, DAPSA = Disease Activity Index for Psoriatic Arthritis, HAQ = Health Assessment Questionnaire, MDA = Minimal Disease Activity, N/A = not applicable, NS = non-significant, PASI = Psoriasis Area and Severity Index, PtGA = patient global assessment, SJC = Swollen Joint Count, TJC = Tender Joint Count, VAS = Visual Analogue Scale. For MDA assessment (a dichotomous, binary measurement), the following were taken into consideration: TJC > 1, SJC > 1, PASI > 1, Tender entheseal points > 1, Patient Pain VAS > 1.5, PtGA > 2, HAQ > 0.5. For DAPSA assessment (a continuous measurement), the following were taken into consideration: TJC, SJC, CRP, PtGA > 2, Patient pain VAS. * Underestimation = physician accidentally thought disease activity was lower than it really was; # Overestimation = physician accidentally thought disease activity was higher than it really was.

4. Discussion

In our study, we found that there is limited agreement between the formal use of composite disease activity measures and physician clinical impression of disease activity in the management of PsA. Tight T2T control using clinical judgement alone was implemented in actuality in about 65.0% of PsA patients when compared to using a validated disease activity measure (MDA or DAPSA).

In searching the literature, we found only a single study by van Mens et al. [29] that compared the use of MDA to clinical judgement in assessing disease activity in PsA in daily life. As in our study, the study by van Mens et al. incorporated an independent rheumatologist to evaluate whether the T2T approach was being implemented by providers, and was able to show that only about 35.0% (88/250) of PsA patients considered by the treating rheumatologist to have "acceptable disease state" actually fulfilled MDA status. Similar to results from our study, factors contributing to this discrepancy were the underestimation of the "subjective" components of the composite measures, such as tender joint count and patient pain and global disease activity scores. Additionally, our study also showed that the tendency to overemphasize "objective" clinical findings, such as the involvement of a single joint or enthesis, by treating physicians relative to PRO categories led to the underappreciation of MDA status when it was met in actuality. Similarly, we previously demonstrated this overemphasis on "objective" measures of disease activity in our study on T2T adherence in RA management [30].

The heterogeneity of PsA and lack of consensus on which validated disease activity measure to use have hampered agreement on the most appropriate target to use in the T2T strategy in PsA, ref. [31] leaving clinicians to individually choose which disease activity measure/s to follow in their attempt at T2T implementation in daily practice. As we and van Mens et al. were able to demonstrate in our respective studies, the lack of use of a pre-specified, simple and validated disease activity measure leaves physicians in daily clinical practice in the position of relying on "objective" disease activity measures which can be quantitatively measured, such as swollen joints or entheses, while overlooking "subjective" patient-reported components of disease activity. We surmise that this tendency to rely on "objective" disease activity measures that can be quantitatively measured while underestimating the significance of PRO categories in assessing disease activity likely stems from the desire by the treating physicians to avoid making changes in treatment regimens based on "subjective" disease activity measures, which may be distorted by the presence of co-existing conditions, such as osteoarthritis or fibromyalgia syndrome (FMS), noted in the literature to have high prevalence in PsA [32,33] and to affect PRO and composite disease activity scores, including MDA and DAPSA [33]. Moreover, compounding the difficulty in assessing disease activity in PsA is the lack of concordance between the clinician and PsA patient perspectives on the definition of low disease activity or remission, as recently shown by Gorlier et al. [34].

Barriers to proper T2T implementation in daily clinical practice may also stem from lack of time for complete clinical evaluation of multiple disease domains in PsA and lack of existence of a single, simple, universally accepted and reliable disease activity score capturing all disease domains of PsA. Indeed, a recent review on challenges in measuring PsA disease activity highlights the difficulty in evaluating 68 joints in PsA rather than 28 joints required by the Clinical Disease Activity Index (CDAI) score used in rheumatoid arthritis (RA) and the need to measure multiple domains for disease activity in PsA [35]. The issue of time constraints was recently highlighted in an online survey of 439 U.S. rheumatologists discussing barriers to implementation of T2T strategy in clinical practice, noting time constraints in daily practice (62.5%) and a sense of inefficiency of having to report metrics in electronic medical records (34.8%) [36]. This issue has even led to the recent suggestion to identify a 'target-to-treat' of a specific aspect or few aspects of disease most significant to each individual PsA patient as an alternative appropriate strategy rather than attempting to cover all disease domains [31].

Given the significant improvements in both PsA disease activity and patient-related outcomes in utilizing a tight T2T approach in the management of PsA as demonstrated by the TICOPA trial [27], there is significance in reaching a consensus on which validated disease activity measure to use in the management of PsA in daily practice.

Limitations of our study include the small number of assessing physicians from only one medical center. In addition, we did not capture axial involvement due to the focus on MDA and DAPSA composite measures, which lack assessment of axial involvement, although axial involvement may have prompted treatment changes. The strengths of our study lie in the relatively large number of consecutive PsA patient visits included in our analysis of real-life implementation of T2T strategy in PsA as evaluated against the use of two different practical composite measures.

5. Conclusions

In our cohort, the T2T concept, using a validated score as the target, was implemented properly in approximately 65.0% of PsA patients due to reliance on physicians' clinical impression of disease activity. The main obstacle we encountered in implementation of the T2T concept was in physicians overlooking the PRO components and over-emphasizing the "objective" components of the scores when using clinical judgement alone. In order to improve treatment outcomes in daily practice, efforts are needed to increase physician awareness regarding the significance of PRO categories of disease activity and the use of validated scores in assessing disease activity.

Key Points

1. The T2T concept is properly implemented in the management of about 65.0% of PsA patients when compared to the use of formal composite disease activity measures in daily clinical practice.
2. Discordance between clinical impression and actual disease activity level lies in physician reliance on "objective" components of disease activity, such as swollen joints and entheses, and disregard of more "subjective" aspects of disease activity assessment, such as PRO.
3. There is an unmet need for having a pre-specified, simple, practical, and valid disease activity score which may be used in the management of PsA patients in daily clinical practice.

Author Contributions: All authors listed on this manuscript contributed to its writing, editing, reviewed its contents and agree for it to be published as written. All authors have read and agreed to the published version of the manuscript.

Funding: No funding was provided for the research reported in this manuscript.

Institutional Review Board Statement: The study was approved by the Institutional Review Board (IRB) of Carmel Hospital CMC 0044-11. All patients signed an informed consent according to the declaration of Helsinki agreeing to participate in this PsA longitudinal cohort. No patient identifiable information is included in this manuscript.

Informed Consent Statement: No patient identifiable information is included in this manuscript.

Data Availability Statement: All data are available upon request.

Conflicts of Interest: The authors declare no conflict of interest.

References

1. Ridker, P.M.; Danielson, E.; Fonseca, F.A.; Genest, J.; Gotto, A.M.; Kastelein, J.J.; Koenig, W.; Libby, P.; Lorenzatti, A.J.; MacFadyen, J.G.; et al. Rosuvastatin to prevent vascular events in men and women with elevated C-reactive protein. *N. Engl. J. Med.* **2008**, *359*, 2195–2207. [CrossRef]
2. Mora, S.; Musunuru, K.; Blumenthal, R.S. The clinical utility of high-sensitivity C-reactive protein in cardiovascular disease and the potential implication of JUPITER on current practice guidelines. *Clin. Chem.* **2009**, *55*, 219–228. [CrossRef]

3. Smolen, J.S.; Breedveld, F.C.; Burmester, G.R.; Bykerk, V.P.; Dougados, M.; Emery, P.; Kvien, T.K.; Navarro-Compán, M.V.; Oliver, S.; Schoels, M.; et al. Treating rheumatoid arthritis to target: 2014 update of the recommendations of an international task force. *Ann Rheum Dis.* **2016**, *75*, 3–15. [CrossRef]
4. Smolen, J.S.; Braun, J.; Dougados, M.; Emery, P.; FitzGerald, O.; Helliwell, P.; Kavanaugh, A.; Kvien, T.K.; Landewé, R.; Luger, T.; et al. Treating spondyloarthritis, including ankylosing spondylitis and psoriatic arthritis, to target: Recommendations of an international task force. *Ann. Rheum. Dis.* **2014**, *73*, 6–16. [CrossRef]
5. Coates, L.C. Treating to target in psoriatic arthritis. *Curr. Opin. Rheumatol.* **2015**, *27*, 107–110. [CrossRef]
6. Dougados, M. Treat to target in axial spondyloarthritis: From its concept to its implementation. *J. Autoimmun.* **2020**, *110*, 102398. [CrossRef]
7. Gladman, D.D.; Antoni, C.; Mease, P.; Clegg, D.O.; Nash, P. Psoriatic arthritis: Epidemiology, clinical features, course, and outcome. *Ann Rheum Dis.* **2005**, *64* (Suppl. 2), ii14–ii17. [CrossRef]
8. Husted, J.A.; Gladman, D.D.; Farewell, V.T.; Long, J.A.; Cook, R.J. Validating the SF-36 health survey questionnaire in patients with psoriatic arthritis. *J. Rheumatol.* **1997**, *24*, 511–517. [PubMed]
9. Coates, L.C.; Helliwell, P.S. Validation of minimal disease activity criteria for psoriatic arthritis using interventional trial data. *Arthritis Care Res.* **2010**, *62*, 965–969. [CrossRef] [PubMed]
10. Coates, L.C.; Kavanaugh, A.; Mease, P.J.; Soriano, E.R.; Acosta-Felquer, M.L.; Armstrong, A.W.; Bautista-Molano, W.; Boehncke, W.-H.; Campbell, W.; Cauli, A.; et al. Group for research and assessment of psoriasis and psoriatic arthritis 2015 treatment recommendations for psoriatic arthritis. *Arthritis Rheumatol.* **2016**, *68*, 1060–1071. [CrossRef] [PubMed]
11. Smolen, J.S.; Schöls, M.; Braun, J.; Dougados, M.; FitzGerald, O.; Gladman, D.D.; Kavanaugh, A.; Landewé, R.; Mease, P.; Sieper, J.; et al. Treating axial spondyloarthritis and peripheral spondyloarthritis, especially psoriatic arthritis, to target: 2017 update of recommendations by an international task force. *Ann Rheum Dis.* **2018**, *77*, 3–17. [CrossRef] [PubMed]
12. Singh, J.A.; Guyatt, G.; Ogdie, A.; Gladman, D.D.; Deal, C.; Deodhar, A.; Dubreuil, M.; Dunham, J.; Husni, E.; Kenny, S.; et al. Special article: 2018 american college of rheumatology/national psoriasis foundation guideline for the treatment of psoriatic arthritis. *Arthritis Rheumatol.* **2019**, *71*, 5–32. [CrossRef] [PubMed]
13. Gossec, L.; Baraliakos, X.; Kerschbaumer, A.; de Wit, M.; McInnes, I.; Dougados, M.; Primdahl, J.; McGonagle, D.G.; Aletaha, D.; Balanescu, A.; et al. EULAR recommendations for the management of psoriatic arthritis with pharmacological therapies: 2019 update. *Ann Rheum Dis.* **2020**, *79*, 700–712. [CrossRef] [PubMed]
14. Mease, P.J.; Coates, L.C. Considerations for the definition of remission criteria in psoriatic arthritis. *Semin Arthritis Rheum.* **2018**, *47*, 786–796. [CrossRef] [PubMed]
15. Mease, P.J. Measures of psoriatic arthritis: Tender and Swollen Joint Assessment, Psoriasis Area and Severity Index (PASI), Nail Psoriasis Severity Index (NAPSI), Modified Nail Psoriasis Severity Index (mNAPSI), Mander/Newcastle Enthesitis Index (MEI), Leeds Enthesitis Index (LEI), Spondyloarthritis Research Consortium of Canada (SPARCC), Maastricht Ankylosing Spondylitis Enthesis Score (MASES), Leeds Dactylitis Index (LDI), Patient Global for Psoriatic Arthritis, Dermatology Life Quality Index (DLQI), Psoriatic Arthritis Quality of Life (PsAQOL), Functional Assessment of Chronic Illness Therapy-Fatigue (FACIT-F), Psoriatic Arthritis Response Criteria (PsARC), Psoriatic Arthritis Joint Activity Index (PsAJAI), Disease Activity in Psoriatic Arthritis (DAPSA), and Composite Psoriatic Disease Activity Index (CPDAI). *Arthritis Care Res.* **2011**, *63* (Suppl. S11), S64–S85.
16. Perruccio, A.V.; Got, M.; Li, S.; Ye, Y.; Gladman, D.D.; Chandran, V. Treating psoriatic arthritis to target: Defining the psoriatic arthritis disease activity score that reflects a state of minimal disease activity. *J. Rheumatol.* **2020**, *47*, 362–368. [CrossRef]
17. Mulder, M.L.M.; van Hal, T.W.; van den Hoogen, F.H.J.; de Jong, E.M.G.J.; Vriezekolk, J.E.; Wenink, M.H. Measuring disease activity in psoriatic arthritis: PASDAS implementation in a tightly monitored cohort reveals residual disease burden. *Rheumatology* **2021**, *60*, 3165–3175. [CrossRef]
18. Mumtaz, A.; Gallagher, P.; Kirby, B.; Waxman, R.; Coates, L.C.; J, D.V.; Helliwell, P.; Fitzgerald, O. Development of a preliminary composite disease activity index in psoriatic arthritis. *Ann. Rheum Dis.* **2011**, *70*, 272–277. [CrossRef]
19. Coates, L.C.; Fransen, J.; Helliwell, P.S. Defining minimal disease activity in psoriatic arthritis: A proposed objective target for treatment. *Ann. Rheum Dis.* **2010**, *69*, 48–53. [CrossRef]
20. Coates, L.C.; Helliwell, P.S. Treating to target in psoriatic arthritis: How to implement in clinical practice. *Ann Rheum Dis.* **2016**, *75*, 640–643. [CrossRef]
21. Gossec, L.; McGonagle, D.; Korotaeva, T.; Lubrano, E.; De Miguel, E.; Østergaard, M.; Behrens, F. Minimal disease activity as a treatment target in psoriatic arthritis: A review of the literature. *J. Rheumatol.* **2018**, *45*, 6–13. [CrossRef]
22. Smolen, J.S.; Schoels, M.; Aletaha, D. Disease activity and response assessment in psoriatic arthritis using the Disease Activity index for PSoriatic Arthritis (DAPSA). A brief review. *Clin. Exp. Rheumatol.* **2015**, *33* (Suppl. S93), S48–S50. [PubMed]
23. Schoels, M.M.; Aletaha, D.; Alasti, F.; Smolen, J.S. Disease activity in psoriatic arthritis (PsA): Defining remission and treatment success using the DAPSA score. *Ann. Rheum Dis.* **2016**, *75*, 811–818. [CrossRef]
24. Aletaha, D.; Alasti, F.; Smolen, J.S. Disease activity states of the DAPSA, a psoriatic arthritis specific instrument, are valid against functional status and structural progression. *Ann. Rheum Dis.* **2017**, *76*, 418–421. [CrossRef]
25. Perrotta, F.M.; Marchesoni, A.; Lubrano, E. Minimal Disease Activity and Remission in Psoriatic Arthritis Patients Treated with Anti-TNF-α Drugs. *J. Rheumatol.* **2016**, *43*, 350–355. [CrossRef] [PubMed]
26. Lubrano, E.; De Socio, A.; Perrotta, F.M. Comparison of Composite Indices Tailored for Psoriatic Arthritis Treated with csDMARD and bDMARD: A Cross-sectional Analysis of a Longitudinal Cohort. *J. Rheumatol.* **2017**, *44*, 1159–1164. [CrossRef]

27. Coates, L.C.; Moverley, A.R.; McParland, L.; Brown, S.; Navarro-Coy, N.; O'Dwyer, J.L.; Meads, D.M.; Emery, P.; Conaghan, P.G.; Helliwell, P.S. Effect of tight control of inflammation in early psoriatic arthritis (TICOPA): A UK multicentre, open-label, randomised controlled trial. *Lancet* **2015**, *386*, 2489–2498. [CrossRef]
28. Haddad, A.; Thavaneswaran, A.; Ruiz-Arruza, I.; Pellett, F.; Chandran, V.; Cook, R.J.; Gladman, D.D. Minimal disease activity and anti-tumor necrosis factor therapy in psoriatic arthritis. *Arthritis Care Res.* **2015**, *67*, 842–847. [CrossRef] [PubMed]
29. van Mens, L.J.J.; Turina, M.C.; van de Sande, M.G.H.; Nurmohamed, M.T.; van Kuijk, A.W.R.; Baeten, D.L.P. Residual disease activity in psoriatic arthritis: Discordance between the rheumatologist's opinion and minimal disease activity measurement. *Rheumatology* **2018**, *57*, 283–290. [CrossRef]
30. Gazitt, T.; Oren, S.; Reitblat, T.; Lidar, M.; Gurman, A.B.; Rosner, I.; Halabe, N.; Feld, J.; Kassem, S.; Lavi, I.; et al. Treat-to-target concept implementation for evaluating rheumatoid arthritis patients in daily practice. *Eur. J. Rheumatol.* **2019**, *6*, 136–141. [CrossRef] [PubMed]
31. Tucker, L.J.; Ye, W.; Coates, L.C. Novel concepts in psoriatic arthritis management: Can we treat to target? *Curr. Rheumatol. Rep.* **2018**, *20*, 71. [CrossRef] [PubMed]
32. Macchioni, P.; Salvarani, C.; Possemato, N.; Gutierrez, M.; Grassi, W.; Gasparini, S.; Perricone, C.; Perrotta, F.M.; Grembiale, R.D.; Bruno, C.; et al. Ultrasonographic and Clinical Assessment of Peripheral Enthesitis in Patients with Psoriatic Arthritis, Psoriasis, and Fibromyalgia Syndrome: The ULISSE Study. *J. Rheumatol.* **2019**, *46*, 904–911. [CrossRef] [PubMed]
33. Brikman, S.; Furer, V.; Wollman, J.; Borok, S.; Matz, H.; Polachek, A.; Elalouf, O.; Sharabi, A.; Kaufman, I.; Paran, D.; et al. The Effect of the Presence of Fibromyalgia on Common Clinical Disease Activity Indices in Patients with Psoriatic Arthritis: A Cross-sectional Study. *J. Rheumatol.* **2016**, *43*, 1749–1754. [CrossRef]
34. Gorlier, C.; Orbai, A.-M.; Puyraimond-Zemmour, D.; Coates, L.C.; Kiltz, U.; Leung, Y.Y.; Palominos, P.; Cañete, J.D.; Scrivo, R.; Balanescu, A.; et al. Comparing patient-perceived and physician-perceived remission and low disease activity in psoriatic arthritis: An analysis of 410 patients from 14 countries. *Ann. Rheum Dis.* **2019**, *78*, 201–208. [CrossRef] [PubMed]
35. Tucker, L.J.; Coates, L.C.; Helliwell, P.S. Assessing disease activity in psoriatic arthritis: A literature review. *Rheumatol Ther.* **2019**, *6*, 23–32. [CrossRef]
36. Curtis, J.R.; Chen, L.; Danila, M.I.; Saag, K.G.; Parham, K.L.; Cush, J.J. Routine Use of Quantitative Disease Activity Measurements among US Rheumatologists: Implications for Treat-to-target Management Strategies in Rheumatoid Arthritis. *J. Rheumatol.* **2018**, *45*, 40–44. [CrossRef]

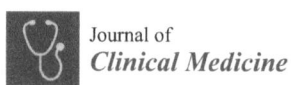

Article

Comparison of Treatment Goals between Users of Biological and Non-Biological Therapies for Treatment of Psoriasis in Japan

Yukari Okubo [1], Ann Chuo Tang [2,*], Sachie Inoue [3], Hitoe Torisu-Itakura [4] and Mamitaro Ohtsuki [5]

1. Department of Dermatology, Tokyo Medical University, 6-1-1 Shinjuku, Shinjuku-ku, Tokyo 160-8402, Japan; yukari-o@tokyo-med.ac.jp
2. Eli Lilly Japan K.K., Akasaka Garden City 13F, 4-15-1 Akasaka, Minato-ku, Tokyo 107-0052, Japan
3. Crecon Medical Assessment Inc., 2-12-15 Shibuya, Shibuya-ku, Tokyo 150-0002, Japan; inoue@crecon.co.jp
4. Eli Lilly Japan K.K., Lilly Plaza One Bldg., 5-1-28, Isogamidori, Chuo-ku, Kobe 651-0086, Japan; itakura_hitoe@lilly.com
5. Department of Dermatology, Jichi Medical University, 3311-1 Yakushiji, Shimotsuke 329-0498, Tochigi-ken, Japan; mamitaro@jichi.ac.jp
* Correspondence: tang_ann_chuo@lilly.com

Abstract: Background: Previously, our cross-sectional observational study in Japan revealed high (68%) discordance within treatment goals between psoriasis patients and their physicians. Objective: This secondary analysis aimed to determine whether patient and physician users of biologics have higher treatment goals than users of non-biologics. Methods: A survey for both patients and physicians on background characteristics, disease severity, treatment goals, treatment satisfaction, and health-related quality of life was conducted at 54 sites. Association between treatment goals and biologic/non-biologic users was assessed using ordinal logistic regression models. Results: In total, 449 patient-physician pairs agreed to participate; 425 completed the survey and were analyzed. More biologic users than non-biologic users reported complete clearance (Psoriasis Area and Severity Index 100) as a treatment goal (patient-reported: 23.6% vs. 16.1%; physician-reported: 26.9% vs. 2.2%). Biologic users were significantly associated with higher treatment goals than non-biologic users (patient-reported: 1.8 (1.15–2.87) (odds ratio (9 5% CI)), $p = 0.01$; physician-reported: 11.0 (5.72–21.01), $p < 0.01$). Among biologic users, higher treatment goals were associated with higher treatment satisfaction (patient- and physician-rated); lower treatment goals were associated with back lesions and increasing patient age (patient-rated) and higher disease severity (physician-rated). Conclusion: Use of biologics among patients with psoriasis was associated with higher treatment goals. Further use of biologics contributed to treatment satisfaction. Appropriate treatment goals that are shared among patients and their physicians may improve treatment outcomes.

Keywords: cross-sectional studies; health care surveys; Japan; psoriasis; biologics; treatment goal

Citation: Okubo, Y.; Tang, A.C.; Inoue, S.; Torisu-Itakura, H.; Ohtsuki, M. Comparison of Treatment Goals between Users of Biological and Non-Biological Therapies for Treatment of Psoriasis in Japan. *J. Clin. Med.* **2021**, *10*, 5732. https://doi.org/10.3390/jcm10245732

Academic Editors: Mayumi Komine and Francesco Lacarrubba

Received: 12 November 2021
Accepted: 29 November 2021
Published: 7 December 2021

Publisher's Note: MDPI stays neutral with regard to jurisdictional claims in published maps and institutional affiliations.

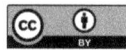

Copyright: © 2021 by the authors. Licensee MDPI, Basel, Switzerland. This article is an open access article distributed under the terms and conditions of the Creative Commons Attribution (CC BY) license (https://creativecommons.org/licenses/by/4.0/).

1. Introduction

Psoriasis is an immune-mediated skin condition that commonly manifests as inflamed, scaly skin lesions [1,2]. Severe symptoms associated with psoriasis are a major contributor to patients' health-related quality of life (HRQOL) [3–6]. Biological therapies have emerged as an effective class of treatment for patients with psoriasis that have a significant effect on disease severity [7,8] and are associated with higher levels of treatment satisfaction compared with other therapies [7]. In Japan, the use of biologics is recommended for patients with poor Health Related Quality of Life, HRQOL (Dermatology Life Quality Index (DLQI) score ≥ 10) [9].

Establishment of treatment goals for patients with psoriasis is considered critical for setting treatment expectations and improving management practices [10]. However, the treatment goals currently recommended in treatment guidelines for psoriasis focus on clinical measures of disease severity and do not take into account other factors such as treatment satisfaction and HRQOL [10,11]. Treatment goals that are aligned between patients and their physicians have the potential to improve treatment outcomes, adherence, and satisfaction [12,13]. Despite this, treatment goals for psoriasis appear to vary widely between patients and their physicians [13,14].

Recently, we conducted a nationwide, cross-sectional observational study in Japan to assess the alignment of treatment goals between patients with psoriasis and their physicians [14]. There was a high level (68%) of discordance of treatment goals between the patient-physician pairs. Factors that contributed most to the discordance were high expectations by patients for complete clearance, and physicians' perceptions that patients had a low understanding of their treatment options. In addition, we found that more patients in the misaligned group than in the aligned group had not received a prescription for a biologic within the past 2 to 3 weeks (78.3% vs. 66.2%, $p = 0.008$), suggesting that patient and physician biologic users are more aligned in their treatment goals.

For this secondary analysis, we hypothesized that patient and physician users of biologics have higher treatment goals than non-biologic users. To test this hypothesis, we examined the associations between treatment goals among paired patients and physicians who used biological therapies to treat psoriasis versus those who did not.

2. Materials and Methods

2.1. Study Design

This nationwide, multicenter, cross-sectional observational study was conducted between October 2015 and May 2016 at 54 sites in Japan [14]. The sites included general practitioners, clinics, university hospitals, and private and public hospitals. The study protocol was reviewed and approved by the Ethics Committee of Jichi Medical University, the Central Institutional Review Board of Medical Corporation Ganka-Koseikai, and the relevant local institution ethics committees of each participating hospital. The study protocol was implemented in accordance with the Declaration of Helsinki (2013), the Guidelines for Good Pharmacoepidemiology Practices (2015), the Ethical Guidelines Concerning Medical Studies in Human Subjects in Japan [15], and ethical principles based on the relevant statutes/standards in Japan.

All treatment decisions and clinical assessments were made at the discretion of the treating physicians. Patients who participated in the study gave written informed consent for the collection and use of their information to be included in this study. Informed consent was obtained from patients after physicians had explained the study protocol to the recruited patients. Only patients who gave their informed consent were given the surveys.

2.2. Study Population

Study participants were patients with physician-reported moderate-to-severe psoriasis and a history of systemic treatments, including biological drugs, and their treating physicians. Dermatologists with experience in oral or biological treatments for psoriasis patients were included. Patients were not included in the study if they were participating in a clinical trial, had completed a clinical trial less than 6 months before the current study, or had pustular psoriasis, erythrodermic psoriasis, or psoriatic arthritis.

2.3. Study Survey

As previously reported [14], the survey comprised 52 questions for patients and 31 questions for physicians. The questions were categorized into background characteristics of patients and physicians, disease severity (Patient Global Assessment (PtGA), Physician Global Assessment (PGA)), treatment goals (same question for both patients and physicians), and treatment satisfaction and HRQOL. Measures used for treatment satisfaction and HRQOL included the Treatment Satisfaction Questionnaire for Medication (TSQM) [16], the Treatment Satisfaction scale (numerical rating scale 0 to 10), the DLQI [17], and the Itch Numeric Rating Scale (Itch NRS) [18]. A DLQI score ≥ 10 was considered as one of the measures for moderate-to-severe psoriasis [19,20]. Treatment goals were categorized from 1 (highest goal) to 7 (lowest goal) where 1 = complete clearance (Psoriasis Area and Severity Index (PASI) 100) [21], 2 = almost complete clearance (PASI 90 to <100), 3 = complete clearance at specific sites (nails, head, genitals, other), 4 = improvement from previous treatment but without complete or almost complete clearance, 5 = relief from itchiness, 6 = other goals, and 7 = no particular goal set.

The ordinal scale for understanding of disease and treatment choice ranged from not at all, to does not understand very well, neither, somewhat understands, understands very well.

Patients who qualified for inclusion were recruited into the study by their physicians. Patients were sent a paper-based survey within 2 weeks of enrollment and returned the surveys by mail. Each patient and their treating physician completed the surveys independently. To minimize the potential for selection bias by physicians, patients were enrolled consecutively.

2.4. Statistical Analysis

Variables for each patient-physician pair were grouped into users of biological therapies (biologic users) and those who did not use biological therapies (non-biologic users), and were examined for associations with treatment goals. Biologic users were defined as patients (and their paired physicians) who were currently using a biological drug for treatment of psoriasis or who had used a biological drug within 3 weeks of completing the survey. Analyses comprised the following: Step 1, variables selected from the survey were categorized into biologic user and non-biologic user groups and were evaluated for differences. Categorical variables were evaluated using the chi-square test; continuous variables were evaluated using the Wilcoxon rank-sum test or Student's t test. Step 2, variables selected from the survey were evaluated by ordinal logistic regression to evaluate any correlations with treatment goals. Step 3, variables that were statistically significant ($p < 0.05$) in Steps 1 and Steps 2 were included as covariates. Step 4, of the variables identified in Step 3, only one variable was selected for the same survey question and included in the final covariates for the further analyses. A clinician was asked to review the variables and select one variable that made the most clinical sense. The reasons for setting this rule were: (1) to avoid too many covariates in a stepwise multivariate model; and (2) to avoid including multiple answers from the same question in the multivariate analyses which would be difficult to interpret.

The ordinal logistic regression models assessed the association between treatment goals (outcome variable) and biologic users and non-biologic users (explanatory variables), and were adjusted for covariates. Associations between treatment goals and use of biological therapies were reported as odds ratios (OR) and 95% CIs. Differences between groups were regarded as statistically significant for $p < 0.05$.

All statistical analyses were performed using SAS® Version 9.4 (SAS Institute Inc., Cary, NC, USA).

3. Results

3.1. Variable Selection

The variables used in the patient-reported analyses included lesion site—symptom on "back" (yes/no), TSQM score (ordinal scale), and DLQI scores (ordinal scale) for daily activities, leisure, and personal relationships. The variables included in the physician-reported analyses included lesion site—symptom on "upper limb" (yes/no), physician's specialty—psoriasis (yes/no), physician's workplace (categorical scale), physician's experience with biologics (ordinal scale), physician's perspective on the patient's understanding of their disease (ordinal scale) and treatment choice (ordinal scale), PGA disease severity (0 to 5 scale), and Treatment Satisfaction (0 to 10 scale). Patient age was included in both patient- and physician-reported models because of its clinical importance. Physicians and patients with missing data for treatment goal or who responded that the treatment goal was "other" or "no setting" were excluded from these analyses. Physicians and patients with missing data for the selected covariates were excluded.

3.2. Study Population

Of the 449 patient-physician pairs that agreed to participate in the study, 425 (94.7% response rate) completed the survey and were analyzed. Of the included patients, most were male and had a reasonably long disease duration (mean, 18.8 years) (Table 1). For most patients, psoriasis predominantly affected the head, neck, and lower limbs, and most had at least 3% of their body surface area (BSA) affected (Table 1). Most patients were currently being treated with topical medication, and 25.6% of patients were being treated with biologics at the time the survey was conducted. Of the included physicians, most had considerable experience treating patients with psoriasis; 69.6% specialized in psoriasis, 86.8% had 10 or more years' experience treating patients with psoriasis, and 75.0% saw 20 or more patients per month (Table 2). Treatment Satisfaction and assessment of disease severity (PtGA, PGA) were similar between patients and physicians (Tables 1 and 2).

Table 1. Patient characteristics.

Variable	Value (n = 414) [5]
Male, %	74.9%
Age (range), y	56.2 ± 13.9 (20.0–93.0)
BMI (range), kg/m^2	24.3 ± 4.6 (16.0–54.9)
Age at disease onset (range), y	37.2 ± 16.2 (0.0–81.0)
Age at disease diagnosis (range), y	40.0 ± 16.2 (4.0–81.0)
Disease duration from onset (range), y	18.8 ± 11.7 (0.0–65.0)
Body part affected (top 3 nominated)	
Lower limbs	78.0%
Head	70.8%
Back	67.1%
Body surface area affected [1]	
<1%	24.4%
1–2%	22.0%
3–10%	37.0%
>10%	16.5%
Current treatment received [2]	
Topical	82.4%
Oral	53.6%
Ultraviolet light	19.1%
Biologic	25.6%
Other	1.4%
Treatment Satisfaction [3]	6.75 ± 2.27
PtGA disease severity [4]	2.54 ± 1.26

[1] Palm size is equivalent to 1%; [2] multiple answers were allowed; [3] 0 = lowest treatment satisfaction, 10 = highest treatment satisfaction; [4] 0 = lowest, 5 = highest severity, all values are mean ± standard deviation unless otherwise indicated. BMI, body mass index; PtGA, Patient Global Assessment; y, year. [5] Out of the total sample (n = 425), 9 pairs were excluded where patient treatment goal information was missing and 2 pairs were excluded where physician treatment goal information was missing.

Table 2. Physician characteristics.

Variable	Value [5] (n = 70)
Male, %	64.3%
Age (range), y	50.6 ± 11.7 (30.0–80.0)
Specialty [1]	
Psoriasis	69.6%
Allergy	40.6%
Other	41.8%

Table 2. Cont.

Variable	Value [5] (n = 70)
Treatment experience with psoriasis [2]	
<2 y	0.0%
2 ≤ 4 y	2.9%
4 ≤ 6 y	5.9%
6 ≤ 8 y	4.4%
8 ≤ 10 y	0.0%
≥10 y	86.8%
Number of patients seen per month [2]	
<5	1.5%
5–9	5.9%
10–14	10.3%
15–19	7.4%
≥20	75.0%
Treatment Satisfaction [3]	6.46 ± 2.08
PGA disease severity [4]	2.51 ± 1.15

[1] Multiple answers were allowed; [2] physician responses with obvious errors and inconsistencies were excluded from the analyses; [3] 0 = lowest treatment satisfaction, 10 = highest treatment satisfaction; [4] 0 = lowest severity, 5 = highest severity. [5] The total number of physicians (n = 70) paired to 425 patients. All values are mean ± standard deviation (range) unless otherwise indicated. PGA, Physician Global Assessment; y, year.

Results by Biologic vs. Non-Biologic Users

When patients and their paired treatment physicians were compared by biologic versus non-biologic users, we found the following results. There were statistically significant differences between biologic users and non-biologic users for both patient-reported and physician-reported characteristics (Table 3). Biologic users had significantly higher treatment satisfaction based on TSQM (global satisfaction score; 68.6 vs. 57.3, p < 0.001) and significantly higher HRQOL scores (lower DLQI scores) than non-biologic users (Table 3). Physicians treating biologic users had significantly greater Treatment Satisfaction (7.8 vs. 6.0, p < 0.001) and significantly lower physician-rated disease severity (PGA disease severity 2.0 vs. 2.7, p < 0.001) (Table 3). Significantly more physician biologic users were psoriasis specialists, who worked in university hospital settings and had more years' experience than non-biologic user physicians.

Table 3. Comparison of patient- and physician-reported characteristics between biologic users and non-biologic users.

Characteristic [1]	Biologic Users	Non-Biologic Users	p [2]
Patient-reported	n [1] = 104	n [1] = 292	
Patient age, y	56.3 ± 15.1	55.9 ± 13.4	0.807
Lesion site, back, n (%)	54 (51.9)	211 (72.3)	<0.001
TSQM score (global satisfaction)	68.6 ± 19.6	57.3 ± 17.1	<0.001
DLQI			
DLQI total score	3.2 ± 5.0	5.0 ± 5.3	<0.001
Daily activities	0.5 ± 1.3	1.0 ± 1.5	<0.001
Leisure	0.5 ± 1.1	0.7 ± 1.3	0.044
Personal relationships	0.2 ± 0.9	0.4 ± 1.1	0.028
Physician-reported	n [2] = 107	n [2] = 309	
Patient age, y	56.9 ± 15.2	56.4 ± 13.8	0.709
Location of lesion (upper limb), n (%)	42 (39.3)	229 (74.1)	<0.001
Physician's specialty—psoriasis, n (%)	99 (92.5)	231 (75)	<0.001
Physician's workplace, n (%)			<0.001
Clinic	35 (32.7)	202 (65.4)	
University hospital	47 (43.9)	81 (26.2)	
Other	25 (23.4)	26 (8.4)	

Table 3. Cont.

Characteristic [1]	Biologic Users	Non-Biologic Users	p [2]
Physician's experience—biologics, n (%)			<0.001
None	0 (0.0)	77 (24.9)	
<1 y	0 (0.0)	10 (3.2)	
1 ≤ 2 y	9 (8.4)	25 (8.1)	
2 ≤ 3 y	4 (3.7)	14 (4.5)	
3 ≤ 4 y	13 (12.2)	19 (6.2)	
4 ≤ 5 y	35 (32.7)	58 (18.8)	
>5 y	46 (43)	106 (34.3)	
Physician's perspective on patient's understanding of disease, n (%)			0.001
Understands very well	42 (39.3)	64 (20.7)	
Somewhat understands	55 (51.4)	215 (69.6)	
Neither	7 (6.5)	27 (8.7)	
Does not understand very well	3 (2.8)	3 (1.0)	
Does not understand at all	0 (0.0)	0 (0.0)	
Physician's perspective on patient's understanding of treatment choice, n (%)			<0.001
Understands very well	45 (42.1)	69 (22.3)	
Somewhat understands	49 (45.8)	209 (67.6)	
Neither	10 (9.4)	27 (8.7)	
Does not understand very well	3 (2.8)	4 (1.3)	
Does not understand at all	0 (0.0)	0 (0.0)	
PGA disease severity	2.0 ± 1.5	2.7 ± 1.0	<0.001
Treatment Satisfaction (0–10 scale)	7.8 ± 1.7	6.0 ± 2.0	<0.001

[1] From the total 425, the number of biologic and non-biologic user pairs that remained in patient-reported analyses was $n = 396$. (The following were excluded: 9 pairs with missing patient treatment goal information, 20 pairs with patients who reported treatment goal as "other" or "no setting"). [2] From the total 425, the number of biologic and non-biologic user pairs in physician-reported analyses was $n = 416$. (The following were excluded: 2 pairs with missing information on treatment goal and 7 pairs who reported that the treatment goal was "other" or "no setting"). Categorical variables were compared using the chi-square test and continuous variables were compared using the t test or Wilcoxon rank-sum test. Data are mean (standard deviation) unless otherwise indicated. DLQI, Dermatology Life Quality Index; PGA, Physician Global Assessment; TSQM, Treatment Satisfaction Questionnaire for Medication; y, years.

Biologic users contributed to a small proportion (13.8%, 8/58) of the total number of patients with DLQI score ≥ 10 (one of the criteria for "moderate-to-severe" psoriasis). For patients with a DLQI score ≥ 10, non-biologic users had more severe disease (3.18 vs. 2.25, PGA disease severity) and lower treatment satisfaction (4.50 vs. 5.88, patient treatment satisfaction) than biologic users. For physicians of patients with a DLQI score ≥ 10, non-biologic users had less experience with biologics than biologic users (36% vs. 12.5% of physicians with ≤2 years of experience).

3.3. Treatment Goals by Biologic vs. Non-Biologic Users

Most patients and physicians reported that their treatment goals were to achieve almost complete clearance, irrespective of whether or not they were biologic users (Figure 1). However, patient and physician biologic users had higher treatment goals than non-biologic users (Figure 1). The percentage of patients reporting complete clearance (PASI 100) as a treatment goal was 23.6% for biologic users and 16.1% for non-biologic users. The percentage of physicians reporting complete clearance (PASI 100) as a treatment goal was 26.9% for biologic users and 2.2% for non-biologic users.

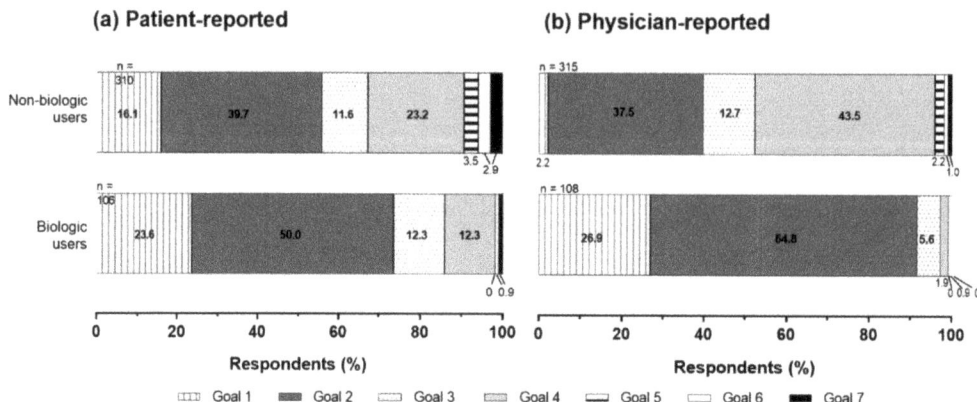

Figure 1. Patient- and physician-reported treatment goals. Goal 1 = complete clearance (Psoriasis Area and Severity Index (PASI) 100) [21], Goal 2 = almost complete clearance (PASI 90 to <100), Goal 3 = complete clearance at specific sites (nails, head, genitals, other), Goal 4 = improvement from previous treatment, but without "complete" or "almost complete clearance", Goal 5 = relief from itchiness, Goal 6 = other goals, and Goal 7 = no particular goal set. (**a**) A larger number of patient (23.6% vs. 16.1%) and (**b**) physician (26.0% vs. 2.2%) among biologic users had higher treatment goals of achieving complete clearance.

3.4. Factors Associated with Treatment Goals by Biologic vs. Non-Biologic Users

Findings from the ordinal analyses showed that patient and physician biologic users were significantly associated with higher treatment goals than their non-biologic user counterparts (Table 4). For patient-reported analyses, biologic users had 1.8-fold higher odds of having higher treatment goals than non-biologic users (OR 1.820 (95% CI 1.154, 2.868), $p = 0.01$). Higher treatment goals were significantly associated with higher patient-rated TSQM scores (global satisfaction) (Table 4). In contrast, lower treatment goals were significantly associated with the presence of back lesions and increasing patient age (Table 4).

For the physician-reported analyses, biologic users had 11.0-fold higher odds of having higher treatment goals than non-biologic users (OR 10.967 (95% CI 5.723, 21.014), $p < 0.001$). Higher treatment goals among biologic users were significantly associated with higher physician-rated Treatment Satisfaction, whereas lower treatment goals were associated with higher PGA disease severity (Table 4).

Table 4. Regression analysis of factors associated with treatment goals.

Variables [1,2]	Odds Ratio (95% CI)	p
Patient-reported variables v [3]	$n = 383$	
Biologic vs. non-biologic	1.820 (1.154, 2.868)	0.010
Age, y	0.983 (0.970, 0.997)	0.016
Lesion site, back	0.544 (0.358, 0.825)	0.004
TSQM score (global satisfaction)	1.014 (1.002, 1.026)	0.021
DLQI score		
Daily activities	1.106 (0.900, 1.360)	0.336
Leisure	1.132 (0.886, 1.446)	0.321
Personal relationships	1.085 (0.858, 1.373)	0.497

Table 4. *Cont.*

Variables [1,2]	Odds Ratio (95% CI)	p
Physician-reported variables [4]	n = 413	
Biologic vs. non-biologic user	10.967 (5.723, 21.014)	<0.001
Patient age, y	1.003 (0.989, 1.017)	0.664
Location of lesion (upper limb)	0.870 (0.549, 1.377)	0.552
Physician's specialty—psoriasis	1.042 (0.602, 1.803)	0.884
Physician's workplace		
University hospital	0.696 (0.429, 1.128)	0.141
Other	0.663 (0.342, 1.284)	0.223
Physician's experience—biologics	1.096 (0.991, 1.212)	0.073
Patient's understanding of disease (physician perspective)	1.390 (0.839, 2.303)	0.202
Patient's understanding of treatment choice (physician perspective)	0.631 (0.386, 1.032)	0.067
PGA disease severity	0.720 (0.584, 0.887)	0.002
Treatment Satisfaction	1.285 (1.139, 1.449)	<0.001

[1] From the n = 396 of Table 3, 383 remained in the analyses (13 pairs that had missing covariate information were excluded). [2] From the n = 416 of Table 3, 413 remained in the analyses (3 pairs that had missing covariate information were excluded). [3] p values for differences in treatment goals between biologic and non-biologic users were calculated using an ordinal logistic regression model adjusted for age (y), lesion site—back (yes/no), TSQM score (ordinal scale), and DLQI scores (ordinal scale). [4] p values for differences in treatment goals between biologic and non-biologic users were calculated using an ordinal logistic regression model adjusted for age (y), lesion site—upper limb (yes/no), Physician's specialty—psoriasis (yes/no), Physician's workplace (yes/no), Physician's experience with biologics (ordinal scale), Physician's perspective of patient's understanding of disease (ordinal scale) and treatment choice (ordinal scale), Physician GA severity (0–5 scale), and Treatment Satisfaction (0–10 scale). DLQI, Dermatology Life Quality Index; PGA, Physician Global Assessment; TSQM, Treatment Satisfaction Questionnaire for Medication; y, years.

4. Discussion

In our previous primary analysis, which focused on treatment goal alignment and showed that there is a high level of discordance between Japanese patients with psoriasis and their physicians, we showed that patients tended to set higher treatment goals than their physicians and had a greater desire for "complete clearance", irrespective of treatment received [14]. We also found that there was more treatment goal misalignment (n = 220, 78.3%) than alignment (n = 88, 66.2%) among non-biological users (i.e., patients who had not had a prescription for a biological drug within the previous 2 to 3 weeks) (p = 0.008) [14]. Hence, we extend these findings to show the characteristics of biologic users and non-biologic users and to examine the treatment goals for both patient and physician biologic users versus non-biologic users, adjusted for other factors. In this subgroup analysis of biologic users versus non-biologic users, complete clearance (PASI 100) was reported as a treatment goal for 23.6% and 26.9% of patient and physician biologic users, respectively, compared with 16.1% and 2.2% of patient and physician non-biologic users, respectively. Both patients and physicians who were biologic users set higher treatment goals than non-biologic users. The results of these secondary analyses may explain the difference in treatment goal alignment and misalignment among recent non-biologic users found in the previous primary analysis. Since the introduction of biologics for treating psoriasis, clinicians' expectations for a successful treatment outcome with biological therapies have increased to "complete" or "almost complete clearance" (PASI > 90) [13]. In addition, patients treated with biologics have greater success achieving their treatment goals [22] and have higher treatment satisfaction compared with other therapies [7,23]. Therefore, given the experience of patients and physicians with biologics, it is likely that both patients and their physicians have higher expectations for treatment success with biologics than with non-biologics.

In our study, there was a larger percentage of male than female patients with psoriasis. In Japan, the higher percentage of males is consistent with the real-world report [1,2,24]. As for how our sample has an even higher percentage of males, it is not known. Although physicians assess the severity of psoriasis based on symptoms and the body area affected, patients can be more focused on the effects of psoriasis on their HRQOL [10,11,25]. Our findings are consistent with this focus on HRQOL in that treatment goals were associated with disease severity and treatment satisfaction for both patient and physician biologic users. At the time this survey was conducted, both patient- and physician-rated disease severity (PtGA, PGA) was lower and treatment satisfaction was higher among biologic users than non-biologic users. This suggests that as disease severity decreases with the use of biologics, treatment satisfaction increases and the clinical improvement experienced by patients translates to greater patient HRQOL.

In the current study, we found that patient biologic users contributed a small proportion (13.8%) of the total number of patients with DLQI scores ≥ 10, a criterion to be recommended for biological therapies in Japan [9]. Many patients who used non-biologics in our study had high DLQI scores ≥ 10 and tended to be less satisfied with their treatment than biologic users. In addition, their physicians tended to have less experience with biologics. Together, these data suggest a large number of patients with psoriasis may be undertreated in Japan, despite being eligible for biological therapy.

In the additional analysis in this study focusing on treatment satisfaction misalignment between patient and physician, we reported that "not changing the treatment goal from start of treatment" was a factor in a patient's treatment satisfaction being higher than that evaluated by the physician [26]. Hence, the importance of the treatment goal leading to satisfactory treatment outcomes would need to be discussed and emphasized.

As this was a nationwide, multicenter, cross-sectional study conducted in real-world clinical practice, the findings are representative of general Japanese patients and their treating physicians. However, there are a few limitations worthy of mention. First, the interpretation of the findings should take into account the cross-sectional design of the study, which limits the strength of any observed associations, the potential for selection bias arising from consecutive enrollment of patients. In a cross-sectional setting, we cannot make an inference on the causal-effect relationships between outcomes of disease state versus setting a high goal and biologics usage. The patient disease state at the time of the survey could have been a result of prior medical interventions. Second, along with setting PASI scores as the treatment goal target, PASI scores would need further validation as a clinically meaningful treatment goal in the future. Although both physicians and patients may consider biologics to have a higher chance of achieving complete or almost complete response, this perspective could be more dominant among physicians. Patients may simply consider the results satisfactory, even being far from complete clearance. Third, as this was a secondary analysis that focused on a comparison between biologic users and non-biologic users, the sample size for some comparisons may not have been sufficiently powered to detect differences between groups. Fourth, since our sample is derived from the Japanese population within the Japanese health care setting, the study should take into consideration that biologics prescribers in Japan are limited to only hospitals or clinics accredited by the Medical Society. Therefore, although patients and their physicians may have higher treatment goals, some prescribers are limited in the use of biologics by this unique Japanese guideline unless there is a solid referral system. In this study, our analysis was to compare "biologic users versus non-biologic users", and not "biologic accredited versus non-accredited institutions". We recognized this Japanese health care situation. Therefore, without including the analyses in the main results, we also looked at how the treatment goals performed in the accredited medical institutions versus those in the non-accredited medical institutions. We found that, similar to results in our previous report (5) and in this report, patients and doctors who were biologics users had higher treatment goals (almost complete or complete clearance) than the non-biologic users even when compared only within the accredited institutions (patients: 73% vs. 52%; doctors: 91.4% vs. 41%). In addition, the treatment goal misalignment was higher among pairs of patients and their treating doctors who were not treated with biologics (75%) vs. those treated with biologics (57%) within the accredited institutions. The rate of misalignment among non-biologic users in the accredited institutions (75%) was comparable to the non-biologic users in the non-accredited institutions (69%). Although we found similar trends of treatment goals when comparing the results by categories of biologic accredited institutions, we did not perform in-depth analyses to control the intended associations with other factors due to sample size limitations. Further studies would be needed to further address the differences of treatment goals by health care settings. Finally, while the patient-centric treatment approach is ideal in clinical settings, we should note that treatment satisfaction related to the use of biologics has financial implications to the patients and the health care system or vice versa. This can be a limitation in some health care systems.

In summary, we found that there were differences between biologic users and non-biologic users such as disease severity, physicians' experience and workplace, and physicians' perspectives on their patients' understanding of disease and treatment options. Patients with psoriasis and their physicians who were users of biological therapies shared higher treatment goals after adjustment for contributing factors. Better understanding of treatment goals between patients and their physicians has the potential to contribute to the development of patient-centered goals that can improve treatment outcomes. The results indicate that availability and experience with biologic treatment are elevating treatment goals for both physicians and patients and are addressing unmet treatment needs.

Author Contributions: All authors (Y.O., A.C.T., S.I., H.T.-I. and M.O.) participated in the interpretation of study results and in the drafting, critical revision, and approval of the final version of the manuscript. Y.O. and A.C.T. were involved in development of the study design, Y.O. and M.O. were investigators in the study and were involved in data collection, and S.I. was involved in data collection and conducted the statistical analysis. All authors have read and agreed to the published version of the manuscript.

Funding: This study was sponsored by Eli Lilly Japan K.K., manufacturer of ixekizumab. Medical writing assistance was provided by Serina Stretton, PhD, CMPP of ProScribe–Envision Pharma Group, and was funded by Eli Lilly Japan K.K. ProScribe's services complied with international guidelines for Good Publication Practice (GPP3). Eli Lilly Japan K.K. was involved in the study design, data collection, data analysis, and preparation of the manuscript.

Institutional Review Board Statement: The study protocol was implemented in accordance with the Declaration of Helsinki (2013), the Guidelines for Good Pharmacoepidemiology Practices (2015), the Ethical Guidelines Concerning Medical Studies in Human Subjects in Japan [15], and ethical principles based on the relevant statutes/standards in Japan.

Informed Consent Statement: Patients who participated in the study gave written informed consent for the collection and use of their information to be included in this study. Informed consent was obtained from patients after physicians had explained the study protocol to the recruited patients. Only patients who gave their informed consent were given the surveys.

Acknowledgments: The authors would like to thank all patients and physicians from the clinics and hospitals across Japan (Appendix A) who generously shared their time to participate in this study.

Conflicts of Interest: Y. Okubo has been a consultant, scientific advisor and/or investigator for Eli Lilly K.K., Kyowa Hakko Kirin Co. Ltd., Mitsubishi Tanabe Pharma Corporation, Maruho Co. Ltd., Celgene K.K., Janssen Pharmaceutical K.K., AbbVie GK, Eisai Co. Ltd., Torii Pharmaceutical Co. Ltd., Leo Pharma A/S, MSD K.K., Boehringer Ingelheim Japan, Inc., Novartis AG, Taiho Pharmaceutical CO., Ltd., and Bristol-Meiers Squibb Company. M. Ohtsuki has been paid as a consultant to AbbVie GK, Boehringer-Ingelheim Japan, Inc., Celgene K.K., Eisai Co. Ltd., Janssen Pharmaceutical K.K., Kyowa Hakko Kirin Co. Ltd., LEO Pharma A/S, Eli Lilly and Company, Maruho Co. Ltd., Novartis AG, Pfizer Inc., Mitsubishi Tanabe Pharma Corporation, Torii Pharmaceutical Co. Ltd., Taiho Pharmaceutical CO., Ltd., Amgen Inc., Sun Pharma Japan Ltd., UCB Japan Co. Ltd., and Bristol-Myers Squibb Company. S. Inoue is an employee of CRECON Medical Assessment Inc.; CRECON Medical Assessment Inc. was paid to conduct the analyses for this report. A.C. Tang is an employee of Eli Lilly K.K. Japan. H. Torisu-Itakura is an employee of Eli Lilly K.K. Japan and is an Eli Lilly stock holder.

Appendix A. List of Participating Institutions

Department of Dermatology, Asahikawa Medical University
Department of Dermatology, Jichi Medical University
Department of Dermatology, Tokyo Women's Medical University
Department of Dermatology, School of Medicine, Teikyo University
Department of Dermatology, Tokyo Medical University
Department of Dermatology, School of Medicine, Tokai University
Department of Dermatology, Graduate School of Medicine, Gifu University
Graduate School of Medical Sciences, Nagoya City University
Department of Dermatology, School of Medicine, Kindai University
Department of Dermatology, Graduate School of Medicine, Osaka City University
Department of Dermatology, Kawasaki Medical School
Department of Dermatology, Faculty of Medicine, Fukuoka University
Department of Dermatology, Tokyo Teishin Hospital
Department of Dermatology, St Luke's International Hospital
Department of Dermatology, Yokohama Chuo Hospital
Public Interest Incorporated Foundation Jiai-kai, Branch of Imamura Hospital
Department of Dermatology, Ina Central Hospital
Department of Dermatology, Iida Municipal Hospital
Department of Dermatology, Osaka Kaisei Hospital
Medical Corporation Kojin-kai, Sapporo Dermatology Clinic
Medical Corporation Kojin-kai, Fukuzumi Dermatology Clinic
Kobayashi Skin Clinic
Department of Dermatology, EST Clinic
Sugawara Dermatology Clinic
Medical Corporation Subaru-kai, Sugai Dermatology Park Side Clinic
Hattori Dermatology Clinic
Medical Corporation Koten-kai, Iidabashi Clinic
Medical Corporation Shohei-kai, Niki Dermatology Clinic
Clinic of Dermatology, Ningyocho
Dr. Mariko Skin & Dermatology Clinic
Tsujimoto Skincare Clinic
Shirosaki Dermatology & Neurology Clinic
Kato Dermatology
Hou Dermatology
Machino Skin Clinique
Yasumoto Dermatology Clinic
Takagi Dermatology Clinic
Fushimi Skin Clinic
Omorimachi Dermatology
Hayashibe Derma Clinic
Hasegawa Dermatology Clinic
Medical Corporation Kojin-kai, Ario Sapporo Dermatology Clinic
Atago Dermatology
Medical Corporation Shotoku-kai, Hino Clinic
Nomura Dermatology Clinic
Zoshiki Dermatology Clinic
Nakatsu Dermatology Clinic
Saruwatari Dermatology Clinic
Kusuhara Dermatology Clinic

Medical Corporation Shimizu Dermatology Clinic
Kokubu Clinic, Abashiri Dermatology Clinic
Nishide Skin Clinic
Kazama Skin Clinic
Shimizu Skin Clinic

References

1. Kubota, K.; Kamijima, Y.; Sato, T.; Ooba, N.; Koide, D.; Iizuka, H.; Nakagawa, H. Epidemiology of psoriasis and palmoplantar pustulosis: A nationwide study using the Japanese national claims database. *BMJ Open* **2015**, *5*, e006450. [CrossRef] [PubMed]
2. Ito, T.; Takahashi, H.; Kawada, A.; Iizuka, H.; Nakagawa, H. Epidemiological survey from 2009 to 2012 of psoriatic patients in Japanese Society for Psoriasis Research. *J. Dermatol.* **2018**, *45*, 293–301. [CrossRef] [PubMed]
3. Hirabe, M.; Hasegawa, T.; Fujishiro, Y.; Kigawa, M.; Fukuchi, O.; Nakagawa, H. Factors associated with quality of life among patients with psoriasis. Comparison between psoriasis-specific QOL measures and generic QOL measures. *Nihon Koshu Eisei Zasshi* **2008**, *55*, 65–74.
4. Mabuchi, T.; Yamaoka, H.; Kojima, T.; Ikoma, N.; Akasaka, E.; Ozawa, A. Psoriasis affects patient's quality of life more seriously in female than in male in Japan. *Tokai J. Exp. Clin. Med.* **2012**, *37*, 84–88. [PubMed]
5. Okubo, Y.; Arai, K.; Fujiwara, S.; Amaya, M.; Tsuboi, R. Assessment of the quality of life of patients with psoriasis using Skindex-16 and GHQ-28. *Jpn. J. Dermatol.* **2007**, *117*, 2495–2505.
6. Okubo, Y.; Natsume, S.; Usui, K.; Amaya, M.; Tsuboi, R. Low-dose, short-term ciclosporin (Neoral®) therapy is effective in improving patients' quality of life as assessed by Skindex-16 and GHQ-28 in mild to severe psoriasis patients. *J. Dermatol.* **2010**, *38*, 465–472. [CrossRef] [PubMed]
7. Florek, A.G.; Wang, C.J.; Armstrong, A.W. Treatment preferences and treatment satisfaction among psoriasis patients: A systematic review. *Arch. Dermatol. Res.* **2018**, *310*, 271–319. [CrossRef] [PubMed]
8. Armstrong, A.W.; Betts, K.A.; Signorovitch, J.E.; Sundaram, M.; Li, J.; Ganguli, A.X.; Wu, E.Q. Number needed to treat and costs per responder among biologic treatments for moderate-to-severe psoriasis: A network meta-analysis. *Curr. Med. Res. Opin.* **2018**, *34*, 1325–1333. [CrossRef] [PubMed]
9. Ohtsuki, M.; Terui, T.; Ozawa, A.; Morita, A.; Sano, S.; Takahashi, H.; Komine, M.; Etoh, T.; Igarashi, A.; Torii, H.; et al. Japanese guidance for use of biologics for psoriasis (the 2013 version). *J. Dermatol.* **2013**, *40*, 683–695. [CrossRef] [PubMed]
10. Armstrong, A.W.; Siegel, M.P.; Bagel, J.; Boh, E.E.; Buell, M.; Cooper, K.D.; Duffin, K.C.; Eichenfield, L.F.; Garg, A.; Gelfand, J.M.; et al. From the Medical Board of the National Psoriasis Foundation: Treatment targets for plaque psoriasis. *J. Am. Acad. Dermatol.* **2017**, *76*, 290–298. [CrossRef]
11. Mrowietz, U.; Kragballe, K.; Reich, K.; Spuls, P.; Griffiths, C.E.M.; Nast, A.; Franke, J.; Antoniou, C.; Arenberger, P.; Balieva, F.; et al. Definition of treatment goals for moderate to severe psoriasis: A European consensus. *Arch. Dermatol. Res.* **2011**, *303*, 1–10. [CrossRef] [PubMed]
12. Radtke, M.A.; Reich, K.; Spehr, C.; Augustin, M. Treatment goals in psoriasis routine care. *Arch. Dermatol. Res.* **2015**, *307*, 445–449. [CrossRef] [PubMed]
13. Brezinski, E.A.; Armstrong, A.W. Strategies to maximize treatment success in moderate to severe psoriasis: Establishing treatment goals and tailoring of biologic therapies. *Semin. Cutan. Med. Surg.* **2014**, *33*, 91–97. [CrossRef] [PubMed]
14. Okubo, Y.; Tsuruta, D.; Tang, A.C.; Inoue, S.; Torisu-Itakura, H.; Hanada, T.; Ohtsuki, M. Analysis of treatment goal alignment between Japanese psoriasis patients and their paired treating physicians. *J. Eur. Acad. Dermatol. Venereol.* **2018**, *32*, 606–614. [CrossRef] [PubMed]
15. Ministry of Education, Culture, Sports, Science and Technology. Ethical Guidelines Concerning Medical Studies in Human Subjects. 2015. Available online: http://www.lifescience.mext.go.jp/files/pdf/n1500_02.pdf (accessed on 18 April 2018).
16. Atkinson, M.J.; Sinha, A.; Hass, S.L.; Colman, S.S.; Kumar, R.N.; Brod, M.; Rowland, C.R. Validation of a general measure of treatment satisfaction, the Treatment Satisfaction Questionnaire for Medication (TSQM), using a national panel study of chronic disease. *Health Qual. Life Outcomes* **2004**, *2*, 12. [CrossRef] [PubMed]
17. Finlay, A.Y.; Khan, G.K. Dermatology Life Quality Index (DLQI)—A simple practical measure for routine clinical use. *Clin. Exp. Dermatol.* **1994**, *19*, 210–216. [CrossRef] [PubMed]
18. Kimball, A.B.; Naegeli, A.N.; Edson-Heredia, E.; Lin, C.Y.; Gaich, C.; Nikaï, E.; Wyrwich, K.; Yosipovitch, G. Psychometric properties of the Itch Numeric Rating Scale in patients with moderate-to-severe plaque psoriasis. *Br. J. Dermatol.* **2016**, *175*, 157–162. [CrossRef] [PubMed]
19. Finlay, A.Y. Current severe psoriasis and the rule of tens. *Br. J. Dermatol.* **2005**, *152*, 861–867. [CrossRef]
20. Okubo, Y. Hands-on practice manual-illustrations & visual- 46: Plaque psoriasis. *Clin. Derma.* **2011**, *13*, 3–6. Available online: http://www.tokyo-med.ac.jp/derma/content/files/topics_okubo_2011clinicalderma.pdf (accessed on 17 June 2018). (In Japanese)
21. European Medicines Agency (EMEA); Committee for Medicinal Products for Human Use (CHMP). Guideline on Clinical Investigation of Medicinal Products Indicated for the Treatment of Psoriasis. 2004. Available online: http://www.ema.europa.eu/docs/en_GB/document_library/Scientific_guideline/2009/09/WC500003329.pdf (accessed on 19 April 2018).

22. Lambert, J.; Ghislain, P.D.; Lambert, J.; Cauwe, B.; Van den Enden, M. Treatment patterns in moderate-to-severe plaque psoriasis: Results from a Belgian cross-sectional study (DISCOVER). *J. Dermatol. Treat.* **2017**, *28*, 394–400. [CrossRef]
23. Ichiyama, S.; Ito, M.; Funasaka, Y.; Abe, M.; Nishida, E.; Muramatsu, S.; Nishihara, H.; Kato, H.; Morita, A.; Imafuku, S.; et al. Assessment of medication adherence and treatment satisfaction in Japanese patients with psoriasis of various severities. *J. Dermatol.* **2018**, *45*, 727–731. [CrossRef] [PubMed]
24. Kamiya, K.; Oiso, N.; Kawada, A.; Ohtsuki, M. Epidemiological survey of the psoriasis patients in the Japanese Society for Psoriasis Research from 2013 to 2018. *J. Dermatol.* **2021**, *48*, 864–875. [CrossRef] [PubMed]
25. Strohal, R.; Prinz, J.C.; Girolomoni, G.; Nast, A. A patient-centred approach to biological treatment decision making for psoriasis: An expert consensus. *J. Eur. Acad. Dermatol. Venereol.* **2015**, *29*, 2390–2398. [CrossRef] [PubMed]
26. Okubo, Y.; Torisu-Itakura, H.; Hanada, T.; Aranishi, T.; Inoue, S.; Ohtsuki, M. Evaluation of treatment satisfaction misalignment between Japanese psoriasis patients and their physicians—Japanese psoriasis patients and their physicians do not share the same treatment satisfaction levels. *Curr. Med. Res. Opin.* **2021**. epub ahead of print. [CrossRef] [PubMed]

MDPI AG
Grosspeteranlage 5
4052 Basel
Switzerland
Tel.: +41 61 683 77 34

Journal of Clinical Medicine Editorial Office
E-mail: jcm@mdpi.com
www.mdpi.com/journal/jcm

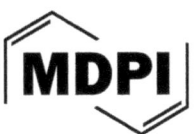

Disclaimer/Publisher's Note: The statements, opinions and data contained in all publications are solely those of the individual author(s) and contributor(s) and not of MDPI and/or the editor(s). MDPI and/or the editor(s) disclaim responsibility for any injury to people or property resulting from any ideas, methods, instructions or products referred to in the content.

www.ingramcontent.com/pod-product-compliance
Lightning Source LLC
LaVergne TN
LVHW070629100526
838202LV00012B/762